THE COMPREHENSIVE GUIDE TO GLUTATHIONE

RESEARCH AND CLINICAL APPLICATIONS

JIMMY GUTMAN, MD FACEP

FOREWORD BY
GUSTAVO BOUNOUS, MD

GSH BOOKS
MONTREAL, CANADA

This book discusses the manufacture and use of glutathione (GSH) by the human body and proposes strategies that, according to scientific research, may benefit us in times of sickness and of health. Knowledge of GSH is very much in its infancy but is evolving in leaps and bounds as new preventive and therapeutic possibilities become apparent. Readers with existing medical conditions, anyone on medication and those undergoing medical treatment of any sort are encouraged to seek the advice of a qualified medical professional before making use of the recommendations in this book.

The authors and publisher expressly disclaim responsibility from the use or application of information described in this book.

THE COMPREHENSIVE GUIDE TO GLUTATHIONE by Jimmy Gutman MD, FACEP

Published in Canada by GSH Books, Montreal
EDITOR, ILLUSTRATION & DESIGN: Stephen Schettini
COVER: Dave Farrant
Printed in Canada

PUBLICATION HISTORY
1st edition, 1998: The Ultimate GSH Handbook
ISBN 0-9687078-0-7
Published in Canada by Gutman & Schettini, Montreal

2nd edition, 2000: Glutathione – Your Body's Most Powerful Healing Agent
ISBN 0-9687078-2-3
Published in Canada by Gutman & Schettini Inc., Montreal

3rd edition, 2002: Glutathione – Your Body's Most Powerful Protector
ISBN 0-9731409-0-9
Published in Canada by Kudo.ca Communications Inc., Montreal
First Impression, November 2002
Second Impression, September 2004

4th edition, 2008: Glutathione – Your Key to Health
ISBN 0-9731409-0-9
Published in Canada by Kudo.ca Communications Inc., Montreal

5th edition, 2019: The Comprehensive Guide to Glutathione
ISBN 978-1-9991788-1-9
Published in Canada by GSH Books Inc., Montreal

WHAT HEALTH PROFESSIONALS ARE SAYING ABOUT THIS BOOK

"Thorough and fascinating"
A thorough and fascinating synopsis of glutathione. Easy to read. Covers the topic completely and backs up all statements with reliable medical references. Stop searching libraries and the internet…it's all here.

JAMES WEISS MD, FCCP
Pulmonary and Internal Medicine
Los Angeles, CA

"Cutting edge"
This book provides access to the cutting edge of one of today's hottest research topics – glutathione in health and illness. Reading it will open up a new world of discovery. I highly recommend this book to everyone from fellow researchers to those interested in improving their health.

DR. JEAN MARCOUX MD, FRCP(C)
Chairman, Advisory Board of the
American Lung Association, Houston

"Highly recommended"
For the growing number of people interested in complementary medicine – a synthesis of alternative and conventional treatments for illness – it will be obvious that this book by Jimmy Gutman and Stephen Schettini is timely. Glutathione plays a pivotal role in the defense against both aging and disease, and this well executed and researched publication makes that very clear. I highly recommend glutathione – your body's most powerful protector to anyone intent on living a healthier life naturally.

PHYLLIS BALCH CNC
Author, "Prescription for Nutritional Healing"
and, "Prescription for Dietary Wellness"

"Most complete, up-to-date and readable"
"Glutathione – Your Body's Most Powerful Protector" is the most complete, up-to-date and readable reference I've yet seen on the essential issue of antioxidant supplementation with GSH. I recommend it.

RONALD KLATZ, MD, DO
President, American Academy of
Anti-Aging Medicine (A4M)
[www.worldhealth.net]

"Demystifies the subject"
Many facts and fantasies exist regarding glutathione – where it works, when it works, how to raise its levels. Given glutathione's impending widespread integration into clinical practice it is refreshing to pick up a source that demystifies the subject.

DR. ROGER D. ANDERSON
Director, Anderson Clinical Research

"Read this book"
How can this one substance address so many health issues? It's because glutathione is the body's 'decision maker' of oxidant-antioxidant balance. Dr. Gutman has compiled the cream

of the latest GSH research and put it between two covers. Read this book and you'll understand the critical importance of GSH to the health of every cell in your body.

DR. BIKUL DAS
Researcher in molecular biology
Author, "The Science Behind Squalene"

"Invaluable"

Firstly, Dr. Gutman's book collects all the tremendously important scientific reports about glutathione into a single source. Secondly, it explains it in plain English. It is an invaluable addition to any health library and to the understanding of this crucial topic.

ALLAN SOMERSALL PHD, MD
Physician, Nutritionist, Chemist
Author, "Breakthrough in Cell Defense"

"World-wide research"

Like the use of antioxidant vitamins and minerals two decades ago, GSH therapy is causing quite a stir among the medical community and patients alike. Researchers are already familiar with the healing power of GSH in chronic illnesses like cancer, viral hepatitis, autoimmune diseases, diabetes and atherosclerosis. Dr. Gutman's book compiles worldwide research findings and details the entire range of ailments caused or exacerbated by low GSH levels. In these pages you will find all the information you need to take advantage of increased glutathione levels.

ZOLTAN P. RONA MD, MSC
Author, "The Joy of Health"
Medical Editor, "Encyclopedia of Natural Healing "

To my wife Susan and our
children Evan and Bianca.
Through the hours, days and
weeks that I have been immersed
in this important project their love
and patience have never wavered.

Acknowledgments

I have worked through hundreds of theoretical papers, laboratory experiments, and clinical studies by Dr. Gustavo Bounous, and had the extraordinary opportunity to speak with him frequently and at great length. With prodigious wit, charm and wisdom Dr. Bounous conveyed to me, and to many other health professionals, the extraordinary powers of glutathione (GSH). Our debt to him is immeasurable.

Dr. Patricia Kongshavn who co-wrote many of the seminal articles on glutathione with Dr. Bounous is in the opinion of many "the great-grandmother of clinical immunology." She wrote the first chapter of the first book on clinical immunology broadly distributed to the medical community. I hold her dear, both as a friend and as a remarkable mentor.

Thanks to Dr. Wulf Droge who continued my education after the passing of Dr. Bounous. His exquisite knowledge of glutathione, the immune system and free-radical biology has advanced the world's knowledge of the aging process immensely.

And finally, thanks to two people I've never met but who have made a profound contribution to our knowledge of glutathione: Alton Meister and Mary Anderson.

To health!

—Jimmy Gutman MD

Table of Contents

PART TWO
GLUTATHIONE IN SICKNESS

PART THREE
GLUTATHIONE IN THE BRAIN & NERVOUS SYSTEM

FOREWORD
by Gustavo Bounous M.D.

In the late 1970's the Department of Medicine at McGill University in collaboration with other Canadian Medical Schools undertook the vast project of Research on Nutrition, including several animal species. My team, then based at the Montreal General Hospital and made up of medical doctors and immunologists, was excited to come up with hard data linking protein ingestion with optimal health.

After exploring the potential benefits of a large array of different protein sources and generating numerous publications, we received a package containing WPC (whey protein concentrate) from a Swiss company inquiring if this powder could be used commercially as food. Whey proteins at this time were largely treated as a surplus byproduct of the dairy industry, and much of it was discarded as a non-food commodity.

To our surprise this particular protein was not only nutritionally adequate but was able to increase the immune response in various animals measuring various parameters. It took yet several more years of research to discover that this batch of protein was rich in the building blocks needed by the body to make glutathione. My team's focus then shifted towards the effect of raising glutathione in the immune system.

Our successes in the lab came to an abrupt stop one day, and I was absolutely at a loss to explain why. After a few months, I encountered some fortuitous news that gave me the answer. The manufacturer of the particular protein we were studying had been obliged to change their production methods by using more aggressive pasteurization methods, including a form of heating. It turned out that the specific proteins needed by the cells to make glutathione, being very sensitive to heat, had been broken down and were no longer effective glutathione precursors.

My advantageous involvement with great scientists was followed by another stroke of good fortune in the form of some individuals with excellent business sense. They aided me in the complex and expensive process of patenting a method of using non-denatured whey protein as a means of raising glutathione. Together, we sourced a North American dairy capable of producing this delicate protein in a way that preserved its biological ability to affect glutathione synthesis.

It was obvious to us all that this was an important breakthrough, but back then, the knowledge of glutathione was not nearly as developed as it is today. Medical science had little knowledge of the broad implications on health of raised glutathione. I've been both overwhelmed and enormously gratified to sift through the literal explosion of glutathione research in the past dozen years.

Dr. Jimmy Gutman has been the leading light in bringing the complex knowledge of this topic to the public at large. He has spent years researching glutathione and its abundant potential clinical applications and has written several books explaining these important findings in simple terms. His background as a physician and as an educator has given him the perfect tools to be able to bring these discoveries to light. These pages contain clear explanations that most non-scientists can understand, but that are also backed up by a plethora of published research findings sufficient to satisfy even the most obsessive-compulsive scientist. I myself have discovered many fascinating facets of glutathione activity by reviewing his manuscripts.

I thank Dr. Gutman for bringing the world of glutathione research to the public eye, and I thank him for his camaraderie, thought-provoking questions and friendship through the years.

—Gustavo Bounous, M.D.

Preface

My first medical specialty was emergency medicine. I spent many long shifts in the E.R. but was also engaged in research, teaching and management. I am what's called an academic clinician. Today I still practice some clinical medicine but my focus is principally on research and development, teaching and writing. This book is the latest in a series of books written on glutathione over the past two decades.

As an emergency doctor I know that it's not easy to make snap decisions with unflappable confidence. It is yet another task to impart this skill to a student. In the end, there is no greater sense of accomplishment than to see a novice initially sickened at the sight of blood turn into a team leader running major trauma codes. Seeing such accomplishment continually reinforces my love of teaching.

This book springs from the same love. I've tried to present the material clearly and concisely, taking care not to overwhelm the reader with technicalities and jargon. Our intention is obviously to reach the broadest possible audience. However, medical science being what it is, a good amount of terminology has crept into the text. We have kept it as brief as possible.

I take the same approach I developed while teaching medical interns and students—I provide the material, but learning it is your responsibility. A book of this size covering so many areas—each one bristling with its own medical specializations—barely skims the surface. To thoroughly understand the remarkable qualities of GSH you may choose to extend your reading beyond this introductory text—and we help you with that too. Following the contents of each chapter you'll find extensive reference lists. I hope you will delve into this material which I consider to be the core of the book.

Having said that, I sincerely hope that this latest edition provides some insight and encourages you to explore the remarkable world of glutathione and the human immune response system. Our mandate is to provide the most up-to-date knowledge of GSH by constantly revising and expanding this book. To do this effectively we rely in part on your feedback. Please let us know what you think, and especially what you would like to see in future editions.

—Jimmy Gutman MD, FACEP

Editor's Note

Back in the spring of 1997 I made a new acquaintance. His name was Jimmy Gutman and he was on fire about something called glutathione. I had to ask him to repeat the word, which makes me smile now because since then I've used it a million times.

I've always been interested in human biology, but the story I heard that day supercharged my interest. We decided to make a book of it, and here we are. Now in its fifth edition, it has become the major project of my publishing career.

It's also been fascinating. The tale of glutathione is one of lifeless molecules fitting into the biochemical jigsaw puzzle as if they know where to go and what to do. The dazzling processes of the immune system demonstrate the body's non-stop, no-holds-barred drive to stay alive. Since learning about glutathione, the idea of an 'optimal immune response' has taken on new significance. It's something I must manage myself. This book demonstrates to the medical world that glutathione therapy lies at the very heart of preventive medicine.

Dr. Gutman has since studied and spread the word of GSH far and wide, with heartening results. His long and critical examination of literally thousands of studies has made him the most widely-read physician in the world on GSH and its role in the body. This book, which began as a slim volume of barely a hundred pages, has grown into a comprehensive reference guide for anyone wanting to know all about glutathione.

If you're looking for someone to explain glutathione I not only commend you to Dr. Gutman but also congratulate you on finding the most qualified person alive for the job. You'll benefit from his unmatched knowledge, his skill in communicating it, and the generosity with which he shares everything to do with glutathione. If you've met Dr Gutman, or just heard him speak, you'll understand when I say that working with him has been the most rewarding relationship of my career.

Dr. Gutman is responsible for the content of this book and I for its delivery. There have been many changes and corrections through these five editions, but few disagreements. Thanks to Dr. Gutman's scrutiny, the scientific rigor of this work has survived the almost endless process of editing. For my part, I am satisfied that anybody who wants to do so can, with a little effort, read and follow any chapter.

I'm not a doctor but I am sometimes a patient, and I've learned over the years that scientific training alone does not necessarily make a good doctor. Like many people today I believe a true healer combines personal integrity and compassion with a rigorous sense of scientific enquiry. Dr. Gutman both teaches that and role-models it. I hope that through studying this book you will come to value him as much as I do.

Good studies!

—Stephen Schettini

Introduction

Pick up a medical journal or health magazine and chances are you'll find yet another article describing the benefits of GSH (glutathione). A computer search of traditional medical literature reveals upwards of 150 thousand scientific articles—this represents over 50 thousand since the last edition of this book! Medical science has known of this tiny molecule for almost a hundred years, so why the recent explosion of interest?

It reflects fascinating new discoveries about GSH and how it so profoundly affects our life.

While scientists are busy with research, North Americans in unprecedented numbers are taking an active role in maintaining their own health. Increasingly, we accept greater responsibility for our own wellbeing and so are learning more and more about preventive maintenance. This feeds a growing industry based on nutritional supplements, fitness and diet.

Our interest is timely but not coincidental. Average age in the industrialized world is on the rise, and our already overburdened health care systems are facing the additional strain of a disproportionately large geriatric population. Then there are environmental problems to contend with: the depletion of the ozone layer, general pollution, the spread of environmental toxins and poisons, increasingly virulent microbes, deteriorated nutritional benefit from our food supply... the list grows longer.

Experts have only an imperfect understanding of these things and the media frightens us with news of infections that are increasingly resistant to present-day antibiotics. Diseases unknown to "baby-boomers" years ago are now household words, such as: Ebola, Zika, AIDS, chronic fatigue syndrome, West Nile disease, fibromyalgia, metabolic syndrome, autism. The inescapable stress of life today fosters cancer, heart disease and gastrointestinal problems. Antibiotics become less effective while microscopic organisms learn to adapt and outwit us. The old attitude of fixing people only when their bodies break is giving way to the realization that it's wiser to prevent health problems than to wait for them. This may sound obvious, but it's a social change that takes time.

Today we see a shift in two directions. On the one hand, we have continuous advances in technology and medical skills. On the other, interest in alternative, or "complementary," medicine is growing. Most exciting of all, medical practitioners are crossing the great divide. After decades of exclusion, complementary regimens and therapies are finally being placed in the scientific spotlight. This is great news for patients and practitioners everywhere.

The result is a shift towards more comprehensive therapies. For the first time in decades, doctors are emphasizing diet, life style, physical exercise and spiritual wellbeing as integral components of health maintenance and therapy. In addition to balanced eating habits and fresh foods, dietary regimes include vitamin supplements and other natural products. These products enhance our health in various ways, many of which are still being discovered. Their contributions to the prevention of the diseases of aging are encouraging.

This book is about GSH (glutathione)—a substance manufactured naturally by the body to battle disease and aging. It demonstrates how GSH defends you against pollution and disease in the twenty-first century, and explains how to elevate your body's glutathione levels.

Doctors and patients alike should develop an open-minded but cautious approach to all possible diagnostic and therapeutic tools. That's the approach we've taken in this book. We have looked at both conventional and alternative ways to elevate GSH levels. All information is based on hard scientific research. To simplify presentation we've avoided the constant intrusion of superscripts and footnotes, for our sources are many. Instead, they're listed at the end of each chapter.

The volume, variety and reliability of research data on glutathione is staggering, and places the importance of glutathione beyond any doubt. We encourage you to study these papers, but not to get bogged down in dry facts. We've included anecdotal stories to show that GSH is not an abstract idea but something that affects your health and wellbeing every day.

Our hope is that this book will help you help yourself and your loved ones. Good reading, and good health!

PART ONE

GLUTATHIONE IN HEALTH

[CHAPTERS 1 TO 4]

Part One describes glutathione in general terms. Its four chapters describe GSH itself, its role in detoxification, the part it plays in immune response, and how to raise your GSH levels.

IMPORTANT NOTE
GLUTATHIONE AS A DIETARY SUPPLEMENT

We must first clarify an important, frequently misunderstood part of the glutathione story. Upon learning about GSH for the first time, many people go to their health store, buy it, and start dosing themselves. However, while GSH is freely available in this form, this sort of oral, ingested glutathione will have negligible effects on your health. The product decomposes rapidly in the digestive system and is quickly removed from the gut. Apart from a few very specific instances, GSH cannot be introduced into the body in this way. It must be made within your cells—which is where it's naturally found. The effective way to stimulate the production of GSH is to provide your body with the basic elements it needs to make glutathione by itself. Some pharmaceutical medications, such as N-acetyl-cysteine (NAC), have been developed to provide these precursors. There are also natural ways to increase glutathione levels, in particular the use of denatured (bioactive) whey proteins. These are discussed throughout this book, and described in detail in Chapter 4.

Possible Clinical Applications of Raised Glutathione

NEUROLOGY
- Parkinson's disease
- Alzheimer's disease
- Seizures
- Multiple sclerosis
- Autism

PULMONARY
- Break up mucus (esp. cystic fibrosis)
- Asthma
- Chronic bronchitis
- Emphysema
- Pulmonary fibrosis

CARDIOVASCULAR
- Prevent heart disease
- Prevent stroke
- Prevent atherosclerosis
- Prevent reperfusion injury

DIGESTIVE SYSTEM
- Inflammatory bowel disease
- Hepatitis
- Malnutrition
- Pancreatitis
- Peptic ulcer

TOXICOLOGY
- Certain drug overdoses
- Tobacco smoke, auto exhaust
- Pollutants including heavy metals, pesticides
- Prevents hearing loss from noise pollution
- Detoxifies many well-known carcinogens

INFECTIOUS DISEASE AND IMMUNOLOGY
- Anti-viral (AIDS, hepatitis, herpes, common cold, etc.)
- Bacterial infection
- Certain autoimmune dysfunction
- Chronic fatigue syndrome
- Immunosuppression

CANCER
- Cancer prevention
- Suppress tumor growth
- Eliminate carcinogens, mutagens
- Retard oxidative damage to DNA
- Prevent wasting disease
- Ease side effects of chemo- and radiotherapy

METABOLIC
- Enhances athletic performance
- Decreases recovery time from physical stress/injury
- Decreases cholesterol and oxidation of LDL
- Supports hemoglobin in kidney failure

EYE DISEASES
- Cataracts
- Macular degeneration
- Glaucoma

1

Glutathione (GSH)

WHEN WE PUBLISHED the first edition of this book, few people had ever heard of glutathione. Now two decades have passed, along with an avalanche of new research, and the word rolls easily off the tongue of most health care professionals, especially those working in nutrition and preventative care. Today researchers and scientists continue to uncover the role of this substance in health and disease. Before long the term will be considered as fundamental to our understanding of health and sickness as 'cholesterol' and 'vitamins.'

Your life depends on glutathione—literally. Without it, your liver would shrivel up and die from the overwhelming accumulation of toxins, your cells would disintegrate from unrestrained oxidative stress and, as if you needed more problems, your body would have little resistance to bacteria, viruses or cancers. Protective systems of the body, including the immune system, rely heavily upon this exceptional molecule. So does the optimal functioning of antioxidants, detoxification pathways and cellular energy production.

The importance of glutathione

Glutathione's importance to your health cannot be overstated. Your immune system is on a constant prowl for pathogens—agents of cellular damage, toxicity and disease. To neutralize them, it needs a ready supply of glutathione. If there's not enough, invaders penetrate the body's defenses, infecting it and contributing to aging, long-term damage—even cancer.

We can't avoid illness and aging altogether (though a few scientists are pursuing the age-old dream of immortality) but by keeping our intracellular glutathione levels up, we also keep our immune system fully loaded. In other words, GSH is a fundamental and critical contributor to the immune response.

Research on glutathione

In the last twenty years the volume of research into GSH has grown enormously. A variety of theoretical papers, bench-top laboratory experiments, epidemiological studies, animal projects and, most importantly, clinical trials on humans, has linked glutathione to a huge variety of illnesses. The list is long and would be hard to believe but for the strength and

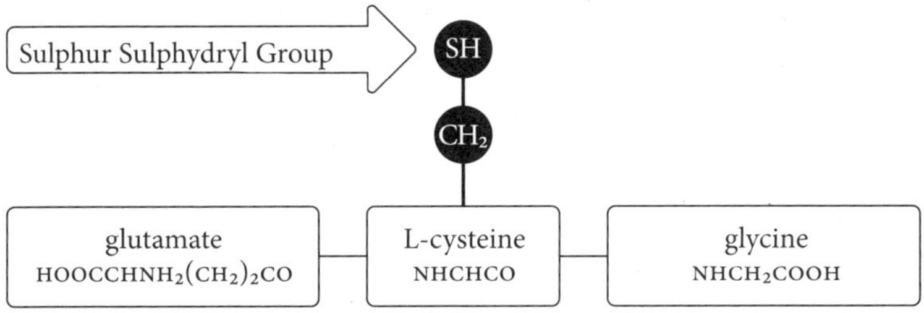

FIGURE 1: *The molecular structure of glutathione*

Enhanced immune function	Protein synthesis
Elimination of toxins	Prostaglandin synthesis
Elimination of carcinogens	Leukotriene synthesis
Antioxidant cell protection	Amino acid transport
Protection against ionizing radiation	Enzyme activation and regulation
DNA synthesis and repair	

TABLE 1: Some metabolic functions of glutathion

credibility of the research. It is now clear that glutathione's role is pivotal. Without it, many bodily processes would fail.

All the information in this book is derived from the scientific reports listed at the end of each chapter. Hundreds of articles have described how elevated glutathione levels help combat the infirmities of aging, including Parkinson's disease, Alzheimer's disease, cataract formation, macular degeneration, and cancers of aging (such as prostate cancer). You will find references to all these subjects and more in the index.

GSH is also known to play a crucial role in the cardiovascular system, helping prevent heart disease, stroke, atherosclerosis and reperfusion injury. In an ideal situation—where the patient is exercising, eating properly, avoiding tobacco and maintaining a good general lifestyle—raising glutathione levels can actually help reverse atherosclerosis (see Chapter 7).

In the digestive system, glutathione helps fight inflammatory bowel disease, hepatitis, malnutrition, pancreatitis and peptic ulcer. Its antioxidant properties and its role in maintaining the immune response have led to exciting new strategies against these all-too-common problems (see Chapter 13).

Overdosing of certain drugs has been treated for some time with a variety of GSH-enhancing drugs that have become mainstays in critical care medicine. However only recently has it been recognized that glutathione is a powerful detoxifier of many other nasty substances—including those released from cigarette smoke and automobile exhaust, pollutants including heavy metals and pesticides, and many well-known carcinogens. Believe it or not, the evidence shows that GSH even helps prevent hearing loss from noise pollution (see Chapter 15).

In infectious disease and immunology, glutathione's anti-viral properties help the body fight AIDS, hepatitis, herpes and the common cold. Its role in combating bacterial infection has also been clearly described. Although raised GSH levels are not a "cure," they elevate and sustain the natural immune response, providing reinforcement, dealing with the threats at hand and minimizing damage. Glutathione also has potential applications against some autoimmune dysfunctions, chronic fatigue syndrome and states of immunosuppression.

The immune system is on constant alert against the threat of cancer. Glutathione helps prevent carcinogenesis (the transformation of normal cells into cancer cells) by eliminating carcinogens and mutagens from the body and by reducing oxidative damage to DNA and other sensitive structures within the cell. In cases of diagnosed cancer, glutathione has been shown to suppress tumor growth, prevent the wasting disease associated with advanced cancer and ease the side effects of chemotherapy and radiotherapy (see Chapter 5).

In pulmonary or respiratory medicine, raised glutathione levels have been used for many years in Europe and are now increasingly used in North America. Glutathione can break up mucus (especially in cystic fibrosis), reduce the danger of asthmatic attacks, aid in both acute and chronic bronchitis and fight emphysema and pulmonary fibrosis. All these mechanisms are described in Chapter 12.

I	Immune Reinforcement: The immune system depends on the GSH for its proper functioning, particularly for the creation and maintenance of white blood cells, the body's first line of defense against infections (see Chapter 3).
D	Detoxifier: The GSH enzyme system eliminates dozens of toxins, including drug metabolites, pollutants, carcinogens and radiation damage. It's no wonder that GSH concentrations are higher in the liver, the body's main detoxifying organ. (See Chapter 2).
E	Energizer: the energy in each cell is produced by small energy generators called "mitochondria." These tiny bio-machines produce both "heat" and "pollution." What keeps them running cool and clean is glutathione.
A	Antioxidant: GSH is the most active of all natural antioxidants in your body. The effectiveness of other antioxidants such as vitamins C and E depends on glutathione. This essential characteristic of glutathione is described in the following pages.

TABLE 2: A good IDEA: the four functions of glutathione

This book also includes chapters on glutathione's many metabolic functions. It plays several roles in the complications of diabetes, in the reduction of cholesterol and in the oxidation of bad cholesterol (LDL), as well as supporting red blood cell levels in patients with kidney failure.

Finally, we present research emphasizing the importance of glutathione in the healthy individual. For the physically active, GSH enhances athletic performance, decreases recovery time from physical stress and aids in immune function. For the average person, its role in health maintenance just can't be overstated. Glutathione modulation is an essential part of staying young, active and healthy (see Chapters 23 and 24).

In his book on antioxidants (What You Should Know About the Super Antioxidant Miracle) Dr. Earl Mindell states, "We literally cannot survive without this miraculous antioxidant." Dr. John T. Pinto of the Sloan Kettering Cancer Center in New York proclaims, "It is the master antioxidant." Jean Carper in her book Stop Aging Now! claims, "You must get your levels of glutathione up if you want to keep your youth and live longer. High levels of GSH predict good health and long life. Low levels predict early disease and death."

In the more staid language of science, we turn to Dr. Gustavo Bounous, a researcher into the raw science of glutathione and a leading authority on GSH and nutrition at Montreal's McGill University. With some prescience he said, "In view of existing scientific data, all we can expect from the environment is continued pollution, ozone depletion, and the increased virulence of infections. I think that enhancing glutathione levels will allow for a better quality of life."

You don't have to be a scientist to understand that as society "progresses" we become increasingly dependent upon technology, and have to live with its many unhealthy

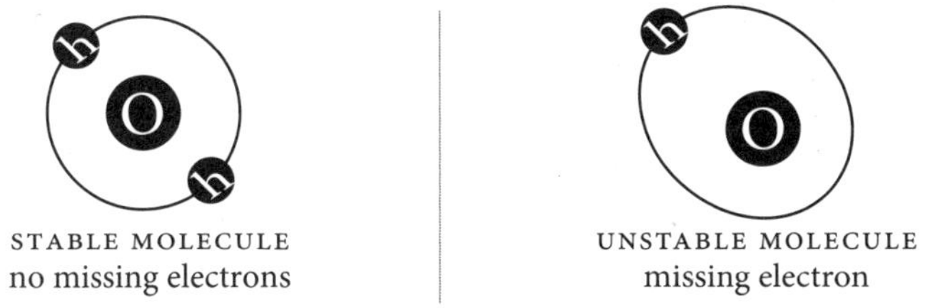

FIGURE 2: An atom loses an electron to become a free radical

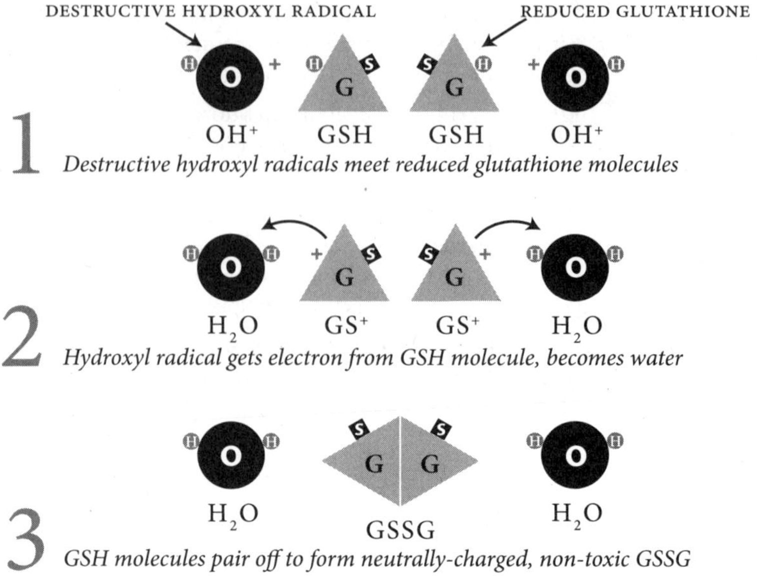

G = Glutathione backbone	S = Sulphydryl group
O = Oxygen	OH = Hydroxyl radical
+ = Missing electron	H_2O = Water
H = Hydrogen electron	GSSG = Paired GSH molecules

Figure 3: Oxidation: a GSH molecule encounters a destructive, positively-charged hydroxyl radical, giving it an electron and turning it into harmless water. The GSH molecule does not become a radical but pairs up with another radicalized GSH molecule. They neutralize each other and form non-toxic GSSG.

by-products. Not all of them are as tangible as toxic waste. There's the stress and pressure of modern life—few of us take the time to listen closely to our bodies' demands, to eat and exercise accordingly, or even to rest when necessary. We are driven by forces that sometimes leave us numb to our spiritual and physical needs. Our whole being is affected.

However, a strong immune system can help us bear the physiological brunt. It just needs regular maintenance and the all-important raw materials to make glutathione.

GSH—the molecule

Glutathione is the general term for glutathione sulfhydryl, abbreviated as GSH. The 'SH' represents the critically active sulfur sulfhydryl group. GSH is a peptide (very small protein) that occurs naturally within the body, where it is assembled by individual cells from its three components.

All three are amino-acids: glycine, glutamate (glutamic acid), and the harder-to-find cysteine. Because it contains three amino acids it is referred to as a tripeptide. Glutathione's molecular structure is shown in Figure 1.

Cysteine, the scarcest of these components, is a sulfur-containing amino acid that contributes the sulfhydryl group to the molecule, making it also the most important. When cells have cysteine, they manufacture GSH efficiently.

Unfortunately, cysteine is in short supply for two reasons: firstly, it is absent or deficient in many diets; secondly, its presence in the diet must be in an accessible form. Most of the cysteine you ingest will not survive the journey through the digestive tract and into your cells. It needs to piggyback on a larger molecule or protein.

Without enough cysteine, cells cannot produce enough GSH and the body suffers on four fronts:

1. the immune system is compromised, leaving you vulnerable to disease;
2. toxins accumulate in the body, causing further damage;
3. energy production within the cell deteriorates;
4. cellular oxidation contributes to general decline and aging.

On the other hand, there are many benefits for the body with elevated glutathione levels. Some of its metabolic functions are shown in Table 1:

All these functions can be summarized under four general categories, shown in Table 2 with the acronym IDEA: Immune booster, Detoxifier, Energizer and Antioxidant.

These four functions are not separate. As far as the immune system is concerned, it is just using glutathione to do its job. A GSH molecule may neutralize a free radical, be recycled by the GSH system and then eliminate a stray toxin. The remainder of Part I describes these functions in detail—including how to maintain them.

Before we look at its antioxidant role we must first describe the processes of oxidation.

Oxidation and Antioxidation

Interest in preventative and anti-aging medicine has grown enormously. Much time and money has been spent on addressing the wear and tear of living, breathing and eating. The non-stop activity of body maintenance places continuous stress on all the cells of the body, each of which either responds effectively or suffers damage. Terms like "oxidation," "free radical," "oxyradical" and "antioxidant" are used to describe these processes. Let's look at what they mean.

Each and every cell in the body is a biological machine that is gradually worn down by the work of staying alive. It's an imperfect system. Like all machines, cells derive their energy from the consumption (oxidation) of fuel (nutrients and oxygen)—but at a price. This process produces waste products (free radicals or oxyradicals) that are harmful. One of a cell's most routine tasks is to neutralize and remove these threats, and the key substance it uses is glutathione. Glutathione is the body's principal antioxidant. When it runs out, oxyradicals proliferate, slowly but surely wreaking havoc. In Part II you will see that severe GSH deficiency is common to many diseases, especially in their advanced, chronic states.

How do oxyradicals form? If you were to look inside a cell, you'd see thousands of tiny chemical reactions that use oxygen to metabolize nutrients and release energy. This oxidation is a necessary process, but it produces harmful byproducts known as oxyradicals (unstable atoms).

An atom is a nucleus orbited by electrons. By working in pairs (like children on a seesaw) electrons maintain a balanced and stable orbit. But oxidation sometimes knocks an electron off its orbit, leaving its partner unbalanced, as shown in Figure 2. The atom spontaneously corrects the imbalance by stealing an electron from a neighboring atom, which then steals from yet another. Imagine a playground full of children jumping from seesaw to seesaw. The resulting chain reaction of disrupted molecules can cause untold damage. Fortunately, cells are equipped with natural antioxidants—agents that neutralize free radicals by giving them an electron, rather as a playground monitor ensures that each child has a partner.

This process of oxidation and antioxidation is always going on. Oxidation isn't a bad thing. It provides energy and is also a frontline defense against bacteria

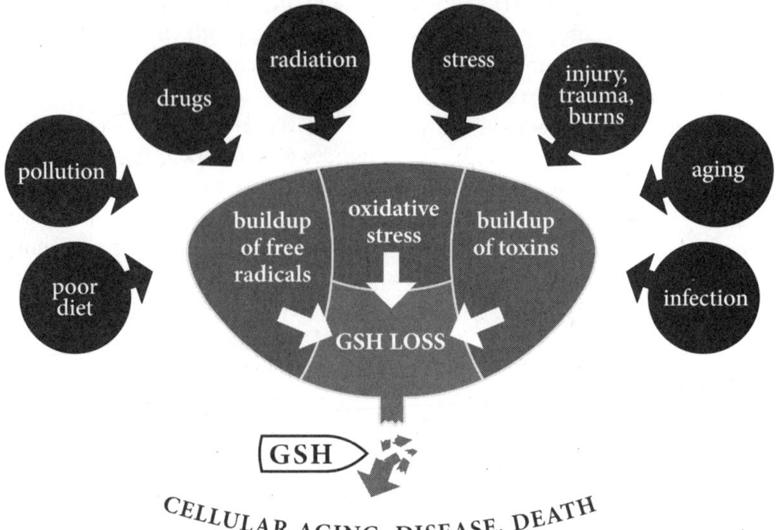

FIGURE 4: Surviving in a hostile world

(ADAPTED FROM KIDD & HUBER, "NATURAL ANTIOXIDANTS—FIRST LINE OF DEFENSE," 1991)

and viruses. But if your diet lacks certain nutrients or vitamins, or if your body experiences excessive oxidative stress and increased production of oxyradicals, individual cells will suffer unwanted consequences. This isn't surprising. After all, oxidation causes metal to rust, apples to rot and butter to turn rancid. It also causes natural aging in humans. But its effects don't end there. Free radicals can damage or destroy cell walls, cause cell death (apoptosis) and disrupt DNA patterns, sometimes leading to cancer.

Lipid peroxidation (a precipitous oxidative chain reaction) is responsible for the breakdown of fats, and produces "bad" cholesterol (LDL-cholesterol). This damages arteries and leads to blocked blood vessels, heart disease and stroke (see Chapter 7). The list of ailments caused by oxidation and free radical formation grows longer every day. In fact, a whole new field of medicine has emerged, called "Free Radical Biology." It studies the diseases and potential damaging effects of oxidative stress. Today there is no doubt that antioxidants can mitigate cell damage, lessen the threat of disease and slow the harmful effects of aging.

Many factors contribute to oxidative stress, including poor diet, pollution, drugs, radiation, stress, trauma, injury, burns, aging and infection by bacteria or viruses. Each time your immune system confronts a threat, free radicals are released. When more energy is used and the rate of oxidation increases, free radicals are created in large numbers. This happens during exercise, and whenever your body encounters fatigue, illness, inflammation, pollution, toxins or radiation.

As you will see in the following paragraphs, glutathione is the body's key natural antioxidant. The best way to minimize oxidative damage is by raising intracellular GSH levels and keeping them there.

GSH: the Immune System Enhancer

A body well-stocked with intracellular glutathione resists illness more effectively than one that depends on exogenous (dietary) antioxidants. GSH helps prevent pathogens from gaining a foothold, and those that do get through are immediately confronted by an enhanced immune response. Glutathione is therefore both preventive and therapeutic. This is mostly because elevated glutathione levels produce more white blood cells, which constitute the most important division of the immune system's ground-troops. Glutathione's overall role in the immune response is discussed in Chapter 3.

Glutathione—the Detoxifier

Toxic substances are everywhere, exacerbated by continuous technological advance. Our cities are congested and polluted. Our food supplies are engineered. Unable to avoid all this, we inhale and ingest natural and synthetic toxins every day.

As long as your body has the health and nourishment it needs, it goes to great lengths to eliminate toxins and protect itself. Your main organ of detoxification is the liver—the largest in the body and the depository of the body's highest concentrations of glutathione. Experimental studies have shown that low glutathione levels lead to poor liver function and result in unnecessarily large amounts of toxins circulating through the body. They continuously damage individual cells and organs. Chapter 2 describes the role of glutathione in detoxification. The liver and its function is described in Chapter 9.

Glutathione—Energy Maintenance for the Cell

Cells require a constant supply of energy to perform their many tasks. Energy production has a downside too—toxic waste products that can interfere with further energy production. This is why glutathione is so critical. It takes part in energy production at: a) a molecular level, b) a cellular level and c) a whole-body level.

a) At the molecular level:
Energy is produced when nutrients are burned in the process of oxidation, producing unwanted by-products like free radicals. Glutathione's job is to mop them up. When there's isn't enough, free radicals act without restraint, breaking chemical bonds, causing general havoc.

b) At the cellular level:
Glutathione enables each cell's power generators (mitochondria) to produce uninterrupted, clean energy.

c) At a whole body level:
Glutathione's role in maintaining physical and mental performance is evident.

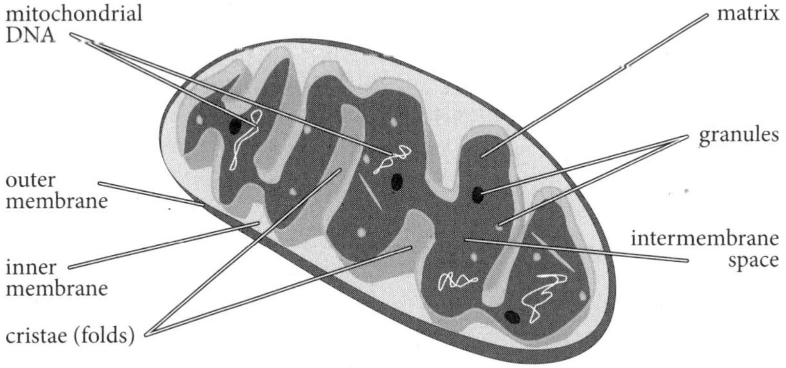

FIGURE 5: Mitochondria are tiny structures in the cell that act like "generators" to provide cellular energy. When these generators "heat up" from free radical accumulation, they can slow down or even burn out. Glutathione is needed to "cool down" these structures.

Glutathione—the Master Antioxidant

How does GSH work with other antioxidants? All have their advantages and disadvantages. You should never stop using established supplements like vitamins C and E, which act synergistically with GSH. This means they enhance each other's effectiveness.

We call GSH the master antioxidant because it replenishes the action of other antioxidants. When vitamins C and E pick up a damaging oxyradical, they hand it off to the GSH system and are then free to go back for others. GSH similarly neutralizes peroxide and lipoic acid. In fact, all of these antioxidants help to neutralize each other, and glutathione is at the center of cellular antioxidation systems. Strictly speaking, it's GSH and not the vitamin that ultimately neutralizes the radical.

Another synergistic antioxidant is selenium. Studies show it to be clinically similar to glutathione and it is an integral component of the important enzyme GSH-peroxidase. For this reason, selenium is considered a GSH booster.

None of these important but lesser antioxidants occur naturally in the cell—only

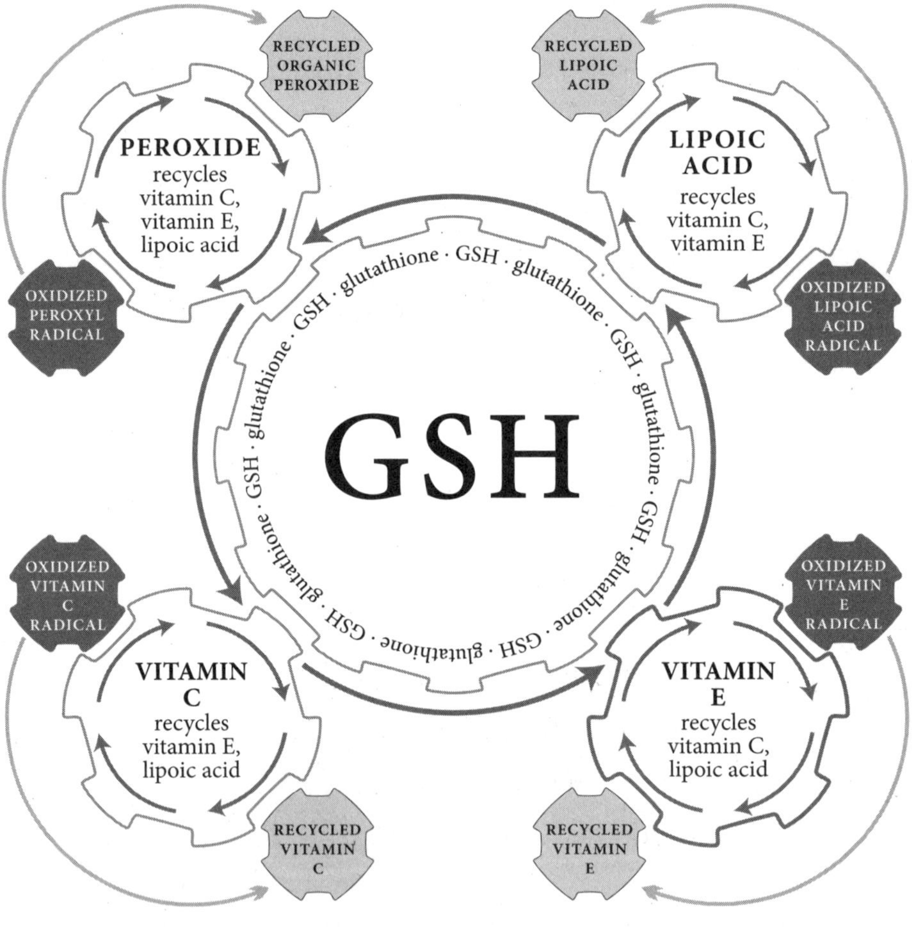

FIGURE 6: Inside each cell the antioxidation gears are driven by GSH as it recycles peroxide, lipoic acid, vitamin C, vitamin E and other antioxidants, getting them back to work

glutathione. All others are derived from the food we eat. Because GSH is a vital, natural component of your cells, it is an "endogenous" antioxidant, meaning that it's manufactured within, from amino acid precursors.

If you want to boost your body's defenses against oxidation, your best bet is to give it the raw materials it needs to produce glutathione. GSH is at the heart of cellular antioxidation. It works in conjunction with the secondary "exogenous" antioxidants such as peroxide, lipoic acid, vitamin C and vitamin E, relieving them of destructively charged ions and freeing them to return to the battle.

Conclusion

Glutathione carries out many crucial functions in the body, of which four stand out by the acronym "IDEA". GSH is **I**: a critical element that sustains the functioning and well-being of our **I**mmune systems, **D**: a key enzyme system for the **D**etoxification of countless noxious substances, **E**: **E**ssential for the maintenance of cellular **E**nergy, and **A**: the most important naturally-occurring **A**ntioxidant in our cells. These four vital roles played by glutathione throughout your body have been established beyond doubt. Considerable research is now underway to discover the full range of clinical applications for the preventative and therapeutic roles of elevated glutathione levels.

GLUTATHIONE

REFERENCES

Bachhawat AK, Kaur A. *Glutathione Degradation.* Antioxid Redox Signal 27(15) :1200-1216, 2017

Beutler E. *Nutritional and metabolic aspects of glutathione.* Annual Review of Nutrition 9:287-302, 1989

Braverman E, Pfeiffer C, Blum K, Smayda R. *The Healing Nutrients Within: Facts, Findings, and New Research on Amino Acids. [ISBN 0-87983-706-3]* Keats Publishing, New Canaan, CT 1987

Bray T, Taylor C. *Enhancement of tissue glutathione for antioxidant and immune functions in malnutrition.* Biochemistry Pharmacology 47:2113-23, 1994

Calabrese G, Morgan B, Riemer J. *Mitochondrial Glutathione: Regulation and Functions.* Antioxid Redox Signal 27(15):1162-1177, 2017

Carper J. *Stop Aging Now! [ISBN 0-06-018355-1]* HarperCollins Publishers, New York, NY, 1995

Commandeur JNM, Stijntjes GJ, Vermeulen NPE. *Enzymes and transport systems involved in the formation and disposition of glutathione S-conjugates.* Pharmacol. Reviews 47: 271-330, 1995

Deneke SM, Fanburg BL. *Regulation of cellular glutathione.* American Physiological Society L163-L173, 1989

Deponte M. *The Incomplete Glutathione Puzzle: Just Guessing at Numbers and Figures?* Antioxid Redox Signal 27(15):1130-1161, 2017

Espinosa-Diez C, Miguel V, Mennerich D, Kietzmann T et al. *Antioxidant responses and cellular adjustments to oxidative stress.* Redox Biol 6:183-97, 2015

Franco R, Schoneveld OJ, Pappa A, Panayiotidis Ml. *The central role of glutathione in the pathophysiology of human diseases.* Arch Physiol Biochem 113(4-5):234-58, 2007

Fraternale A, Brundu S, Magnani M. *Glutathione and glutathione derivatives in immunotherapy.* Biol Chem 398(2):261-275, 2017

Fahey, RC.`Protection of DNA by Thiols. *Pharmac. Therapeut. 39: 101-108, 1988*

Garcia-Giménez JL, Roma-Mateo C et al. *Role of glutathione in the regulation of epigenetic mechanisms in disease.* Free Radic Biol Med 112: 36-48, 2017

Go YM, Jones DP. *Redox theory of aging:implications for health and disease.* Clin Sci (Lond) 131(14):1669-1688, 2017

Homma t, Fujii J. *Application of Glutathione as Anti-Oxidative and Anti-Aging Drugs.* Curr Drug Metab 16(7):560-71, 2015

Kidd PM. Glutathione: *Systemic protectant against oxidative and free radical damage.* Alternative Medicine Review 2:155-176, 1997

Kidd PM, Huber W. *Natural antioxidants – First line of defense in Living with the aids virus: A strategy for long term survival.* PMK Biomedical-Nutritional Consulting: 115-142, 1991

Lomaestro B, Malone M. *Glutathione in health and disease: Pharmacotherapeutic Issues.* Annals of Pharmacotherapy 29:1263-73, 1995

Meister A. *Glutathione metabolism.* Methods in Enzymology 252:3-7, 1995

Meister A, Anderson ME. *Glutathione.* Ann Revue Biochemistry 52:711-60, 1983

Mindell E. *What you should Know About the Super Antioxidant Miracle. [ISBN 0-87983-721-7]* Keats Publishing, New Canaan, Connecticut, 1996

Pressman AH. *The GSH Phenomenon. [ISBN 0-312-15135-7]* St. Martin's Press, New York NY. First Edition, 1997

Poprac P, Jomova K, Simunkova M et al. *Targeting Free Radicals in Oxidative Stress-Related Human Diseases.* Trends Pharmacol Sci 38(7):592-607, 2017

Wu G, Fang YZ, Yang et al. *Glutathione metabolism and its implications for health.* J Nutr 134(3):489-92, 2004

2

GSH & Detoxification

Toxins, glutathione and health

Medical science and public health measures have notably reduced death rates and prolonged the average life span, especially in developed countries. But development has its downside. Our environment contains tens of thousands of confirmed toxic substances, and the pace of life, combined with consumer-oriented marketing, promotes poor lifestyle habits that, to some extent, we all adopt. In the twenty-first century we can expect a longer life span than our ancestors but one potentially burdened by chronic ailments. The full promise of longevity is blunted.

It's remarkable that we don't all succumb to the daily onslaught of toxins in our food, air and water. We have our body's defense mechanisms to thank, especially the GSH detoxification process. But like all biological systems, this can be overwhelmed by extensive or prolonged attack, and may eventually begin to function poorly.

Although GSH was discovered in 1888 by the French scientist Joseph de Rey-Pailhade, it was almost a century later, in the 1970s, that its detoxifying role was identified. Over the past thirty years a detailed understanding of this process unfolded slowly, but the huge growth of interest in preventive medicine and in GSH is reenergizing research and leading to new discoveries. The major organs of detoxification and elimination are the liver and the kidneys. They have the body's highest levels of intracellular GSH (see Table 3).

Organ	GSH (µ-mol/g)
Liver	7.3
Kidney	4.0
Lung	2.9
Heart	2.4
Brain	1.5

Table 3: Organ GSH content in lab animals

GSH is the most important thiol[1] in living systems. It plays a critical role not only in humans but in all life, including insects, plants and micro-organisms.

Jones, Brown and Sternberg, a team of biochemists from Emory School of Medicine in Atlanta, wrote, "GSH has multiple functions in detoxification and its depletion has been associated with an increased risk of chemical toxicity." They continue, "GSH can be depleted by different agents (and GSH) plasma levels vary with gender, age, race and dietary habits." This suggests that an individual's risk of environmental toxic damage can be determined by monitoring glutathione levels.

Lew and Quitanihila at the University of California confirmed the upside of this discovery. The increased liver GSH levels seen in actively trained, physically fit individuals render them better equipped to handle toxic threats from substances like acetaminophen. Flanagan and Meridith at the Poisons Unit of Guy's Hospital in London reviewed the use of the GSH-enhancing drug N-acetylcysteine (NAC) as a detoxifying agent. They believe that besides, its common use against acetami-

[1] Sulfur-containing amino-acid

arsenic	cadmium	copper	lead	selenium	tin
arsine	chromium	gold	mercury	silver	vanadium
bismuth	cobalt	iron	nickel	thallium	zinc

TABLE 4: *A list of potential heavy metal toxins*

nophen overdose, research will demonstrate its potential to detoxify the body of carbon monoxide, carbon tetrachloride, chloroform, and other harmful compounds.

Over the years, and sometimes in large doses, we're exposed to many organic and inorganic toxins. As long as there's sufficient glutathione they are removed from the body, but if there's a shortage they can push the body into a gradual or rapid decline. Fortunately, this process may be reversed by raising GSH with pharmaceutically-induced or even dietary supplementation, as illustrated by the following stories:

Case studies

LARA, A 28-YEAR-OLD TECHNICAL WRITER, *did what she could to live a healthy lifestyle. She exercised regularly but was finding it increasing difficult to satisfy herself nutritionally. Foods she'd previously enjoyed—including dairy and meat products—left her bloated, cranky and fatigued. She started taking various supplements to round off her dietary needs, but still felt "left short." In addition, trips downtown were fraught with episodes of itchy, runny eyes and nose, headaches and shortness of breath. Because perfumes, auto exhaust and other odors made her feel 'sick,' she avoided crowds. Fortunately, her job being what it was, she could do most of her work at home. After visiting a local clinic she was diagnosed as agoraphobic, but this made no sense to her. She loved going out. Then a nutritionist suggested that she was in fact suffering from multiple chemical sensitivity, and prescribed the GSH-enhancing drug NAC as a detoxifier. After a few weeks of cramps, diarrhea, sweating and considerable urination she began to improve. She started cautiously reintroducing previous favorites back into her diet. She remains on her low dose of NAC and her ability to tolerate odors is getting better.*

LINDA WAS A RECENTLY UNEMPLOYED, *24 year-old office manager whose common-law husband had abruptly moved out of their apartment. Distressed, she drank two bottles of wine and swallowed 30 to 40 tablets of extra strength (500 mg) acetaminophen (paracetamol). After the alcohol had worn off, she showed up next morning at the emergency department of the local hospital. Her stomach wasn't pumped because too much time had passed since she'd taken the pills. Her acetaminophen blood level was at 150 micrograms per milliliter (µg/ml)—enough to damage the liver if left untreated—and her initial liver enzyme profile was already showing abnormalities. She was treated immediately with NAC (N-acetylcysteine), and thereafter every four hours for the next three days. Oral charcoal was also used on day one, and although her liver enzyme abnormalities worsened over the first forty-eight hours, they eventually returned to normal. Linda suffered nausea and cramps during her hospital stay, but was glad to be alive. After being cleared by the psychiatric consultant, she was sent home.*

Prevention

A serious shortcoming of traditional medicine is its focus on treatment rather than prevention. This isn't without cause. The need to see people who are sick or suffering is always more pressing than the good intention to meet those in good health. And there's no lack of disease out there—if anything, there's a shortage of doctors. It's fallen to other branches of the healing arts to address the issues of prevention and general well-being.

Nutrition-sensitive approaches can teach us a great deal, but the heart and soul of health maintenance is self-awareness. We must study for ourselves, pay attention to our bodies and learn to manage the conditions that affect our well-being. As much as possible, we need to know what harmful influences to avoid and identify the unavoidable ones. Then we can provide our body with the resources it needs to fight them.

Smoking and tobacco

Medically, statistically and economically, one of the greatest risks to health in North America is tobacco. A huge body of evidence accumulated over decades leaves no doubt that cigarette smoking profoundly increases the risk of contracting cancer, as well as chronic obstructive pulmonary disease (COPD), including asthma, chronic bronchitis and emphysema, as well as cardiovascular disease. After years of successful lobbying and denial, the tobacco industry finally admitted what the medical community knew for ages—cigarettes kill.

Cigarette smoke releases thousands of different chemicals, each puff containing trillions of free radicals. The smoke literally burns away antioxidant vitamins like C and E along with other nutrients. Even worse, it triggers inflammation of the lungs—the principal source of oxidative stress. The degree of lung inflammation and injury is directly related to the extent of oxidation caused by cigarette smoke. On top of all this, tobacco tar contains potent carcinogens that—as well as lung cancer—cause all sorts of other tumors. GSH is well known to scavenge these free radicals and also to neutralize the tobacco-based toxins through binding and eliminating them from the body. If you're not ready to quit smoking or if you can't avoid second-hand smoke, elevated GSH levels will help protect you.

Many studies have outlined the role of GSH in preventing or suppressing the damage caused by smoking. Clinicians have even used glutathione-enhancing drugs like NAC to actually treat some of these consequences, and not just to try and prevent them. A more detailed analysis and review of clinical studies is found in Chapter 12.

Radiation

Ionizing radiation is a known cause of cancer, and that's not the only harm it does. One of the most extensively studied of all carcinogens, it accounts for about three percent of all cancers. Some radiation comes from natural sources such as cosmic rays and natural radioactive minerals. The most common is the ultraviolet radiation of sunlight, a threat that's increased by the depletion of the protective ozone layer. Other sources include nuclear waste from energy plants, industrial waste, weapons test residue and certain building materials. X-rays from radiographs, mammograms, CT-scans and other medical test equipment are weak but not insignificant. They have a cumulative effect over time.

Exposure to radiation results in the formation of hydroxyradicals—the most reactive of all free radicals. Many studies have shown that GSH is key to neutralizing them. Some physicians are now raising GSH levels of patients prior to radiation therapy. This tends to reduce side-effects, and has also been seen to enhance the effectiveness of the therapy itself.

At the Swiss Institute for Experimental Cancer Research, Applegate conducted studies on human cells cultured in the laboratory. First, his team depleted their glutathione levels with the drug BSO. Then they exposed the cells to radiation. What they found was a significantly higher ratio of DNA mutations, meaning an increased risk of cancer. Navarro and a team in Spain showed that humans exposed to radiation suffered from significant GSH abnormalities.

In India, Bhattathiri led a research team studying patients with oral cancer. Each patient's GSH levels were measured before radiation therapy, and then compared to the side-effects of the therapy. It was clear that the lower their initial GSH levels, the more injury they suffered. Following these tests the team felt able to identify in advance the susceptibility of any patient to radiation damage, simply by measuring their GSH levels. They recommended that treatment dosages be adapted to the individual's ability to withstand the therapy.

A group of genetic researchers at Germany's Nurnberg University studied the potential of NAC to protect human white blood cells from X-ray damage. Cells pretreated with NAC clearly had a protective advantage over untreated ones. Glutathione's role in cancer, chemotherapy, and radiotherapy is discussed in Chapter 5.

Enhanced GSH levels can also reduce the damaging effects of sunburn. It is believed that skin damaged by sunburn can develop various forms of skin cancer. Chapter 21 reviews some important studies relating to sun exposure, ultraviolet-radiation damage and glutathione's protective role.

Heavy metal toxicity

Heavy metals are metals from periodic table groups 2A through 6A. The semi-metallic elements boron, arsenic, selenium, and tellurium are often included. Many are essential in small quantities but toxic at high levels. Absorbed from the environment and food chain, they accumulate in both plant and animal tissues and can become a significant health hazard. Some metals like arsenic are actually used as poisons. Nutritional supplements like iron, and medications like bismuth, are helpful or essential in appropriate doses, but they too can be toxic at high levels.

Heavy metals influence all sorts of living tissue and interfere with many bodily functions. The nervous system, the renal (kidney) system, the cardiovascular (heart and circulation) system, the hematological (blood) system, the gastrointestinal (digestive) system and many others are impacted one after another. Heavy metals exact their damage by generating free radicals and also by sabotaging the biochemistry of normal metabolic functions.

Glutathione and its associated enzymes help regulate and eliminate many of these metals. Clinical studies have outlined the role of GSH in heavy metal toxicology. Its role has been examined in the way cells process arsenic, arsine, bismuth, cadmium, chromium, cobalt, copper, gold, iron, lead, mercury, nickel, selenium, silver, thallium, tin, vanadium and zinc. Of all these substances, mercury appears to deplete GSH the most.

Mercury toxicity

Mercury is a heavy metal and an insidious, potent toxin that warrants special attention. It's commonly found in our environment and is the subject of considerable controversy—especially when it comes to mercury amalgams (dental fillings). I've seen usually staid and sober medical and dental professionals coming close to blows over this issue at educational conventions. However, one of the tenets of the Hippocratic oath is, "Above all, do no harm." Ample clinical evidence supports a much closer look into how this significant neurotoxin is used in clinical applications.

Mercuric substances can be either organic or inorganic. Inorganic forms include pure or elemental mercury (quicksilver), or the salts of mercury (mercuric chloride, mercuric oxide and others), all of which may be inhaled or ingested. That brings a high risk to occupations such as dentistry; manufacture of batteries, explosives and jewelry; development of photographic film and taxidermy. Organic mercury comes in many forms,

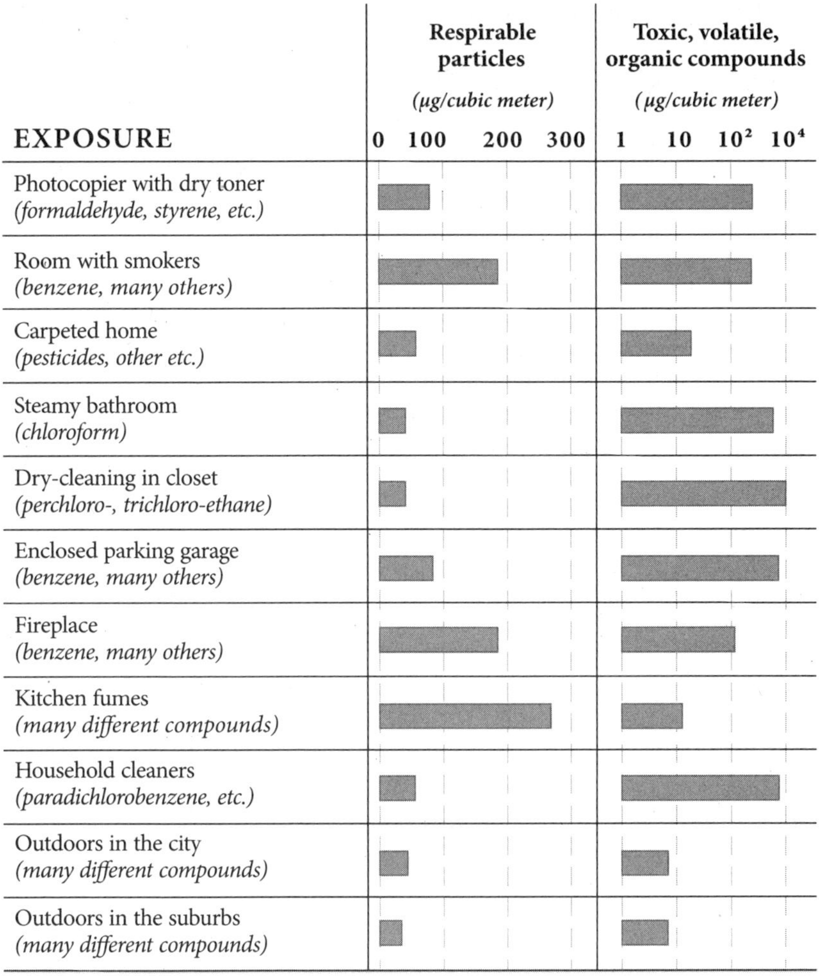

TABLE 5: Everyday toxins (you're better off outdoors!)

[Source: Ott and Roberts, "Everyday exposure to toxic Pollutants" Scientific American 278(2);86-91, 1998]

methyl-mercury being the most common. It's highly toxic. Poisoning by this form usually follows accidental ingestion. Farm workers, embalmers and those who produce or use pesticides, fungicides, insecticides, bactericides, drugs and preservatives are all at risk.

Although primarily a neurotoxin (nerve poison), mercury can cause a broad range of problems, including kidney failure, severe nausea and vomiting, diarrhea, oral lesions (stomatitis), lung inflammation (pneumonitis) and rashes. It affects the nervous system with such symptoms as emotional instability, anxiety, memory loss, and lethargy. The expression "mad as a hatter" has an interesting basis in fact. Hat-makers in the nineteenth century used elemental mercury to form and weigh down their hats, and often paid a high neurological price for repeatedly handling this toxin. Serious mercury poisoning includes tingling or loss of sensation in the extremities, poor coordination, tremors, slurred speech and tunnel vision. These symptoms may lead to paralysis, coma and death.

Traditional treatment of mercury toxicity

requires binding of the metal to larger organic molecules, a process called chelation. Chelating agents may be administered either orally (e.g. D-penicillamine), intramuscularly[2] (e.g. Dimercaprol, BAL) or intravenously.[3] Once chelated, the mercury complex is carried out of the body through normal excretion of urine or stool.

It's been long known that glutathione is a primary cellular defense against mercury toxicity. It begins by effectively quenching the formation of free radicals. Then, crucially, it binds directly to mercuric compounds, expelling them from the cell and enabling the body to excrete them.

A recent article from the International Archives of Occupational and Environmental Health measured the impact of mercury exposure on glutathione levels. Forty-two workers from a chloralkali[4] factory exposed to elemental mercury were compared to seventy-five workers from a lime production plant, where there is no mercury. As expected, blood levels of mercury were higher in mercury workers—and so were levels of lipid peroxidation. This evidence suggests that mercury significantly decreases the detoxifying effects of glutathione peroxidase.

In the laboratory, many studies have shown glutathione to protect cells from toxicity. By raising GSH levels, a team of toxicologists from the University of Arizona was able to decrease mercury-induced kidney damage. An Argentinian team had equal success using NAC to preserve renal (kidney) function. Similar positive results were found using glutathione monoester, selenium, and other agents to enhance GSH levels.

Experiments on tissues from the liver, nerve and small intestine—and even from developing fetuses—have verified that mercury lowers glutathione levels and leads to increased toxic damage. They also confirmed that elevating or sustaining glutathione levels significantly protects cells against mercury poisoning.

Dental amalgams

Quite a controversy surrounds the alleged ill-effects of mercury in dental fillings (amalgams). Mercury is used in so-called 'silver' fillings, making them them malleable and strong, and has been a mainstay of dentistry for many decades. Studies show that for people not otherwise exposed to mercury, these fillings are their main source of exposure. The same studies also note that urinary mercury excretion is significantly higher in people with these fillings, and that excretion levels correspond to the amount of filling in their mouths. A German study determined that the long-term excretion of mercury could be cut to one-fifth by removing amalgams. A recent study from the Journal of Dental research by Sandborgh-England concluded that, "...the process of removing amalgam fillings can have a considerable impact on Hg (mercury) levels in biological fluids."

The big question is whether or not this higher level of mercury exposure is enough to produce ill-effects. A recent study by the Australian Blumer looked at 80 patients with dental amalgams who also showed symptoms of chronic mercury toxicity. Using the chelator EDTA to flush mercury from the body, it was found that the urine of patients with fillings had significantly higher levels of mercury. The fillings were removed and patients continued to take oral chelators along with selenium supplementation (to raise glutathione peroxidase). After three months, patients were either symptom-free or greatly improved. Regardless of the controversy, more and more dentists are switching from mercury-based amalgams to newer and safer compounds for fillings.

Proponents of the amalgam-toxicity school of thought wish to detoxify both patients and

[2] into muscles
[3] into the bloodstream
[4] a process that produces chlorine, sodium hydroxide and other industrial chemicals

the dental professionals who are exposed daily to mercury vapors. Merely removing the exposure is not enough. Like all heavy metals, mercury lodges deep within cells unless/until it is properly chelated (removed).

NAC (N-acetylcysteine) raises GSH levels and has been used to detoxify organic mercury (organomercury). Researchers from the Department of Environmental Medicine at the University of Rochester, NY showed that oral NAC profoundly accelerates urinary methylmercury excretion—as much as ten times more than usual. NAC is able to detoxify mercury compounds.

One of the foremost scientists dealing with heavy metal and mercury toxicity is Dr. David Quig of Chicago. After tracing the interplay of mercuric compounds, glutathione, cysteine and other metallothioneins[5] he suggested that the long-term effects of constant low-level mercury exposure have been underestimated. According to him, the most effective way to eliminate these toxins from deep tissue (like the brain) is by eating high-quality, cysteine-rich whey protein. Although the bioactivity of natural whey can easily be denatured, good quality whey protein can have significant GSH-enhancing properties. Studies using undenatured whey protein are currently underway by several research groups. The protein precursors of GSH act here as oral chelating agents.

High levels of mercury poisoning are often treated by emergency dialysis (blood filtration). Wishing to improve this treatment, American military doctors at the Health Sciences Department of Pharmacology at Bethesda, Maryland experimented with ten different chelating agents to remove mercury from blood fluid. The results surprised these kidney specialists, and were revealing. NAC was such an effective chelating agent that it surpassed all traditional ones. Clinicians are now starting to integrate this knowledge, using GSH therapy as a complement to their usual emergency treatments.

Case study

SHERYL, A 32-YEAR-OLD MOTHER OF FOUR, fell ill after the caesarian delivery of her last child. This was two years earlier and the surgical incision was taking far too long to heal. Puzzled, her gynecologist noted some muscular atrophy. She experienced such profound weakness that she was sometimes bedridden for days. Over the next 18 months this fatigue recurred until she was admitted to hospital. Various diagnoses were considered—including multiple sclerosis and chronic fatigue syndrome—but treatment for these conditions was ineffective. When her dentist suggested that mercury toxicity might be a contributing factor, she had her mercury amalgams removed. Then, to rid her of residual mercury herbal supplementation was used, and her symptoms improved modestly. After further internet research, the dentist was led to NAC (N-acetylcysteine). He suggested it to Sheryl and she concurred. Within five days she was markedly stronger. After ten days she walked without pain. Two weeks later she rode her bike for the first time in 2½ years. Three weeks later, other than some mild nausea she felt "almost back to normal." She still feels well and continues to raise an active family.

Lead poisoning

Plumbism, or lead poisoning, is a public health problem that dates back to Roman times. 'Plumbium' is Latin for lead, a metal that for centuries was used in plumbing. Other forms of exposure have been common for just as long, through cooking and eating utensils, pottery, and lead-based paints, now fortunately discontinued. Moonshine liquor is sometimes prepared using automobile radiators, pipes and barrels that are soldered with lead. Mechanics, battery manufacturers, solderers and other tradespeople using lead

[5] Organic metal-sulfur compounds

are subject to occupational exposure.

Lead poisoning symptoms may be subtle and non-specific. They are often hard to diagnose. Acute lead poisoning may be accompanied by severe nausea and vomiting, diarrhea, kidney failure, seizures, coma, paralysis, and death. Continuous, repeated exposure leads to anemia, weakness, aches and pains and irritability—not to mention a host of intellectual disabilities that can profoundly affect learning and behavior. Treatment includes removing the source of lead exposure, and chelation therapy.

Like mercury, lead is detoxified cell by cell with the glutathione enzyme system. The pro-oxidant effect of lead is counterbalanced by the antioxidant capabilities of GSH, and the lead molecule itself can be conjugated (bound) to glutathione and removed from the body.

Lead toxicity affects many tissues, including the central and peripheral nervous system, the liver, the kidneys and red blood cells. Depleted stores of GSH usually indicate increased severity of the problem. Restoration of glutathione levels is protective and helps eliminate lead. Raising GSH levels with agents like NAC and selenium have been a useful complement to traditional therapies, acting at the level of the liver, kidney, red blood cells and even the lens of the eye to counteract the deleterious effect of lead poisoning.

The anemia (loss of red blood cells) that is characteristic of lead toxicity is caused by several different factors. High levels of oxidative stress lead to lipid peroxidation of the red blood cell membrane, followed by cell disruption. A Japanese research group studied workers with high occupational lead exposure by measuring their lipid peroxidation levels, lead concentration and glutathione peroxidase activity. The results show that lead levels and peroxidation levels seem to be directly related, and levels of the essential GSH-peroxidase enzymes fell as lead levels rose.

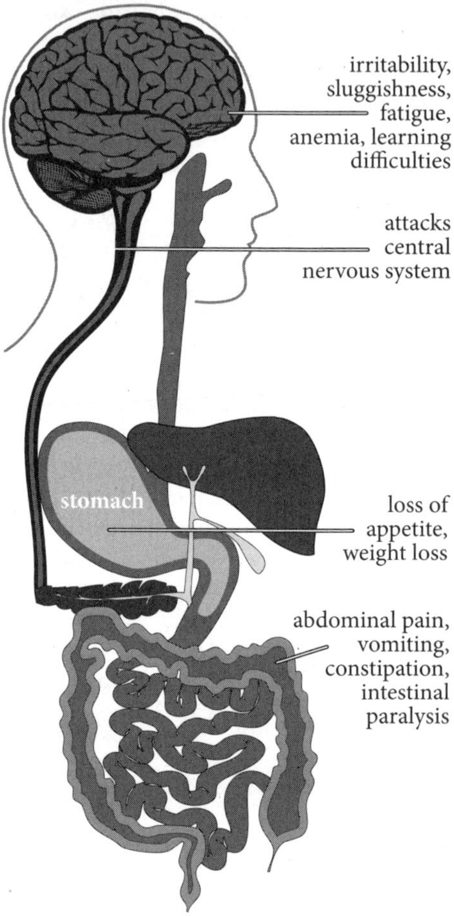

FIGURE 7: Some effects of lead toxicity

Environmental illness

Chronic exposure to xenobiotics (substances foreign to the body) may lead to subtle and hard-to-pinpoint changes in health, and to the full-blown syndromes of Environmental Illness (EI). These often reveal themselves as an unpredictable combination of minor complaints—such as headaches, fatigue and lethargy—that tend to confuse diagnosis. They may be quite profound—as is the case of MCS (multiple chemical sensitivity), which has only recently been recognized as a diagnosable condition. For similar reasons, it was years before the medical community recognized Gulf War Syndrome as a specific illness.

At home, there's plenty of xenobiotic

Acetaminophen (Tylenol, Atasol, others)	**Benzopyrenes** (barbecued foods, fuel exhaust, cigarettes, etc.)
Other pharmaceuticals (Adriamycin, etc.)	**Heavy metals** (lead, mercury, cadmium, cobalt, copper, etc.)
Acetone (common solvent, cleaner, industrial agent)	**Organophosphate pesticides** (parathione, others)
Aflatoxin B1 (natural toxin, carcinogen from moldy nuts etc.)	**Peroxides** (lipid peroxides, cholesterol peroxides, others)
Aliphatic hydrocarbons (vinyl chloride, hexachlorohexane, plastics etc.)	**Isothiocyanates** Carbamates, thiocarbamates
Aromatic hydrocarbons (solvents, fuels, bromobenzenes, chlorobezenes, etc.)	**Arylamines, arylhalides** (industrial exposures, etc.)
Nitrosamines (smoked foods, salami, hot dogs, etc.)	**Sulfates, nitrocompounds, naphthalene** (fuel, fuel by-products, etc.)

TABLE 6: A short list of substances detoxified by GSH conjugation (there are countless more)

exposure. Carpets pick up pesticides from footwear; steamy bathrooms contain chloroform when chlorine in the water reacts with organic matter; dry-cleaned clothes hanging in your closet shed fumes of perchloro-ethane and trichloro-ethane; open fireplaces produce benzene; household cleaners contain paradichlorobenzene.

In the office, photocopy toner releases formaldehyde, styrene and other chemical pollutants. Enclosed parking garages are another source of benzene and other chemicals. Outdoors air in the city and even the country contains many different compounds that we should ideally avoid. And of course, rooms in which people are smoking tobacco contain dozens of carcinogens and other toxic chemicals.

Take care when using mildew removers, mothballs, scented detergents, fabric softeners, lawn fertilizers, pesticides, solvents and cleansers, paints, heating fuels, certain insulation materials and even products used to manufacture mattresses and furniture. A brief list of substances detoxified by GSH conjugation is shown in Table 5. Fortunately, a wealth of published information is available to help you track these substances and where they're used. There are excellent guides online and at your local bookstore describing how to set up an environmentally "safe" home.

Pollutants in the general environment are large in number and widely distributed. Exposure is unavoidable. Add to that the high concentration of specific substances found in various workplaces and the need for protection becomes clear. Writing about chemical toxicity in industrial workers, Parke and Sapota made a powerful statement about the sorts of threats that can be counteracted by GSH. In their report, they claim that many industrial workers with symptoms of systemic inflammation are often misdiagnosed with rheumatoid arthritis, viral infections, connective tissue diseases and similar maladies. Physicians need to be informed more thoroughly about the way chemical pollutants imitate inflammatory diseases.

Exposure to certain chemicals in the workplace has been connected to the onset of cancer. Ross and his colleagues at the University of Southern California linked a deficiency of GSH enzymes to bladder cancer in workers exposed to arylamines[6]—which are also present in cigarette smoke.

[6] Present in oxidants, epoxy polymers, explosives, fungicides, pesticides, colorants, polyurethanes; used in rubber, pharmacology, cosmetics, and other chemical industries

Chronic Fatigue Syndrome, Gulf War Syndrome and Multiple Chemical Sensitivity

These three health problems are dealt with together here for several reasons. They are mutually connected to a threefold combination: environmental exposure to toxins, inappropriate immunological response and genetic predisposition. Not only are symptoms intermittent, they also vary from one person to another, so doctors are hesitant to offer firm clinical diagnoses. Even the names and definitions of these diseases have only been accepted by the medical community with reluctance. There are still physicians who feel these conditions are manifestations of a psychological disorder.

Multiple chemical sensitivity is an environmental disease in which the buildup of toxins reaches a dangerous threshold before symptoms appear. Contact with additional toxins may then trigger a cascade of symptoms that often mimic other diseases. These circumstances make diagnosis very difficult. The onus is on the patient to avoid further exposure, and the health practitioner must suggest detoxification strategies. I have no doubt that, in the near future, glutathione-enhancing treatments will become a standard treatment.

An article in the American Journal of Medicine by Bell, Baldwin and Schwartz at the University of Arizona set out to summarize the connection of chronic fatigue syndrome to chemical sensitivity. They determined that severe chemical sensitivity is a factor in about one-fifth to one-half of chronic fatigue patients, and in about 5% of the American population. Between 15% and 30% of the general population report at least minor problems with chemical intolerances.

A paper entitled "Gulf War Illnesses: complex medical, scientific and political paradox," published by the Institute for Molecular Medicine in California, also linked chemical sensitivity to chronic fatigue syndrome. There is a higher incidence of CFS among Gulf War Veterans than in the general population. Once again, it may mimic other chronic multi-organ or immunological dysfunctions, and may be misdiagnosed and mistreated.

Scientists at the Center for Environmental Hazards Research in New Jersey have determined that, even when chronic fatigue syndrome and multiple chemical sensitivity syndrome are diagnosed among Gulf War Veterans, their symptoms differ substantially from the CFS and MCS diagnoses in the population at large. Discrepancies are found in immunological parameters, demographics and prognosis.

A discussion of chronic fatigue syndrome (CFS), also called chronic fatigue/immune dysfunction syndrome (CFIDS), myalgic encephalomyelitis (ME) or systemic exertion intolerance disease (SEID), would not be out of place in our chapter on immunology (Chapter 3). Looking at its causes, CFS appears to be less of a toxicological problem than an immune disorder. It is best classified as a post-viral or post-infectious syndrome. The causal sequence often begins with an acute viral illness, usually followed by an overactive lymphatic response—swollen glands or lymph node enlargement (a symptom of "glandular fever"). For unknown reasons, some people develop an abnormal immunological and neuro-endocrinological response. This inability to fight threats combines with an imbalance in the body's hormonal secretions to introduce the symptoms of CFS.

Rheumatologists have now better defined the syndrome to enable more accurate diagnosis. It is characterized by persistent fatigue, musculo-skeletal pain, sleep disturbance and cognitive and psychological abnormalities. A clear test for CFS does not yet exist, but researchers are trying to elaborate the many subtle biochemical and physiological changes that characterize it. One such group is led by Dr. Paul Cheney, one of the first clinicians to describe the syndrome in the late 1980's and early 90's. Founder and director of the Cheney Clinic in North Carolina, his research has been on the cutting edge of our understanding of chronic fatigue. He believes that, although the initial event may be viral, it is subsequent abnormalities in protein synthesis and enzyme production that lead to liver failure and the inability of cells to detoxify themselves.

Cheney initially used oral glutathione or injectable glutathione, and later the GSH precursor drug NAC (N-acetylcysteine), all with modest success. When bioactive, undenatured whey protein became available, many of his patients responded with dramatic results. This dietary source of GSH precursors is described in Chapter 4.

The recognized German immunochemist Dr. Wulf Droge has coined the term "Low CG Syndrome" to describe a number of disease states associated with a depletion of cysteine and glutathione. These include chronic fatigue syndrome, AIDS, certain cancers, sepsis, Crohn's disease, ulcerative colitis, major trauma and others.

Case study

William, a lawyer from Alabama, noticed a change in his health at age 39. His initial visits to a number of physicians were neither conclusive nor accurate in their diagnoses. None of their treatment options proved helpful. Unable to carry his usual heavy workload, he was forced to end his law practice in 1994. His own research led him to a local CFS support group, where he learned about a prestigious southeastern clinic specializing in chronic fatigue. Initial treatment with vitamins, nutrients and dietary changes proved minimally successful. The head of this clinic was investigating the use of undenatured whey protein and after 12 weeks, William's improvement was noticeable. Three months later, he woke up one morning and "felt well again." That day he picked up his golf clubs for the first time in five years. Months later he was shooting in the low 90's and planning to restart his practice.

Conclusion

The number of toxins our bodies deal with every day is truly remarkable. To cope with this burden a fit, rested, well-fed person must maintain adequate immunological and biochemical defenses. The role played by GSH in these defense systems cannot be overstated. Glutathione detoxifies a large number of pollutants, carcinogens, heavy metals, herbicides, pesticides and radiation. We are exposed every day to toxins like cigarette smoke, automobile exhaust, food preservatives and dental amalgam and our body depends on GSH for their removal. Substances that raise GSH levels are being used with increasing frequency in the field of toxicology with considerable success.

GSH & DETOXIFICATION

REFERENCES

Abt G, Vaghef H, Gebhart E, et al. *The role of n-acetylcysteine as a putative radioprotective agent on X-ray-induced dna damage as evaluated by alkaline single-cell electrophoresis.* Mutation Research 384: 55-64, 1997

Adenuga AA, Wright ME, Atkinson DB. *Evaluation of the reactivity of exhaust from various biodiesel blends as a measure of possible oxidative effects: A concern for human exposure.* Chemosphere 147:396-403, 2016

Ahmed T, Pathak R, Mustafa MD et al. *Ameliorating effect of N-acetylcysteine & curcumin on pesticide-induced oxidative DNA damage in human peripheral blood mononuclear cells.* Environ Monit Assess 179(1-4):293-9, 2011

Applegate LA, Lautier D, Frenk E, Tyrrell RM. *Endogenous glutathione levels modulate the frequency of both spontaneous & long wavelength ultraviolet induced mutations in human cells.* Carcinogenesis 13: 1557-1560, 1992

Aust SD, Chignell CF, Bray TM, Kalyanaraman B. Mason RP *Free radicals in toxicology.* Toxicology & Applied Pharmacology 120:168-178, 1993

Awasthi YC, Dao DD. *Glutathione-mediated detoxification mechanisms of human placenta.* Placenta Suppl. 3: 289-301, 1981

Baker DH, Czarnecki-Mauldon GL. *Pharmacological role of cysteine in ameliorating or exacerbating mineral toxicities.* American Institute of Nutrition 117:1003-1010, 1987

Baker MA, Dillard CJ, Tappel AL. *Effect of gold on selenium & glutathione peroxidase activities in rat tissues.* Drug Nutr. Interact. 3: 141-152, 1985

Ballatori N. *Glutathione mercaptides as transport forms of metals.* Adv. Pharmacol. 27: 271-298, 1994

Ballatori N, Lieberman MW, Wang W. *N-acetylcysteine as an antidote in methylmercury poisoning.* Environ. Health Perspect. 106: 267-271, 1998

Ballatori N, Wang W, Lieberman MW. *Accelerated methylmercury elimination in gamma-glutamyl transpeptidase-deficient mice.* American J. Pathol. 152: 1049-1055, 1998

Barbaro G, Di Lorenzo G, Ribersani M, et al. *Serum ferritin & hepatic glutathione concentrations in chronic hepatitis C patients related to the hepatitis C genotype.* J. Hepatol. 30: 774-782, 1999

Barcelos GR, Grotto D, de Marco KC et al. *Polymorphisms in glutathione-related genes modify mercury concentrations & antioxidant status in subjects environmentally exposed to methylmercury.* Sci Total Environ 463:319-25, 2013

Bell IR, Baldwin CM, Schwartz GE. *Illness from low levels of environmental chemicals: relevance to chronic fatigue syndrome & fibromyalgia.* American J. Med. 105(3A): 74S-82S, 1998

Bergerow J, Zander D, Freier I, Dunemann L. *Long-term mercury excretion in urine after removal of amalgam fillings.* Int. Arch. Occup. Environ. Health 66: 209-212, 1994

Bhattathiri VN, Sreelekha TT, Sebastien P, et al. *Influence of plasma GSH level on acute radiation mucositis of the oral cavity.* Int. J. Radiat. Oncol. Biol. Phys. 29: 383-386, 1994

Biaglow JE, Varnes ME, Epp ER, et al. *Role of GSH & other thiols in cellular response to radiation & drugs.* Drug Metabolism Review 20:1-12, 1989

Blair PC, Thompson MB, Bechtold M, et al. *Evidence for oxidative damage to red blood cells in mice induced by arsine gas.* Toxicology 63: 25-34, 1990

Blumer W. *Mercury toxicity in dental amalgam fillings.* J. Adv. In Med. 11: 219-221, 1998

Bose S, Mukhopadhyay B, Chaudhury S, Bhattacharya S. *Correlation of metal distribution, reduced GSH & metallothionine levels in liver & kidney of rat.* Indian J. Exp. Biol. 32:679-681, 1994

Bowatte G, Lodge CJ et al. *Do Variants in GSTs Modify the Association between Traffic Air Pollution & Asthma in Adolescence?* Int J Mol Sci 17(4):485, 2016

Bowatte G, Lodge CJ, Perret JL et al. *Interactions of GST Polymorphisms in Air Pollution Exposure & Respiratory Diseases & Allergies.* Curr Allergy Asthma Rep 16(12):85, 2016

Bounous G, Molson J. *Competition for glutathione precursors between the immune system & the skeletal muscle: pathogenesis of chronic fatigue syndrome.* Med Hypotheses 53(4):347-9, 1999

Breton CV, Salam MT, Vora H, Gauderman WJ, Gilliland FD. *Genetic variation in the glutathione synthesis pathway, air pollution, & children's lung function growth.* Am J Respir Crit Care Med 183(2):243-8, 2011

Bulat P, Dujic I, Potkonjak B, Vidakovic A. *Activity of glutathione peroxidase & superoxide dismutase in workers occupationally exposed to mercury.* Int. Arch. Occup. Environm. Health 71 Suppl: S37-S39, 1998

Bump EA, Brown JM. *Role of GSH in the radiation response of mammalian cells in vitro & in vivo.* Pharmacology & Therapeutics 47:117-136,1990

Burton CA, Hatelid K, Divine K, et al. *Glutathione effects on toxicity & uptake of mercuric chloride & sodium arsenite in rabbit renal cortical slices.* Environ. Health Perspect. 103 Suppl 1: 81-84, 1995

Cabaña-Muñoz ME, Parmigiani-Izquiero JM, Bravo-González LA et al. *Increased Zn/Glutathione Levels & Higher Superoxide Dismutase-1 Activity as Biomarkers of Oxidative Stress in Women with Long-Term Dental Amalgam Fillings: Correlation between Mercury/Aluminium Levels (in Hair) & Antioxidant Systems in Plasma.* PLoS One 10(6):e0126339, 2015

Castro-Giner F, Künzli N, Jacquemin B et al *Traffic-related pollution, oxidative stress genes, & asthma (ECHRS).* Environ Health Perspect 117(2):1919-24, 2009

Chatterjee A. *Reduced glutathione: a radioprotector or a modulator of DNA-repair activity?* Nutrients 5(2):525-42, 2013

Chaudhari A, Dutta S. *Alterations in tissue GSH & angiotensin converting enzyme due to inhalation of diesel engine exhaust.* Journal of Toxicology & Environmental Health 9:327-337, 1982

Chen BY, Chen CH, Chuang YC et al. *Schoolchildren's antioxidation genotypes are susceptible factors for reduced lung function & airway inflammation caused by air pollution.* Environ Res 149:145-

150, 2016

Chen CY, Huang YL, Lin TH. *Lipid peroxidation in liver of mice administered with nickel chloride: with special reference to trace elements & antioxidants.* Biol. Trace Elem. Res. 61: 193-205, 1998

Chen TS, Richie JP Jr, Lang CA. *Life span profiles of glutathione & acetaminophen detoxification.* Drug Metab. Dispos. 18: 882-887, 1990

Chhabra SK, Hashim S, Rao AR. *Modulation of hepatic glutathione system of enzymes in suckling mouse pups exposed translactationally to malathione.* J. Appl. Toxicol. 13: 411-416, 1993

Cross CE, Halliwell B, Borish ET, et al. *Oxygen radicals & human disease.* Annals of Internal Medicine 107:526-545, 1987

Colovic MB, Vasic VM, Djuric DM, Krstic DZ. *Sulphur-containing Amino Acids.* Curr Med Chem 25(3):324

Colovic MB, Vasic VM, Djuric DM, Krstic DZ. *Sulphur-containing Amino Acids: Protective Role Against Free Radicals & Heavy Metals* Curr Med Chem 25(3):324-335, 2018

Daggett DA, Nuwaysir EF, Nelson SA, et al. *Effects of triethyl lead administration on the expression of glutathione S-transferase isoenzymes & quinone reductase in rat kidney & liver.* Toxicology 117: 61-71, 1997

Daggett DA, Oberley TD, Nelson SA, et al. *Effect of lead on rat kidney & liver: GST expression & oxidative stress.* Toxicology 128: 191-206, 1998

DeLeve LD, Kaplowitz N. *GSH metabolism & its role in hepatotoxicity.* Pharmacology & Therapeutics 52:287-305, 1991

Delfino RJ, Stainer N, Tjoa T et al. *Air pollution exposures & circulating biomarkers of effect in a susceptible population: clues to potential causal component mixtures & mechanisms.* Environ Health Perspect 117(8):1232-8, 2009

De Luca C, Raskovic D, Pacifico V, Thai JC, Korkina L. *The search for reliable biomarkers of disease in multiple chemical sensitivity & other environmental intolerances.* Int J Environ Res Public Health 8(7):2770-97, 2011

De Luca C, Scordo MG, Cesareo E et al. *Biological dfinition of multiple chemical sensitivity from redox state & cytokine profiling & not from polymorphisms of xenobiotic-metabolizing enzymes.* Toxicol Appl Pharmacol 248(3):285-92, 2010

Droge W, Holme E. *Role of cysteine & glutathione in hiv infection & other diseases associated with muscle wasting & immunological dysfunction.* FASEB. J. 11: 1077-1089, 1997

Eke BC, Vural N, Iscan M. *Combined effects of ethanol & cigarette smoke on hepatic & pulmonary xenobiotic metabolizing enzymes in rats.* Chem. Biol. Interact. 102: 155-167, 1996

Elbini Dhouib I, Jallouli M, Annabi A et al. *A minireview on N-acetylcysteine: An old drug with new approaches.* Life Sci 151:359-363, 2016

El-Ebiary AA, Elsharkawy RE, Soliman NA et al. *N-acetylcysteine in Acute Organophosphorus Pesticide Poisoning: A Randomized, Clinical Trial.* Basic Clin Pharmacol Toxicol 119(2):222-7, 2016

Ercal N, Treeratphan P, Hammond TC, et al. *In vivo indices of oxidative stress in lead-exposed C57BL/6 mice are reduced by treatment with meso-2,3-dimercaptosuccinic acid or N-acetyl-cysteine.* Free Radic. Biol. Med. 21: 157-161, 1996

Ercal N, Treeratphan P, Lutz P, et al. *N-acetylcysteine protects Chinese hamster ovary (CHO) cells from lead-induced oxidative stress.* Toxicology 108: 57-64, 1996

Ferguson CL, Cantilenia LR Jr. *Mercury clearance from human plasma during in vitro dialysis: screening systems for chelating agents.* J. Toxicol. Clin. Toxicol. 30: 423-441, 1992

Flanagan RJ, Meredith TJ. *Use of n-acetylcysteine in clinical toxicology. American J.* Med. 91(3C): 131S-139S, 1991

Fuertes E, Brauer M, MacIntyre E et al. *Childhood allergic rinitis, traffic-related air pollution, & variability in the GSTP1, TNF, TLR2, & TLR4 genes: results from the TAG Study.* J Allergy Clin Immunol 132(2):342-52, 3012

Geier DA, Carmody T, Kern JK, King PG, Geier MR. *A significant dose-dependent relationship between mercury exposure from dental amalgams & kidney integrity biomarkers: a further assessment of the Casa Pia children's dental amalgam trial.* Hum Exp Toxicol 32(4):434-40, 2013

Garner M, Reglinski J, Smith WA, Stewart MJ. *The interaction of colloidal metals with erythrocytes.* J. Inorg. Biochem. 56: 283-290, 1994

Giannini L, Vannacci A, Missanelli A et al. *Amatoxin poisoning: a 15-year retrospective analysis & follow-up evaluation of 105 patients.* Clin Toxicol (Phila) 45(5):539-42, 2007

Gugliandolo A, Gangemi C, Calabro C et al. *Assessment of glutathione peroxidase-1 polymorphisms, oxidative stress & DNA damage in sensitivity-related illnesses.* Life Sci 145:27-33, 2016

Gilford FT, Hope J. *Deficient glutathione in the pathophysiology of mycotoxin-related illness.* Toxins (Basel) 6(2):608-23, 2014

Girardi G, Elias MM. *Effectiveness of n-acetylcysteine in protecting against mercuric chloride-induced nephrotoxicity.* Toxicology 67: 155-164, 1991

Girardi G, Elias MM. *Effect of different renal glutathione levels on renal mercury disposition & excretion in the rat.* Toxicology 81: 57-67, 1993

GOSHORN RK. *Chronic fatigue syndrome: a review for clinicians.* Semin. Neurol. 18: 237-242, 1998

GRAF P, SIES H. *Hepatic uptake of cadmium & its biliary release as affected by dithioerythritol & glutathione.* Biochem. Pharmacol. 33: 639-643, 1984

GSTRAUNTHALER G, PFALLER W, KOTANKA P. *Glutathione depletion & in vitro lipid peroxidation in mercury or maleate induced acute renal failure.* Biochem. Pharmacol. 32: 2969-2972, 1983

GURER H, OZGUNES H, NEAL R, ET AL. *Antioxidant effects of n-acetylcysteine & succimer in red blood cells from lead-exposed rats.* Toxicology 128: 181-189, 1998

GYURASICS A, KOSZORUS L, VARGA F, GREGUS Z. *Increased biliary excretion of glutathione is generated by the glutathione-dependant hepatobiliary transport of antimony & bismuth.* Biochem. Pharmacol. 44:1275-1281, 1992

HALL MN, NIEDZWIECKI M, LIU X ET AL. *Chronic arsenic exposure & blood glutathione & glutathione disulfide concentrations in Bangladeshi adults.* Environ Health Perspect 121(9):1068-74, 2013

HANADA K, SAWAMURA D, TAMAI K, HASHIMOTO I, KOBAYASHI S. *Photo-protective effect of esterified GSH against ultraviolet B induced sunburn cell formation in the hairless mice.* Journal of Investigative Dermatology 108:727-730, 1997

HASAN M, HAIDER SS. *Acetyl-homocysteine thiolactone protects against some neurotoxic effects of thallium.* Neurotoxicology 10: 257-261, 1989

HERNANDEZ-ESCOBAR SA, AVILA-CASADO MC ET AL. *Cytological damage of nasal epithelium associated with decreased glutathione peroxidase in residents from a heavily polluted city.* Int Arch Occup Environ Health 82(5):603-12, 2009

HIROTA Y. *Effect of methylmercury on the activity of glutathione peroxidase in rat liver.* Am. Ind. Hyg. Assoc. J. 47: 556-558, 1986

HOUSER MT, MILNER LS, KOLBECK PC, ET AL. *Glutathione monoethyl ester moderates mercuric chloride-induced acute renal failure.* Nephron 61: 449-455, 1992

HSU JM. *Lead toxicity as related to GSH metabolism.* Journal of Nutrition 101:26-33, 1981

HULTBERG B, ANDERSON A, ISSAKSON A. *Alterations of thiol metabolism in human cell lines induced by low amounts of copper, mercury or cadmium ions.* Toxicology 126: 203-212, 1998

HULTBERG B, ANDERSON A, ISSAKSON A. *Alterations of thiol metabolism in human cell lines induced by low amounts of copper, mercury or cadmium ions.* Toxicology 126: 203-212, 1998

HWANG BF, YOUNG LH, TSAI CH ET AL. *Fine particle, ozone exposure, & asthma/wheezing: effect modification by glutathione S-transferase P1 polymorphisms.* PLoS One 8(1):e52715, 2013

ISLAM T, BERHANE K, MCCONNELL R ET AL. *Glutathione-S-transferase (GST) P1, GSTM1, exercise, ozone & asthma incidence in school children.* Thorax 64(3):197-202, 2009

JAMES SJ, SLIKKER W 3RD, MELNYK S ET AL. *Thimerosal neurotoxicity is associated with glutathione depletion: protection with glutathione precursors.* Neurotoxicology 26(1):1-8, 2005

JAMMES Y, STEINBERG JG, MAMBRINI O ET AL. *Chronic fatigue syndrome: assessment of increased oxidative stress & altered muscle excitability in response to incremental exercise.* J Intern Med 257(3):299-310, 2005

JAN AT, ALI A, HAQ Q. *Glutathione as an antioxidant in inorganic mercury induced nephrotoxicity.* J Postgrad Med 57(1):72-7, 2011

JAYAPRAKASH K. *Mercury vapor inhalation & its effect on glutathione peroxidase in goldsmiths exposed occupationally.* Toxicol Ind Health 25(7):463-5, 2009

JOMOVA K, VALKO M. *Advances in metal-induced oxidative stress & human disease.* Toxicology 283(2-3):65-87, 2011

JOZEFCZAK M, TEMANS T, VANGRONSVELD J, CUYPERS A. *Glutathione is a key player in metal-induced oxidative stress defenses.* Int J Mol Sci 13(3):3145-75, 2012

JONES DP, BROWN LA, STERNBERG P. *Variability in glutathione-dependant detoxification in vivo & its relevance to detoxification of chemical mixtures.* Toxicology 105: 267-274, 1995

KAMADA F, MASHIMO Y ET AL. *The GSTP1 gene is a susceptibility gene for childhood asthma & GSTM1 gene is a modifier of the GSTP1 gene.* Int Arch Allergy Immunol 144(4):275-86, 2007

KARIMI R, VACCHI-SUZZI C, MELIKER JR. *Mercury exposure & a shift toward oxidative stress in avid seafood consumers.* Environ Res 146:100-7, 2016

KASPERCZYK S, DOBRAKOWSKI M, KASPERCZYK A, MACHNIK G, BIRKNER E. *Effect of N-acetylcysteine administration on the expression & activities of antioxidant enzymes & the malondialdehyde level in the blood of lead-exposed workers.* Environ Toxicol Pharmacol 37(2):638-47, 2014

KASPERCZYK S, DOBRAKOWSKI M, KASPERCZYK A ET AL. *Effect of N-acetylcysteine administration on homocysteine level, oxidative damage to proteins, & levels of iron (Fe) & Fe-related proteins in lead-exposed workers.* Toxicol Ind Health 32(9):1607-18, 2016

KASPERCZYK S, DOBRAKOWSKI M, KASPERCZYK A ET AL. *The administration of N-acetylcysteine reduces oxidative stress & regulates glutathione metabolism in the blood cells of workers exposed to lead.* Clin Toxicol (Phila) 51(6):480-6, 2013

KATAWA M, SUZUKI KT. *The effect of cadmium, zinc or copper loading on the metabolism of amino acids in mouse liver.* Toxicology Letters 20:149-154, 1984

KELLY GS. *Clinical applications of n-acetylcysteine.* Altern. Med. Rev. 3: 114-127, 1998

KEOGH JP, STEFFEN B, SIEGERS CP. *Cytotoxicity of heavy metals in the human small intestinal epithelial cell line I-407: the role of glutathione.* J. Toxicol. Environ. Health 43: 351-359, 1994

KIDD PM. *GSH: Systemic protectant against oxidative & free radical damage.* Alternative Medicine Review 2:155-176, 1997

KIDD PM. *The free radical oxidant toxins of polluted air. in: Levine SA, Kid PM.* Antioxidant Adaptation – Its role in free radical pathology 69-103, 1985

KIM JH, HONG YC. *GSTM1, GSTT1, & GSTP1 polymorphisms & associations between air pollutants & markers of insulin resistance in elderly Koreans.* Environ Health Perspect 120(10):1378-84, 2012

KOBAL AB, PREZELJ M, HORVAT M, KRSNIK M, GIBICAR D, OSREDKAR J. *Glutathione level after long-term occupation elemental mercury exposure.* Environ Res 107(1):115-23, 2008

KRETZSCHMAR M, KLINGER W. *The hepatic GSH system – influences of xenobiotics.* Experimental Pathology 38:145-164, 1990

KUMAR J, MONICA LIND P, SALIHOVIC S ET AL. *Influence of persistent organic pollutants on oxidative stress in population-based samples.* Chemosphere 114:303-9, 2014

LASH LH, ZALUPS RK. *Alterations in renal cellular glutathione metabolism after in vivo administration of a subtoxic dose of mercuric chloride.* J. Biochem. Toxicol. 11: 1-9, 1996

LEE TC, WEI ML, CHANG WJ, ET AL. *Elevation of glutathione levels & glutathione S-transferase activity in arsenic-resistant Chinese hamster ovary cells.* In Vitro Cell Dev. Biol. 25: 442-448, 1989

LEE DH, JACOBS DR JR. *Hormesis & public health: can glutathione depletion & mitochondrial dysfunction due to very low-dose chronic exposure to persistent organic pollutants be mitigated?* J Epidemiol Community Health 69(3):294-300, 2015

LESLIE EM. *Arsenic-glutathione conjugate transport by the human multidrug resistance proteins (MRPs/ ABCCs).* J Inorg Biochem 108:141-9, 2012

LEVINSSON A, OLIN AC, MODIG L, DAHGAM S ET AL. *Interaction effects of long-term air pollution exposure & variants in the GSTP1, GSTT1 & GSTCD genes on risk of acute myocardial infarction & hypertension: a case-control study.* PLoS One 9(6):e99043, 2014

LEW H, QUINTANILHA A. *Effects of endurance training & exercise on tissue antioxidative capacity & acetaminophen detoxification.* Eur. J. Drug Metab. Pharmacokinet. 16: 59-68, 1991

LI Y, NIE J, BEYEA J, RUDRA CB ET AL. *Exposure to traffic emissions: associations with biomarkers of antioxidant status & oxidative damage.* Environ Res 121 :31-8, 2013

LIVARDJANI F, LEDIG M, KOPP P, ET AL. *Lung & blood superoxide dismutase activity in mercury vapor exposed rats: effect of n-acetylcysteine treatment.* Toxicology 66: 289-295. 1991

LÓPEZ O, HERNÁNDEZ AF, RODRIGO L, GIL F ET AL. *Changes in antioxidant enzymes in humans with long-term exposure to pesticides.* Toxicol Lett 171(3):146-53, 2007

LUND ME, BANNER W JR, CLARKSON TW, BERLIN M. *Treatment of acute methylmercury ingestion by hemodialysis with n-acetylcysteine (Mucomyst) infusion & 2, 3-dimercaptopropane sulfonate.* J. Toxicol. Clin. Toxicol. 22: 31-49, 1984

MACINTYRE EA, BRAUER M, MELÉN E, BAUER CP ET AL. *GSTP1 & TNF Gene variants & associations between air pollution & incident childhood asthma: the traffic, asthma & genetics (TAG) study.* Environ Health Perspect 122(4):418-24, 2014

MADDEN MC, STEVENTS T, CASE M ET AL. *Diesel exhaust modulates ozone-induced lung function decrements in healthy human volunteers.* Part Fibre Toxicol 11 :37, 2014

MADRIGANO J, BACCARELLI A, MITTLEMAN MA ET AL. *Prolonged exposure to particulate pollution, genes associated with glutathione pathways, & DNA methylation in a cohort of older men.* Environ Health Perspect 119(7):977-82, 2011

MINELLI C, GRANELL R, NEWSON R ET AL. *Glutathione-S-transferase genes & asthma phenotypes: a Human Genome Epidemiology (HuGE) systematic review & meta-analysis including unpublished data.* Int J Epidemiol 39(2):539-62, 2010

MINELLI C, WEI I, SAGOO G ET AL. *Interactive effects of antioxidant genes & air pollution on respiratory function & airway disease: a HuGE review.* Am J Epidemiol 173(6):603-20, 2011

MOLIN M, BERGMAN B, MARKLUND SL, ET AL. *Mercury, selenium, & glutathione peroxidase before & after amalgam removal in man.* Acta Odontol. Scand. 48: 189-202, 1990

MOLIN M, MARKLUND SL, BERGMAN B, NILSSON B. *Mercury, selenium, & glutathione peroxidase in dental personnel.* Acta Odontol. Scand. 47: 383-390, 1989

MORRIS G, ANDERSON G, DEAN O ET AL. *The glutathione system: a new drug target in neuroimmune.* Mol Neurobiol 50(3):1059-84, 2014

NARAIN U, ET AL. *The Cost of Air Pollution – Strengthening the Economic Case For Action.* World Bank & Institute for Health Metrics & Evaluation. University of Washington, Seattle. 2016

NATELSON BH, MAO X, STEGNER AJ ET

AL. *Multimodal & simultaneous assessments of brain & spinal fluid abnormalities in chronic fatigue syndrome & the effects of psychiatric comorbidity.* J Neurol Sci 375:411-416, 2017

NAVARRO J, OBRADOR E, PELLICER JA, ET AL. *Blood glutathione as an index of radiation-induced oxidative stress in mice & humans.* Free Radic. Biol. Med. 22: 1203-1209, 1997

NEAL R, COOPER K, GURER H, ERCAL N. *Effects of n-acetylcysteine & 2, 3-dimercaptosuccinic acid on lead induced oxidative stress in rat lenses.* Toxicology 130: 167-174, 1998

NICOLSON GL, NICOLSON NL. *Gulf War illnesses: complex medical, scientific & political paradox.* Med. Confl. Surviv. 14: 156-165, 1998

ORNAGHI F, FERRINI S, PRATI M, GIAVINI E. *The protective effects of N-acetyl-L-cysteine against methyl mercury embryotoxicity in mice.* Fundam. Appl. Toxicol. 20: 437-445, 1993

OTHMAN AI, EL MISSIRY MA. *Role of selenium against lead toxicity in male rats.* J. Biochem. Mol. Toxicol. 12: 345-349, 1998

OTT WR, ROBERTS JW. *Everyday exposure to toxic pollutants.* Scient. Ameri. 278(2):86-91, 1998

PARKE DV, SAPOTA A. *Chemical toxicity & reactive oxygen species.* Internat. J. of Occupational Med. & Environmental Health 9:331-340, 1996

PLANAS-BOHNE F, ELIZALDE M. *Activity of glutathione-S-transferase in rat liver & kidneys after administration of lead or cadmium.* Arch. Toxicol. 66: 365-367, 1992

PLACENTINI S, POLIMANTI R, MOSCATELLI B ET AL. *Glutathione S-transferase gene polymorphisms & air pollution as interactive risk factors for asthma in a multicentre Italian field study: A preliminary study.* Ann Hum Biol 37(3):427-39, 2010

POLLET C, NATELSON BH, LANGE G, ET AL. *Medical evaluation of Persian Gulf veterans with fatigue &/or chemical sensitivity.* J. Med. 29: 101-113, 1998

PUJARI G, BERNI A, PALITTI F, CHATTERJEE A. *Influence of glutathione levels on radiation-induced chromosomal DNA damage & repair in human peripheral lymphocytes.* Mutat Res 675(1-2) :23-8, 2009

QUEIROZ ML, PENA SC, SALTES TS, ET AL. *Abnormal antioxidant system in erythrocytes of mercury-exposed workers.* Human Exp. Toxicol. 17: 225-230, 1998

QUIG D. *Cysteine metabolism & metal toxicity.* Altern. Med. Rev. 3: 262-270, 1998

RAWAL S, KIM JE, COULOMBE R JR. *Aflatoxin B1 in poultry: toxicology, metabolism & prevention.* Res Vet Sci 89(3):325-31, 2010

REDDY P, NAIDOO RN ET AL. *GSTM1 & GSTP1 gene variants & the effect of air pollutants on lung function measures in South African children.* Am J Ind Med 55(12):1078-86, 2012

REA WJ ET AL. *Food & chemical sensitivity after environmental chemical overexposure.* Annals of Allergy 41:101-110, 1987

REHMAN K, NARANMANDURA H. *Arsenic metabolism & thioarsenicals.* Metallomics 4(9):881-92, 2012

REICKS M, RADER JI. *Effects of dietary tin & copper on rat hepatocellular antioxidant protection.* Proc. Soc. Exp. Biol. Med. 195:123-128, 1990

ROMIEU I, RAMIREZ-AGUILAR M, SIENRA-MONGE JJ ET AL. *GSTM1 & GSTP1 & respiratory health in asthmatic children exposed to ozone.* Eur Respir J, 28(5):953-9, 2006

ROSS RK, JONES PA, YU MC. *Bladder cancer epidemiology & pathogenesis.* Seminars in Oncology 23:536-545, 1996

RUBINO FM. *Toxicity of Glutathione-Binding Metals: A Review of Targets & Mechanisms.* Toxics 3(1):20-62, 2015

SAAD-HUSSEIN A, NOSHY M ET AL. *GSTP1 & XRCC1 plymorphisms & DNA damage in agricultural workers exposed to pesticides.* Mutat Res 819, 20-25, 2017

SAMIR AM, AREF WM. *Impact of occupational exposure to elemental mercury on some antioxidative enzymes among dental staff.* Toxicol Ind Health 27(9):779-86, 2011

SANDBORGH-ENGLAND G, ELINDER CG, LANGWORTH S, ET AL. *Mercury in biological fluids after amalgam removal.* J. Dental Res. 77: 615-624, 1998

SANDHIR R, GILL KD. *Effect of lead on lipid peroxidation in liver of rats.* Biol. Trace Elem. Res. 48: 91-97, 1995

SARAFIAN TA, BREDESEN DE, VERITY MA. *Cellular resistance to methylmercury.* Neurotoxicity 17: 27-36, 1996

SARKAR D, DAS D, BHATTACHARYA S. *Role of exogenous reduced glutathione on time dependant 203Hg distribution in liver & kidney of a freshwater teleost, Anabas testudineus.* Biomed. Environ. Sci. 10: 60-64, 1997

SASAKURA C, SUZUKI KT. *Biological interaction between transition metals (Ag, Cd, Hg), selenide/sulfide & selenoprotein* P. J. Inorg. Biochem. 71: 159-162, 1998

SEARS ME. *Chelation: harnessing & enhancing heavy metal detoxification—a review.* ScientificWorldJournal 2013:219840, 2013

SELIG C, NOTHDURFT W, FLIEDNER TM. *Radioprotective effect of N-acetylcysteine on granulocyte/macrophage colony-forming cells of human bone marrow.* J. Cancer Res. Clin. Oncol. 119: 346-349, 1993

SHI X, FLYNN DC, LIU K, DALAL N. *Vanadium (IV) formation in the reduction of vanadate by GSH reductase/NADPH & the role of molecular oxygen.* Ann. Clin. Lab. Sci. 27: 422-427, 1997

SHUNGU DC, WEIDUSCHAT N ET AL. *Increased ventricular lactate in chronic fatigue syndrome. III. Relationships to cortical glutathione & clinical symptoms implicate oxidative stress in disorder pathophysiology.* NMR Biomed 25(9):1073-87, 2012

SINGH S, KUMAR V, SINGH P ET AL. *Genetic polymorphisms of GSTM1, GSTT1 & GSTP1 & susceptibility to DNA damage in workers occupationally exposed to organophosphate pesticides.* Mutat Res 725(1-2), 2011

SINGHAL RK, ANDERSON ME, MEISTER A. *Glutathione, a first line defense against cadmium toxicity.* FASEB J. 1: 220-223, 1987

SMITH CV, JONES DP, GUENTHNER TM, LASH LH, LAUTERBERG BH. *Compartmentalization of GSH: implications for the study of toxicity & disease.* Toxicology & Applied Pharmacology 140:1-12, 1996

SMITH TK. *Dietary modulation of the glutathione detoxification pathway & the potential for altered xenobiotic metabolism.* Adv. Exp. Med. Biol. 289: 165-169, 1991

STOHS SJ, BAGCHI D. *Oxidative mechanisms in the toxicity of metal ions.* Free Radic. Biol. Med. 18: 321-336, 1995

SU MVV, TSAI CH, TUNG KY. *GSTP1 is a hub gene for gene-air pollution interactions on childhood asthma.* Allergy 68(12):1614-7, 2013

SUGAWARA E, NAKAMURA K, MIYAKE T, ET AL. *Lipid peroxidation & concentration of glutathione in erythrocytes from workers exposed to lead.* Br. J. Ind. Med. 48: 239-242, 1991

THOMPSON AM. *The oxidizing capacity of the Earth's atmosphere: Probable past & future changes.* Science 256: 1157-1165, 1992

VALLIS KA. *GSH deficiency & radiosensitivity in aids patients.* Lancet 337:918-919, 1991

VIJAYALAKSHMI K, SOOD PP. *Ameliorative capacities of vitamins & monothiols post therapy in the restoration of methylmercury altered glutathione metabolism.* Cell. Mol. Biol. 40: 211-224, 1994

VOS O, ROOS-VERHEY WSD. *Endogenous versus exogenous thiols in radioprotection.* Pharmacology & Therapeutics 39:169-177, 1988

WALTHER UI, MUCKTER H, FICHTI B, FORTH W. *Influence of glutathione on zinc-mediated cellular toxicity.* Biol. Trace Elem. Res. 67: 97-107, 1999

WEDEEN RP. *Were the hatters of New Jersey "mad"?* Am J Ind Med 16(2):225-33, 1989

WEICHENTHAL S, CROUSE DL ET AL. *Oxidative burden of fine particulate air pollution & risk of cause-specific mortality in the Canadian Census Health & Environment Cohort (CanCHEC).* Environ Res 146:92-9, 2016

WENTEN M, LI YF, LIN PC ET AL. *In utero smoke exposure, glutathione S-transferase P1 haplotypes, & respiratory illness-related absence among schoolchildren.* Pediatrics 123(5):1344-51, 2009

WONG RH, CHANG SY ET AL. *Polymorphisms in metabolic GSTP1 & DNA-repair XRCC1 genes with an increased risk of DNA damage in pesticide-exposed fruit growers.* Mutat Res 654(2):168-75, 2008

WU S, WANG B, YANG D ET AL. *Ambient particulate air pollution & circulating antioxidant enzymes : A repeated-measure study in healthy adults in Beijing, China.* Environ Pollut 208:16-24, 2016

WU VV, PEDEN DB ET AL. *Glutathione-S transferase M1 regulation of diesel exhaust particle-induced pro-inflammatory mediator expression in normal human bronchial epithelial cells.* Part Fibre Toxicol 9:31, 2012

WOODS JS, ELLIS ME. *Up-regulation of glutathione synthesis in rat kidney by methyl mercury.* Biochem. Pharmacol. 50: 1719-1724, 1995

WRIGHT LS, KORNGUTH SE, OBERLY TD, SIEGEL FL. *Effects of lead on glutathione S-transferase expression in rat kidney: a dose-response study. Relationship to mercury-induced oxidative stress.* Toxicol. Sci. 46: 254-259, 1998

XIE J, FUNAKOSHI T, SHIMADA H, KOJIMA S. *Comparative effects of chelating agents on pulmonary toxicity of systemic nickel in mice.* J. Appl. Toxicol. 16: 317-324, 1996

YILDIZ D, CAKIR Y. *Efflux of glutathione & glutathione complexes from human erythrocytes in response to inorganic arsenic exposure.* Biol Trace Elem Res 150(1-3):451-9, 2012

ZALUPS RK, BARFUSS DW. *Participation of mercuric conjugates of cysteine, homocysteine, & n-acetylcysteine in mechanisms involved in the renal tubular uptake of inorganic mercury.* J. American Soc. Nephrol. 9: 551-561, 1998

ZEPEDA-ARCE R, ROJAS-GARCIA E ET AL. *Oxidative stress & genetic damage among workers exposed primarily to organophosphate & pyrethroid pesticides.* Environ Toxicol 32(6):1754-1764, 2017

ZHANG Q, ZHOU XD, DENNY T, ET AL. *Changes in immune parameters seen in Gulf War veterans but not in civilians with chronic fatigue syndrome.* Clin. Diagn. Lab. Immunol. 6: 6-13, 1999

3

GSH & the Immune System

The immune system

It's amazing how many people still believe that catching a cold is the result of sitting in a draft or going out with wet hair. It is a simple and well-proven fact that the common cold is a contagious, transmittable disease. We don't catch colds from cold air—despite the disease's name. Although both the expression and the misconception are deeply ingrained in our culture, what actually causes the illness is exposure to the cold virus.

People sometimes blame a cold on being stressed out, overworked or having exercised too much—and in fact they're closer to the truth. Although these factors are not the root cause (the virus is), they do lend the cold virus a helping hand by temporarily diminishing immune resources. By overdoing it, these patients have become more susceptible.

Most visits to the doctor follow the immune system's failure to deal with a particular threat. However, there is good news: the immune system can be reinforced.

Few people are aware of this—even those who work most conscientiously on their well-being. Many people know how to look after their heart and muscles. Only a few give the immune system the attention it deserves. However, it's your front line and best defense against all infectious and destructive attacks.

To maintain a good immune response you should exercise regularly (45 to 60 minutes, 3 times weekly), eat regularly and enjoy a varied diet. You must maintain a good body weight, sleep regularly (8 hours for young adults, less for the elderly), supplement your diet with vitamins, minerals and micronutrients, avoid undue stress and—funnily enough—laugh a lot. You should also avoid radiation and toxins, abuse of tobacco, alcohol and caffeine and the unnecessary use of antibiotics and steroids. See Table 7.

The immune defense system is extraordi-

DO	DON'T
Exercise regularly (45-60 min., 3 times weekly)	Abuse tobacco
Eat regular & varied meals	Abuse alcohol
Maintain ideal body weight	Abuse caffeine
Sleep regularly (8 hours for young adult, less for elderly)	Use antibiotics inappropriately
Supplement your diet with vitamins, minerals & micronutrients	Use steroids inappropriately
Avoid undue stress	Expose yourself to radiation
Laugh a lot	Expose yourself to toxins

Table 7: Do's and don'ts of immune system maintenance

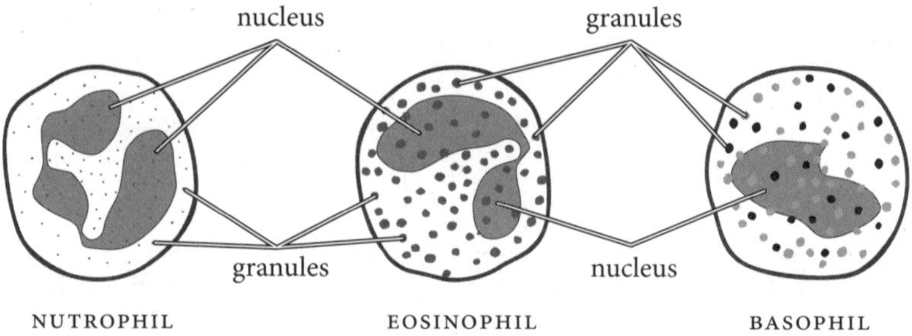

· *shock troops of the immune system*
· *first response against pathogens*
· *the body's most abundant immune cells*

· *carry microbial weapons & enzymes*
· *phagocytic (devour pathogens)*
· *repertoire of weapons/strategies*

FIGURE 8: Three types of polymorphonuclear immune cells, and their shared features

narily sophisticated—and it needs to be. A microscopic examination of any part of the human body shows it teeming with microorganisms that include bacteria, parasites and fungi—and that's just what's inside us. The environment around us—where we find air, water and food—is also saturated with microorganisms. Not all are threatening, but enough are. It's amazing we survive at all.

Usually, we only consult a physician after we get sick. The doctor launches an offensive 'attack,' using antibiotics, antiviral compounds or chemotherapy to destroy the invader. This strategy has saved countless lives and is effective despite a wide variety of side-effects and other drawbacks, including antibiotic resistance. It's the best way we've found to fight the war, even when it leads to collateral damage.

How about avoiding it altogether? After all, the battleground's your body. The side-effects of drugs and chemotherapy are like the random destruction of war that kills innocent bystanders and degrades life for survivors.

If you prevent invaders from gaining a foothold in the first place, you avoid widespread damage. This is the holy grail of preventive medicine, and explains why you can never overstate the value of the body's own resources. The best prevention practice is to care for your immune system just as you do the rest of your body.

The immune response

The immune response seeks out, identifies, and attacks threatening microorganisms, allergens, cancer cells and grafted tissue. These carry on them molecules called "antigens." It is these molecules that trigger the body's immune reaction, which is called an "antigen response."

When an antigen enters the blood stream, immune cells are activated. There are two types of immune response: general and adaptive. General immunity is managed by polymorphonuclear cells (the cells that make up pus). These are large cells that simply engulf pathogens and digest them.

The adaptive immune response involves lymphocytes. These are another type of immune cell. They're much smaller than polymorphonuclear cells, but they're also more sophisticated. They're said to be adaptive because they design a specific defense for each pathogen. The two main types of lymphocytes, B-cells and T-cells, work in unison.

B-cell lymphocytes identify pathogens and tag them. T-cell lymphocytes target them, and come in several forms. Helper T-cells alert other immune cells that the battle is on, killer T-cells destroy the intruder, and suppressor T-cells switch off the immune response afterwards.

The various lymphocyte cells and their cooperative ways are marvels of biology. However, a healthy immune response is by no means guaranteed. If there aren't enough immune cells, the response falls short. The immune cells themselves may be incompetent, or they may be outmatched by a new or more aggressive pathogen. Adaptive immune cells remember specific pathogens so that if they encounter them again, they no longer need a heads-up from the B-cells—they attack immediately. Sometimes this leads to partial or complete immunity. For example, you only catch the measles once; even if you're exposed to the virus again, it's highly unlikely to infect you again.

The immune system is impressive but far from infallible. It treats some threats as if they aren't threats at all, allowing them to infect the body. On the other hand, immune cells may treat normal structures as if they're threats, and attack the body. This is "autoimmune" disease, some of which are shown in Table 8. There are over a hundred autoimmune diseases.

Ideally we want the immune response to prevent infection, ignore harmless

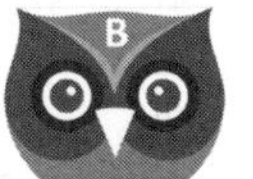

B-cells (lookouts):
- tag intruders
- alert T-cells

T-cells (soldiers):
- target intruders
- destroy threats
- recruit more immune cells
- retire when complete

FIGURE 9: Adaptive immune cells (FIGURE 10:) are of two types

substances, accept transplanted organs, not attack its own organs and protect the body against carcinogenesis and tumor growth. What we want to avoid is: recurrent infection, allergic response to harmless substances, rejection of transplanted organs, auto-immune disease and cancer.

The two most common glitches with the immune system are autoimmune disease and allergies. In autoimmune disease the body mistakes normal tissue for a foreign antigen and attacks it, destroying healthy tissue. In the case of allergies, the immune system mistakes a harmless substance for a potentially dangerous one and reacts with an aggressive response that can be deadly.

The immune system and GSH

Glutathione plays a central role in the functioning of immune cells. Groundbreaking GSH researcher Dr. Gustavo Bounous said, "The limiting factor in the proper activity of our lymphocytes is the availability of glutathione."

This is strikingly clear in the example of the human immunodeficiency virus (HIV) which destroys helper T-cells, leaving killer T-cells cut off and powerless. HIV doesn't in fact destroy the body. It simply leaves it defenseless. As a result, invading microorganisms that the body would normally shrug off are able to cause the severe infections of AIDS (see Chapter 12).

AIDS is essentially a T-cell dysfunction. Patients suffer from low GSH levels, notably in circulating T-cells. Several studies have

Lupus	Polymyositis
Myasthenia gravis	Scleroderma
Chronic fatigue syndrome	Lou Gehrig's disease (ALS)
Rheumatoid arthritis	Grave's disease
Multiple sclerosis	Crohn's Disease

TABLE 8: Some autoimmune diseases

shown that the level of GSH found in AIDS patients predicts their chances of survival and quality of life.

The healthy growth and activity of immune cells depends upon the availability of GSH. Through experiments that lower GSH levels, we know that the ability of cells to fight pathogens is severely diminished, leaving the door wide open to disease. Numerous studies have shown that the level of GSH within lymphocytes corresponds directly to the effectiveness of the immune response. Put simply, GSH is a crucial supply—essentially a sort of 'food' for the immune system.

In autoimmune diseases such as rheumatoid arthritis, lupus (SLE) and in normal aging (Chapter 6), the response of T-cell lymphocytes to antigens is weakened. Furthermore, chronic inflammatory conditions have been associated with low serum and red blood cell GSH concentrations.

Glutathione levels and activity have been measured in many different autoimmune phenomena besides lupus and rheumatoid arthritis. Low GSH levels have been implicated in idiopathic thrombocytopenia purpura (ITP), diabetes, multiple sclerosis, autoimmune liver diseases, Sjögren's syndrome and others. The Italian group led by the Drs. Perricone has looked extensively into the role of glutathione in autoimmune disease. They describe how GSH diminishes inflammation and free radical damage, and inhibits inflammatory cytokines.

Although we say that glutathione "boosts" the immune system, it's essential to point out that it doesn't simply make it "stronger." At times it deliberately slows it down in order to limit inflammation. This regulatory function is particularly important when it comes to autoimmune disease and allergic reactions.

GSH's role in allergic reactions has been a subject of intense review. Oxidative stress in the allergic response can get out of hand in a vicious cycle of activity that promotes further inflammation, with unfortunate consequences such as allergic asthma.

It's important to note that elevating GSH in transplanted tissue, such as a donor kidney or heart, could risk the immune system rejecting the tissue. However, in an "autograft" procedure, the patient's own tissues are used (for example skin grafts from one part of the body to another). In this case, there's no danger of rejection since the tissue is not foreign but familiar.

A lymphocyte attacks a pathogen by releasing powerful oxidizing chemicals such as peroxide. To do this, it protects itself against these chemical weapons with its own GSH. While all this happens, lymphocytes continue to replicate themselves (monoclonal expansion) until they have covered the full extent of the threat. This consumes oxygen and releases more oxidants. To manage monoclonal expansion efficiently—and with minimal collateral damage—GSH neutralizes the negative effects of oxidation.

This shows that GSH is consumed in two ways as it fights against infection—by stabilizing free radicals and by stimulating immune cell growth. This is well described in acute infections like bacterial pneumonia. In chronic infections such as hepatitis C or AIDS, GSHdepletion is even more pronounced. Recent research has demonstrated that elevated GSH levels help the immune system address these infections more effectively.

Doctor Bounous and his McGill University team tested the immune response of laboratory animals fed a carefully-prepared diet of bioactive whey protein isolate rich in GSH precursors. The animals demonstrated both higher intracellular GSH levels and a heightened response to immune challenge. Interestingly, animals fed a similar diet of cysteine-enriched casein (see Chapter 4) did not benefit from the same effects.

This demonstrates once again that the protective activity of GSH is twofold: it enhances the activity of immune cells and also functions as an antioxidant within them.

An alarming variety of antibiotic-resistant bacterial infections—such as flesh-eating disease, vancomycin-resistant enterococcus (VRE), and methicillin-resistant staphylococcus aureus (MRSA)—have made their way into our hospitals and communities. Some

	Desired response	Undesired response
Infectious agent	Protective immunity	Recurrent infection
Harmless substance	No response	Allergy
Transplant organ	Acceptance	Rejection
Self organ	Self-tolerance	Auto-immune disease
Tumor	Tumor immunity	Cancer

TABLE 9: Desired and undesired immune responses

health professionals believe that viruses such as those causing AIDS and Hepatitis C are just the tip of a pandemic iceberg, and that a wave of newly emerging pathogens is on its way. Old foes like tuberculosis, previously thought to be eliminated, are back with a vengeance, no longer susceptible to previously successful treatments. Enhanced GSH levels are a practical precaution against this trend.

An excellent review of glutathione and infection was published in 2013 by Morris et al. The report details the protective effects of GSH and also suggests it for therapeutic interventions. Many articles examine the treatment potential of glutathione on bacterial, viral, fungal and parasitical infection. A newer field of infectious disease focuses on "biofilms"—microbial communities of bacteria reproduce rapidly on biological surfaces, such as the lining of the mouth, vagina, teeth and other exposed tissues. Dimicola analyzed studies using the glutathione precursor NAC in the treatment of biofilms (see Figure 36 in the dentistry chapter). They promote the notion that raising glutathione has unfulfilled potential clinical use.

Conclusion

The immune system coordinates a variety of specialized cells to fight off infection and other threats. The healthy growth and activity of these cells depends upon the availability of GSH. Glutathione is at the heart of most immune functions, explaining why low GSH levels are seen in many diseases. This is best exemplified by AIDS, which is characterized by a severely compromised immune system.

Raising and maintaining GSH levels can minimize the risk of these diseases. Although only very ill people are severely deficient in GSH, those in good or fair health will benefit from GSH supplementation, especially considering the environmental toxins and drug-resistant bacteria we're exposed to these days. The use of GSH supplementation to fight specific diseases is discussed in Part 2 of this book.

Without question, the best type of preventive medicine is an optimized immune system, and a critical means to optimize it is by feeding it glutathione.

GSH AND THE IMMUNE SYSTEM

REFERENCES

ANDERSON ME. *GSH & GSH delivery systems. Advances in Pharmacology 38:65-78, 1997*

BOUNOUS G, BATIST G, GOLD P. *Immunoenhancing property of dietary whey proteins in mice: role of glutathione.* Clinical & Investigative Medicine 12:154-161, 1989

BOUNOUS G, GOLD P. *The biological activity of undenatured dietary whey protein in mice: role of glutathione.* Clinical & Investigative Medicine 14:296-309, 1991

BOUNOUS G, KONGSHAVN P. *Influence of dietary proteins on the immune system of mice.* Journal of Nutrition 112:1747-1755, 1982

BOUNOUS G, KONGSHAVN P. *Differential effect of*

dietary protein type on B-cell & T-cell immune responses in mice. Journal of Nutrition 115:1403-1408, 1985

DINICOLA S, DE GRAZIA S, CARLOMAGNO G, PINTUCCI JP. *N-acetylcysteine as powerful molecule to destroy bacterial biofilms. A systematic review.* Eur Rev Med Pharmacol Sci 18(19):2942-8, 2014

DROGE W, POTTMEYER-GERBER C, SCHMIDT H, NICK S. *Glutathione augments the activation of cytotoxic T lymphocytes in vivo.* Immunobiology 172:151-156, 1986

FRATERNALE A. ET AL. *GSH & analogs in antiviral therapy.* Mol Aspects Med 30(1-2):99-110, 2009

FRATERNALE A. ET AL. *Antiviral & immunomodulatory properties of new pro-glutathione (GSH) molecules.* Curr Med Chem 13(15):1749-55, 2006

FRATERNALE A, BRUNDU S, MAGNANI M. *Glutathione & glutathione derivatives in immunotheraphy.* Biol Chem 398(2):261-275, 2017

FIDELUS RK, GINOUVES P, LAWRENCE D, TSAN MF. *Modulation of intracellular glutathione concentrations alters lymphocyte activation & proliferation.* Experimental Cell Research 170:269-275, 1987

FIDELUS RK, TSAN MF. *Glutathione & lymphocyte activation: a function of aging & autoimmune disease.* Immunology 61:503-508, 1987

FITZPATRICK AM, TEAGUE WG, BURWELL L, BROWN MS, BROWN LA. *NIH/NHLBI Severe Asthma Research Program. Glutathione oxidation is associated with airway macrophage functional impairment in children with severe asthma.* Pediatr Res 69(2):154-9, 2011

FITZPATRICK AM, TEAGUE WG, HOLGUIN F, YEH M, BROWN LA; *Severe Asthma Research Program. Airway glutathione homeostasis is altered in children with severe asthma: evidence for oxidant stress.* J Allergy Clin Immunol 123(1):146-152, 2009

FITZPATRICK AM, JONES DP, BROWN LA. *Glutathione redox control of asthma: from Molecular mechanisms to therapeutic opportunities.* Antioxid Redox Signal 17(2):375-408, 2012

FURUKAWA T, MEYDANI SN, BLUMBERG JB. *Reversal of age associated decline in immune responsiveness by dietary glutathione supplementation in mice.* Mechanisms of Aging & Development 38:107-117, 1987

GMUNDER H, DROGE W. *Differential effects of glutathione depletion of T-cell subsets.* Cellular Immunology 138:229-237, 1991

GUO CH, LIU PJ, LIN KP, CHEN PC. *Nutritional supplement therapy improves oxidative stress, immune response, pulmonary function, & quality of life in allergic asthma patients: an open-label pilot study.* Altern Med Rev 17(1):42-56, 2012

HAMILOS DL, WEDNER HJ. *The role of glutathione in lymphocyte activation.* Journal of Immunology 135:2740-2747, 1985

HOFFMAN S, NOLIN J, MCMILLIAN D, WOUTERS E, JANSSEN-HEININGER Y, REYNAERT N. *Thiol redox chemistry: role of protein cysteine oxidation & altered redox homeostasis in allergic inflammation & asthma.* J Cell Biochem 116(6):884-92, 2015

HUGHES MM, MCGETTRICK AF, O'NEILL LA. *Glutathione & Glutathione Transferase Omega 1 as Key Posttranslational Regulators in Macrophages.* Microbiol Spectr 5(1), 2017

KAFFE ET, RIGOPOULOU EI, KOUKOULIS GK, DALEKOS GN, MOULAS AN. *Oxidative stress & antioxidant status in patients with autoimmune liver diseases.* Redox Rep 20(1):33-41, 2015

KAMHIEH-MILZ J, BAL G, STERZER V, KAMHIEH-MILZ S, ARBACH O, SALAMA A. *Reduced antioxidant capacities in platelets from patients with autoimmune thrombocytopenia purpura (ITP).* Platelets 23(3):184-94, 2012

KARLSSON H. ET AL. *N-acetyl-L-cysteine increases acute graft-versus-host disease & promotes T-cell-mediated immunity in vitro.* Eur J Immunol 41(4):1143-53, 2011

KIDD PM. *Glutathione: Systemic protectant against oxidative & free radical damage.* Alternative Medicine Review 2:155-176, 1997

LAI ZW. ET AL. *N-acetylcysteine reduces disease activity by blocking mammalian target of rapamycin in T cells from systemic lupus erythematosus patients: a randomized, double-blind, placebo-controlled trial.* Arthritis Rheum 64(9):2937-46, 2012

LUKAN N, RACZ O, MOCNEJOVA I, TKAC I. *Monitoring antioxidant enzymes in red cells during allergen immunotherapy.* J Physiol Biochem 64(2):143-8, 2008

MORRIS D. ET AL. *Glutathione & infection.* Biochim Biophys Acta 1830(5):3329-49, 2013

MORRIS D. ET AL. *Glutathione supplementation improves macrophage functions in HIV.* J Interferon Cytokine Res 33(5):270-9, 2013

PERRICONE C. ET AL. *Inhibition of the complement system by glutathione: molecular mechanisms & potential therapeutic implications.* Int J Immunopathol Pharmacol 24(1):63-8, 2011

PERRICONE C, DE CAROLIS C, PERRICONE R. *Glutathione: a key player in autoimmunity.* Autoimmun Rev 8(8):697-701, 2009

ROTILIO G, KNOEPFEL L, STEINKUHLER C, PALMARA AT, CIROLO MR, GARACI E. *Effects of intracellular redox status on cellular regulation & viral infection.* in: Oxidative Stress, Cell Activation & Viral Infection, C. Pasquier et al (eds.), 1994

STAERCK C. ET AL. *Microbial antioxidant defense enzymes.* Microb Pathog 110:56-65, 2017

TAN KS. ET AL. *Glutathione deficiency in type 2 diabetes impairs cytokine responses & control of intracell. bacteria.* J Clin Invest 122(6):2289-300, 2012

4

Raising GSH Levels

If glutathione is manufactured within the body, what can we do to maintain or increase GSH levels? Some pharmaceutical drugs can do it, and so can some natural nutrients. There are many ideas about how to raise GSH levels in the body but only a few actually work and some of them have side effects. To take full advantage of the great potential of GSH in health and disease you must know the myths as well as the facts. This requires an understanding of the biochemical make-up of this important protein.

GSH is a tripeptide—a protein made up of three amino acids—in this case, glycine, glutamate (glutamic acid), and cysteine. The chemical structure[1] of GSH is easily destroyed by the human digestive system. Unlike most laboratory animals, the human gut has unusually high levels of the enzyme GGT (gamma-glutamyl-transferase), which attacks the GSH molecule. This brings us to the first great myth of glutathione—that eating it provides the same benefits to humans as to laboratory animals. Many studies have demonstrated the efficacy of oral glutathione on mice and rats, and yet decades of human studies have failed.

Each cell in the human body manufactures the glutathione it needs within the cell itself. GSH is assembled using the three building blocks (precursors) it obtains from dietary nutrients. Figure 10 shows sources of the three amino acids required to make glutathione. Two of them—glycine and glutamate—are readily available in North American diets, but sources containing the third building-block—cysteine, especially in its biologically active form—are much harder to come by.

Cysteine is a thiol[2]—a sulfur-containing amino acid that is responsible for the biological operations (bioactivity) of the whole molecule. Like GSH, cysteine faces a difficult journey from the mouth into each cell. It too is broken down or physically altered

[1] The arrangement of chemical bonds within the molecule
[2] Any organic compound containing a sulfhydryl (SH) group

Drugs	**Natural Products**	**GSH co-factors**
NAC	oral glutathione	selenium
SAM	cysteine	vitamin B_1
OTC	methionine	vitamin B_2
OTZ	melatonin	vitamin B_6
procysteine	glutamine	vitamin B_{12}
GSH monoesters	lipoic acid	folate, folic acid
GSH diesters	silymarin (milk thistle)	vitamin C
	bioactive whey proteins	vitamin E
		...other nutrients

TABLE 10: GSH-promoting substances described in this chapter

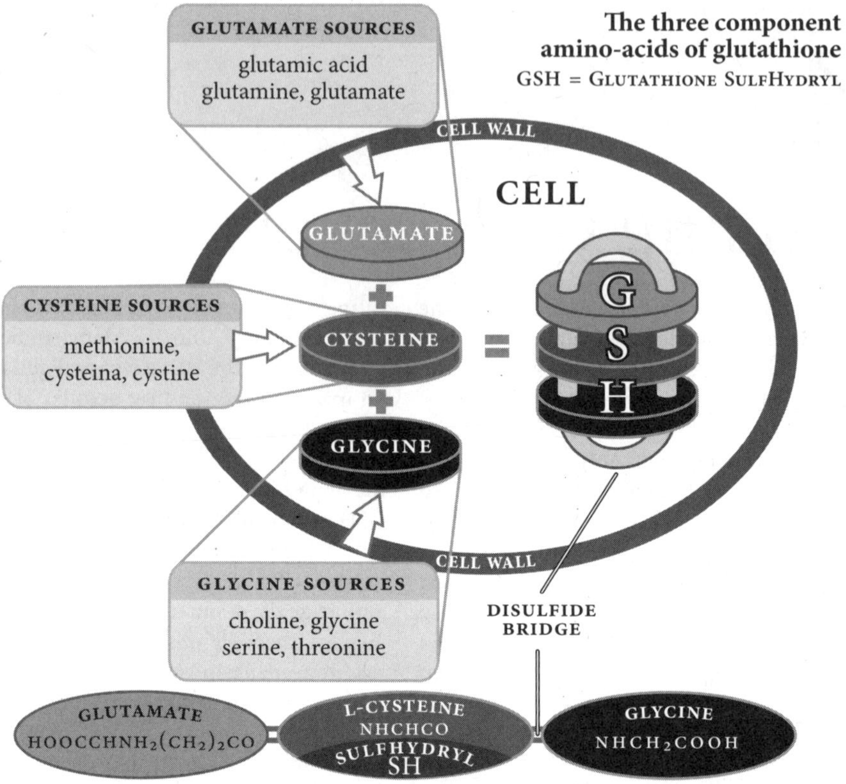

Figure 11: GSH is manufactured in each cell of the body from three amino acid precursors (building blocks)—glutamate, glycine, and harder-to-find cysteine, which contains the biologically active sulfhydryl group (SH).

both in the digestive tract and in the bloodstream. Without these sulfur-containing amino acids, cells can't make GSH. Fortunately, one particular—rather delicate—form of cysteine can make it through. This is cystine (with only one 'e'). Like cysteine and methionine, cystine is a thiol amino acid. It is also said to be a "disulfide" amino acid because it contains two cysteine molecules connected by their sulfur atoms—a 'disulfide bridge.' This physical connection enables cystine to safely travel the digestive and circulatory systems and into individual cells (see Figure 10.)

Cystine is not generally found as a free amino acid. Methionine may serve as a glutathione building block, but it has the tendency to convert into homocysteine, a risk factor for heart disease.

There are several ways to raise GSH levels. All those described in this chapter are listed in Table 10. We also explain how GSH works with other nutrients ("co-factors").

GSH precursors & cellular manufacture

No matter their source, all three building blocks (precursors) of glutathione—glutamate, cysteine and glycine—must be in a form that can travel from the mouth, through the digestive and blood systems, and into individual cells. There, the precursors are combined into GSH. Glutamate is derived from food sources containing uncooked glutamic acid, glutamine and glutamate, and is found in undenatured whey protein. Cysteine comes mainly from protein sources such as eggs, raw milk and undenatured whey protein. They

Substance	Form	Strong	Positive	Weak	None
Glutathione	*Oral*			✓	
	Liposomal			✓	
	Intravenous		✓		
	Sublingual			✓	
	Patches				✓
	Inhaled		✓		
	Nasal			✓	
Whey	*Denatured*			✓	
	Undenatured	✓			
N.A.C.		✓			
L-Cysteine				✓	
RibCis					✓
Lipoic acid				✓	
Milk Thistle				✓	
Sulforaphane			✓		

TABLE 11: Agglomerated evidence for effectiveness of glutathione improvement strategies in humans

are found in other foods too, though in small amounts. The amino acid methionine can break down into cysteine. Various pharmaceutical drugs serve as cysteine delivery systems. Glycine is found in foods rich in the amino acids choline, glycine, serine and threonine.

Pharmaceutical drugs

Many of the research studies described in this book used pharmaceutical drugs to raise GSH levels in test subjects. These drugs are described first. Afterwards, we discuss natural GSH-promoting substances.

NAC (N-ACETYLCYSTEINE)

NAC is a powerful glutathione precursor that for years has been available as a drug (Mucomist, Parvolex, etc.) and on the shelves of health supplement stores. It is a variant of the amino acid L-cysteine, with an added "acetyl" molecule. This greatly enhances the bioavailability (usefulness) of cysteine by delivering it into individual cells. Normally, L-cysteine is almost entirely oxidized during digestion. NAC allows about 15% to avoid oxidation—enough for the cells to make GSH.

For many years NAC has been a mainstay of clinical glutathione therapy. It is routinely used to break up mucus in lung diseases such as cystic fibrosis, chronic bronchitis, asthma and emphysema, and remains the standard treatment for acetaminophen overdose. Most GSH studies on humans have been conducted with NAC. Alongside animal and laboratory experiments, they measured the effectiveness of NAC against a host of diseases that share three characteristics: the presence of oxidative stress, the formation of free radicals and the depletion of glutathione. Such diseases include infection by AIDS/HIV, cancer, heart disease, tobacco damage and heavy metal poisoning.

Its use in cancer therapy is exciting because it can substantially raise glutathione levels and has emerged as a promising anticarcinogen, especially for smokers and others at high risk for cancer. It is also known to have direct anti-tumor effects. Furthermore, its ability to detoxify normal cells helps minimize the harmful side-effects of chemotherapy and radiotherapy. However, its usefulness depends on circumstances, and it should be used wisely. Cancer patients wishing to take NAC must discuss it with their oncologist.

NAC has been used in AIDS research since the early 1990s, when it was found that HIV patients become profoundly glutathione deficient. Much data has resulted from studies at the National Institute of Health, Stanford University, and many other highly respected institutions around the world.

NAC therapy has two common problems: firstly, it is a pharmaceutical drug and carries a certain toxicity itself; secondly, NAC-induced GSH levels reach a rapid peak and decline within hours. The drug is thus described as having a short "half-life." Rapid peaks are often followed by a rapid decline, often below normal levels. To maintain constantly elevated GSH levels, NAC must be swallowed or injected several times per day, and this is very hard on the body. Many people eating NAC report such side-effects as a rash, wheezing, nausea, vomiting, cramps and diarrhea. Others find the smell and taste unacceptable. Although rare, death has been reported in association with NAC. Nevertheless, it is still the most commonly used drug for the job.

Treating drug overdoses or acute pulmonary disease with NAC is a delicate task, requiring careful monitoring by health professionals. Suggested non-prescription oral doses range from 200-2,400 mg/day depending on one's condition. Scientists are modifying the original NAC formulation to improve efficacy and tolerability. New forms include NACA (N-acetylcysteine amide), SNACET (S-nitroso-N-acetylcysteine ethyl ester), NACET (N-acetyl-L-cysteine ethyl ester), and others.

SAM (S-adenosyl-methionine)

SAM is a form of methionine (see page 41) already partially converted to cysteine. It is useful in the treatment of cirrhosis and cholestasis, and is used in Europe as a mood stabilizer. In America, its possible use as an antidepressant is being explored. SAM is expensive to synthesize and may react poorly with other antidepressants. In therapeutic doses its possible side effects include dry mouth, agitation and gastrointestinal problems.

OTC and OTZ

OTC (ornithine decarboxylase, procysteine) and OTZ (oxothiazolidine carboxylate) are synthetic delivery sources—a substrate for the enzyme 5-oxyprolinase. This enzyme participates in glutathione metabolism by first converting the substrate to s-carboxy-cysteine, and then hydrolyzing it to cysteine, which the liver then uses to make GSH. However, since this enzyme is not always present, the usefulness of OTC/OTZ is limited. Most studies have used either laboratory animals or human tissue cultures. Small studies have been conducted with AIDS and cancer patients, and further work is in progress. These drugs are not readily available to doctors or the general public.

GSH monoesters, GSH diesters

These are synthetic compounds that effectively deliver GSH, but they may also be metabolized into alcohol, which potentially depletes GSH. Very few studies have been carried out on humans, but well-recognized GSH researchers such as the late Alton Meister and Mary Anderson have spoken optimistically about further clinical applications. However, the long-term safety of these artificial products remains in question.

Natural Products

Oral & Liposomal glutathione

Why not just eat GSH? It is freely available in fresh fruits, vegetables and meats. It is also sold in pill form or powder by a variety of chemical producers. However, pre-manufactured GSH is not helpful to the body. If bound to certain proteins, a small amount of reduced GSH may make it into the blood stream, but most is lost to the digestive process and does not effectively raise intracellular GSH levels. Researchers describe oral GSH as "not readily bioavailable"[3]—especially in the liver where it is most needed. Flagg and his team at Emory University, Atlanta have even suggested that blood GSH levels might fall after eating GSH-containing foods that trigger "down-regulation."[4] In medical terms, the usefulness of oral GSH is negligible.

Obviously glutathione is a "natural" substance, but where do most glutathione supplements come from? Since glutathione is difficult to extract from plant or animal sources, an alternative resource has been developed. Most of the commercial GSH used in the nutritional and pharmaceutical industries is derived from either bacterial or fungal cultures.

The most commonly used are yeasts like Candida, Sacchromyces and Hansenula; other types are being developed. The DNA of these yeasts is engineered to alter its normal coding in ways that produce more glutathione. These bioengineering techniques include enzymatic cleavage as well as exposure to focused radiation.

An increasingly popular way to make glutathione is by genetically engineering bacteria—including E. Coli (Escherichia coli). Recently, Chinese researchers cloned E. Coli with another bacteria, Actinobacillus succinogenes, to significantly increase GSH yields.

A paper often referenced to prove that oral glutathione is in fact effective in humans, was published by JP Richie and his colleagues in the European Journal of Nutrition (2015). This study was funded by an industrial supplier of glutathione, and the report was criticized by Richie's medical peers as inconsistent with the results of hundreds of other studies that tried and failed to replicate their findings.

Liposomes are tiny spheres (much smaller than cells) that can be modified to deliver pharmaceutical drugs to precise locations in the body. These state-of-the-art delivery systems have been employed for glutathione as well, although results have been mostly disappointing. Nevertheless, a single paper published in 2018 claimed success, its main author being the same JP Richie who claimed benefits from oral glutathione that his peers were unable to replicate (see preceding paragraph). In this case too, the paper was published in the European Journal of Nutrition, and the research was funded by a large producer of liposomal GSH.

Other glutathione supplement producers have funded studies in an effort to demonstrate the efficacy of oral GSH—all without success. A large study done on 40 healthy adults used 500mg of glutathione twice a day for a month. Following this randomized placebo-controlled clinical trial, the authors reported, "No significant changes were observed in biomarkers of oxidative stress, including glutathione status."

It is the general consensus of glutathione researchers that oral forms of glutathione do not effectively raise GSH levels.

Intravenous (IV) Glutathione

Intravenous glutathione has repeatedly shown success in the human body. However, there is still debate about whether the GSH molecule really does travel through cell membranes and into the cell itself. It could be that it is broken down into its constituent parts, which then pass through the membrane and, once back inside, are reconstituted into GSH.

The future of Intravenous glutathione therapy faces challenges. First, it is expensive. Secondly, like any intravenous medication it comes with the risk of pain and infection, and must be monitored by medical professionals. Thirdly, its effectiveness is short-lived.

As far back as 1980, European researchers determined that the "half-life" of intravenous glutathione in the human body was under two minutes. The term "half-life" is a pharmacological measure of how long the

[3] The proportion of a drug or other substance that reaches the circulation when introduced into the body and so is able to have an active effect.

[4] A negative feedback loop in which the cell thinks there is too much glutathione.

body takes to rid itself of half the substance in question. This "half-life" helps scientists to calculate how often a drug must be administered to maintain therapeutic levels. This is why some drugs can be taken once a day, while others must be taken four times. The most successful intravenous glutathione studies have used multiple dosing—or better still, a continuous drip.

Recent research has shown that higher doses of intravenous glutathione last longer, some reaching a half-life of 20 minutes. This explains why very dramatic effects can be witnessed in Parkinson's patients, who may rise from a wheelchair after an infusion, but suffer their usual disability by the time they get home.

Sublingual GSH, Orobuccal GSH

There are other methods of delivery besides swallowing and injecting. Both sublingual ("under the tongue") and orobuccal ("in the cheek") may introduce substances directly through the mucosal lining of the mouth, thus bypassing the harsh conditions of the gastrointestinal tract. This enables glutathione to enter the body without having to pass through the intestines and liver, which break it down.

Less than a handful of articles have demonstrated any success with this strategy. Although the delivery works fine—glutathione levels rise in the bloodstream after sublingual or orobuccal administration—the free glutathione in the bloodstream suffers the same brief fate as intravenous glutathione: its half-life is measured in minutes.

Transdermal Glutathione, Patches

Several forms of topical glutathione are available. Some are in a cream form, others as a patch or a spray. The glutathione molecule is readily absorbed into the outer layers of skin, but not any deeper into the dermis or the bloodstream. Since the effects of topical or patched glutathione are entirely local, only the skin under the patch may benefit.

Aerosolized, Nebulized, Inhaled Glutathione

Even though glutathione lasts only a short time after entering the bloodstream, it still can be effective when in direct contact with certain tissues. Glutathione inhalation treatments were first explored in the early 1990s. Successful studies appeared rapidly, and since then positive outcomes have been demonstrated in patients suffering from asthma, pulmonary fibrosis, HIV/AIDS, cystic fibrosis—and even in patients exposed to air pollution.

A detailed discussion of glutathione in lung disease is found in chapter 12.

Nasal Glutathione

Like sublingual and orobuccal methods, intranasal (though the nose) delivery enables the glutathione to bypass glutathione breakdown in the gut. An additional possible advantage lies in the close proximity of nasal tissue to the brain. Researchers have good reason to believe that intranasal glutathione can raise brain glutathione levels.

Washington researchers led by Mischley have actively pursued this avenue. Focusing on Parkinson's disease, they first set out to establish the safety of a GSH nasal spray. When they surveyed patients taking GSH nasal spray for various reasons, about 12% reported adverse effects. Most were mild.

Using a new technique to measure brain glutathione, patients applied the spray while being scanned with magnetic resonance spectroscopy.[5] Brain GSH levels increased, but only for an hour. This is consistent with intravenous applications of glutathione, in which the short half-life of GSH is also problematic. These results were confirmed in a subsequent study, following patients who administered GSH nasal spray thrice daily for three months. No clinical improvements were observed.

---

[5] Magnetic resonance spectroscopy using an MRI machine. While magnetic resonance imaging (MRI) identifies the inner structure the body, MR spectroscopy compares normal with abnormal brain tissue, to detect tissue changes.

Cysteine (L-cysteine)

The availability of cysteine in each cell determines how much GSH the body can synthesize. This non-essential amino acid is the hardest-to-find glutathione precursor. It does raise intracellular GSH to a small degree and is available without prescription, so why not just eat it?

The problem is that when used as a dietary supplement cysteine can be overdosed, resulting in hypercysteinemia and potential toxicity. Cysteine is readily oxidized in the digestive tract, so very little of it gets through to the bloodstream and cells. What does reach the blood is additionally oxidized there, sometimes into the highly reactive hydroxyl radical—a very harmful oxidant. This clearly defeats the intended role of cysteine as an anti-oxidant.

This was clinically proven by Montreal researchers Drs. Gustavo Bounous and Gerry Batist, who showed that even in mice dietary cysteine has a negligible effect upon immune response. Some were fed a bioactive whey-protein while others ate a simple cysteine/casein combination. The latter group showed no positive response.

Also in question are the raw materials used to manufacture cysteine. They may be "natural," but they have raised eyebrows. Not long ago most cysteine was processed from human hair collected from Chinese barbershops and salons. Since then, the preferred source is Chinese duck feathers and American chicken feathers. It's still natural, but the extraction process involves complex chemistry.

Ribose-L-Cysteine (RibCys)

RibCys is substantially similar to NAC (N-acetylcysteine). Both reduce the amount of cysteine that's oxidized by adding a molecule to the cysteine to "protect" it—the acetyl group in the case of NAC, a ribose molecule for RibCys. For over 30 years Dr. Herb Nagasawa has led research on RibCys. There are upwards of two dozen studies suggesting its potential. Unfortunately, there are no published clinical trials demonstrating that RibCys works in humans.

Methionine (L-methionine)

Methionine—an essential amino acid present in many foods—has been identified as a GSH precursor. It is also available from pharmacological supply outlets and health food stores. The metabolic transformation of methionine into GSH is dependent on many other factors. For example, methionine levels are very low when liver disease is present, and non-existent in newborns. Above certain doses it can be toxic. Of great concern, methionine is also a precursor of homocysteine, a known high risk factor in the development of atherosclerosis (hardening of the arteries) and heart disease.

Melatonin

Melatonin is a hormone, naturally manufactured deep within the brain by the pineal gland. It is a derivative of the amino acid tryptophan and the neurotransmitter serotonin. It has long been recognized for its role in the regulation of sleep and waking cycles and has gained popularity as a supplement for the treatment of jet lag, insomnia and other sleep disturbances.

Like most hormones, melatonin's activity is not confined to a single function. Recently, research papers have described a great number. These include potential anti-aging effects, applications against Alzheimer's disease and cluster headaches, prevention and treatment of cancer, and immunostimulation. Melatonin is a powerful antioxidant in its own right and promotes other antioxidants too.

Apart from its ability to function independently as an antioxidant, melatonin has been shown to effectively raise glutathione levels in many tissues including the brain, liver, muscle and blood serum.[6] Some of its positive benefits have been ascribed specifically to its role in glutathione pathways.

[6] A transparent yellow fluid; the blood without white or red cells, or a clotting factor

An interesting scientific study compared melatonin and glutathione levels during sleep. The research team at the University of Texas showed that subjects given melatonin doubled their brain glutathione levels within 30 minutes. Like GSH anywhere in the body, brain glutathione eliminates toxic hydroxyl radicals, but its effectiveness here is further enhanced by sleep. It seems that melatonin's protective effect on brain and nerve tissue may be due to its GSH-enhancing ability. Several European studies have supported these findings. This same team in Texas led by Reiter has published many papers linking melatonin to GSH production. In a sports physiology experiment, levels of glutathione in muscle were compared before and after extended exercise. Subjects pre-treated with melatonin avoided the usual significant decrease in GSH levels.

The long term safety of melatonin has not yet been established and response to it varies from person to person. This product should only be used in consultation with an appropriate health professional.

Glutamine

Glutamine (GAM) is the most abundant free amino acid in the body. It is common in both blood and muscle tissue, and is the second most common amino acid in the brain after glutamic acid (GA). These three—glutamine, glutamic acid and gamma-aminobutyric acid (GABA)—are closely related and classified as "glutamate"[7] amino acids.

Dr. Eric Braverman called them, "the brain's three musketeers." GAM, GA, and GABA appear close in name and category, but are quite different in function. In the brain, GABA serves as an inhibiting (calming) neurotransmitter while GA is an excitatory one. GAM is mainly a source of energy, and a mediator between GA and GABA. Some proponents of glutamine have called it "brain fuel."

These three amino acids usually fall into the same discussion because they have the ability to metabolize into one another. For example, when the brain registers a lack of glutamic acid, it may draw glutamine from the muscles into the bloodstream, pass it through the blood-brain barrier and transform it into glutamic acid or glutamate.

Nitrogen is a critical component of all amino acids and is released as they break down. Unfortunately free nitrogen easily converts into ammonia, which is especially toxic to nerve tissue in the body and brain. The liver converts nitrogen into urea for excretion though the urine, but this is labor-intensive. Fortunately, its burden is relieved when the nitrogen attaches itself to glutamic acid, forming glutamine—the only amino acid with two nitrogen molecules. In this way, glutamic acid serves as a "sponge" to soak up free nitrogen and protect many tissues from harm.

Glutamine is crucial to the metabolism and maintenance of muscle. It is also the primary nutrient for cells lining the intestinal tract. In periods of stress or severe illness when glutamine levels may fall it is a useful supplement for such diverse groups as athletes and surgical patients, those suffering from the muscle wasting of AIDS or cancer, and people with various gastrointestinal disorders.

Glutamine can also boost the immune system, act as a cancer preventative and treatment, detoxify the body and support liver metabolism. Dr. Ronald Klatz of the American Academy of Anti-Aging Medicine (A4M) describes glutamine as a 'growth-hormone releaser' and an anti-aging agent. The overlap of the possible clinical applications of glutamine and glutathione is no coincidence. Glutamine is the body's source of glutamate (glutamic acid), the second most important component of GSH after cysteine.

Whether taken orally or intravenously, glutamine supplementation raises glutathione concentrations. Harward in Florida and Basoglu in Turkey conducted similar studies to measure the fortifying effect of glutamine on GSH levels in the gut. Levels of lipid peroxidation and oxidative stress both

[7] A salt of glutamic acid

fell in these experiments. Cao in Arkansas found a three-fold increase in intestinal GSH after glutamine supplementation.

Denno and Rounds of Harvard University conducted a study on parenteral[8] nutrition. This is very important during long surgical procedures and under other special circumstances. They showed that when glutamine was included, plasma glutathione levels rose significantly and supported liver functions. With the same team, Hong showed that glutamine supplementation improved survival odds against such toxic threats as acetaminophen overdose by preserving glutathione stores in the liver.

Glutamine also plays a role in cancer therapy. Tumor cells often steal glutamine from other parts of the body, leading to muscle wasting and atrophy. Finding high levels of glutamine in tumors, cancer therapists used to fear that giving patients glutamine only fed the cancer. It is now known that just the opposite is true. Glutamine promotes GSH production, heightening the immune system's defense against tumor cells and making it easier for normal tissue to tolerate chemotherapy and radiotherapy.

Another University of Arkansas study led by Rouse showed how oral glutamine supplementation could lower glutathione in tumors, making them more susceptible to chemotherapy. At the same time the supplements raised glutathione in healthy cells, making them more resistant to chemotherapy. Yoshida and Kalbara conducted similar experiments in Japan and concluded that glutamine supplementation prevents deficiencies of glutamine and glutathione and improves protein metabolism in cancer victims.

Glutamine is found in many plant and animal foods, but is easily destroyed by cooking. Raw spinach and parsley are good sources. Chicken, fish, pork and beef are high in glutamine. However, eating raw meats carries certain health risks. Braver individuals may eat sushi, carpaccio, kibbi, or steak tartar—all uncooked animal products.

Glutamine is widely researched as a nutritional supplement for certain hospitalized patients, but more research is still needed. The appropriate dosage for various conditions is still unclear, especially during periods of physical stress. Store-bought tablets contain as little as one-half gram (500 mg). It also comes in powder form and is dispensed in daily doses of 4 or 5 grams. In extreme situations—following a bone marrow transplant, for example—doses as high as 40 grams per day have been given. Supplemental glutamine must be kept absolutely dry or it will degrade into ammonia.

Completely healthy individuals don't need supplemental glutamine. It can provoke such side effects as gastrointestinal upset. Older people and patients with impaired kidney and liver function should be cautious. Any serious use of this supplement should be monitored by a health professional.

Lipoic acid

Also called alpha-lipoic acid or thioctic acid, lipoic acid is a disulfide compound that acts as an effective antioxidant, a neutralizer of various toxins including some heavy metals, and an important co-enzyme for recycling other antioxidants, including vitamin C, vitamin E and glutathione. Lipoic acid occurs naturally in your body but has also recently appeared on the shelves of health food stores. It is being actively investigated by the scientific community for its medical merits.

Research has revealed the benefits of lipoic acid in such conditions as diabetes, HIV infection and AIDS, liver disease, lead and cadmium toxicity, cataracts, poisoning by amanita mushrooms,[9] reperfusion injury (following stroke and heart attack) and vitamin E deficiency. Lipoic acid also extends body builders' endurance and speeds recovery from injury. You may notice that its advantages entirely overlap those of glutathione. Lipoic acid is vital for converting glutathione to and from its oxidized (GSSG)

---

8 Intravenous administration of nutrition avoiding stomach and gut.

9 Amanita muscaria (also known as fly agaric): a psychoactive mushroom

to its reduced (GSH) form (see Figure 3 in Chapter 1). It regenerates vitamin C, vitamin E and coenzyme Q10. It can also provide redox support to other sulfur groups and NADPH energy reactions.

Although lipoic acid has been described by many researchers as an antioxidant in its own right, scientists such as Bast and Haenen from the Department of Pharmacochemistry in the Netherlands believe that lipoic acid principally contributes to the fight against lipid peroxidation by keeping GSH in its reduced (non-oxidized) state, so that GSH is the active antioxidant. In fact,. they showed that lipoic acid in the absence of glutathione actually promotes oxidation—the opposite of what was expected. One reason glutathione has been called the "master antioxidant" is because glutathione-reductase—the molecule's critical enzyme—maintains lipoic acid in its reduced (non-oxidative) state.

The ability of lipoic acid to enhance GSH function has been demonstrated by other scientists. In Germany, the researcher Buses established that lipoic acid elevated glutathione levels, improved cell viability and protected against radiation damage.

Some leading American researchers in lipoic acid, headed by Packer at the University of California in Berkeley, have said that lipoic acid provides intact cystine, making cysteine available to the cells. It is clinically significant that lipoic acid helps restore glutathione when it is deficient. Recommended dosages range from 100 to 200 mg per day.

Silymarin (milk thistle)

The milk thistle plant Silybum marianum has been used by herbalists for centuries to treat a variety of liver disorders, including hepatitis, alcoholic cirrhosis, jaundice and gallbladder disease. It has also been employed against a number of toxins, including amanita poison mushrooms. The active ingredient of milk thistle is silymarin, a compound made up of the bioflavonoids[10] silybin, silydianin, and silychristin. Silymarin is found in the seeds.

Many clinicians have studied this herbal extract and its use in toxicology and liver disease. It seems to stimulate the growth and regeneration of injured liver cells. However, the primary contribution of its bioflavonoids seems to be free radical scavenging. They also support detoxification enzyme pathways.

Further studies describing this action have demonstrated silymarin's impressive ability to promote glutathione production. Administering it clearly prevents lipid peroxidation and maintains GSH levels. Silybin has a protective effect on acetaminophen overdoses—traditionally treated with the drug NAC. In certain glutathione-deficient states silymarin can increase GSH by as much as 35%, thus accelerating the detoxification of xenobiotics.[11]

Recommended doses vary greatly, from 50 to 500 milligrams thrice daily. Toxic reactions may include gas, cramps and diarrhea. Liver disease should never be treated without the advice of a health professional.

Whey proteins

Whey is a large group of proteins and a constituent of all mammal's milk, including human milk. The most commonly available source of whey is cow's milk. Raw milk contains 5 to 10% protein, of which 80% is casein and 20% whey. Casein is a mainstay of cheese production. For a long time whey was treated as an insignificant byproduct of the dairy industry. However its advantages as a nutritional supplement have changed attitudes and prompted new interest.

Milk derivatives and whey products are marketed to health-conscious people. It is big business and getting bigger. These products are extremely variable in their protein content, their concentration, the forms of proteins present, and other factors which determine their bio-effectiveness—including the level of protein denaturation.

Denaturation refers to a breakdown in the protein structure[12] that may not affect its food

---

[10] Flavonoids are yellow or red/blue pigments found in flowers, fruits and vegetables.

[11] Xenobiotics are chemical substances found within, but not native to, an organism.

[12] The arrangement of chemical bonds within the molecule.

Concentration of total protein	Types of proteins
Degree of denaturization (breakdown)	Fat content
Lactose content	Bioavailability
Biological Activity	Contaminants, toxins
Whey protein variables	

TABLE 12: Whey protein variables

value but that can affect its biological action (bioactivity) in the body. Many nutritionists point out that the fat or lactose content of milk products may still be high enough to cause concern. Others have reservations about the milk industry and its liberal use of antibiotics and steroids to boost production. And we cannot ignore the very real issue of fat-soluble and water-soluble environmental toxins passing into the milk.

Fresh milk whey contains potent GSH precursors such as lactoferrin, beta-lactalbumin, and serum albumin. All are subject to denaturation. When consumed as-is, they are easily digested and their constituent breakdown products delivered into the bloodstream as cysteine and cystine delivery systems. From there they are carried to individual cells, where these precursors are transported through the cell wall and metabolized into GSH.

The GSH precursors in whey protein are fragile, and the molecular bonds that are so important to their passage through the digestive system are easily broken down by heating (as in pasteurization) or by physical stress (such as shaking and churning). By the time most milk products reach your table their bioactivity is entirely lost. Nevertheless, their food value remains. Milk products are usually pasteurized several times to guard against bacterial contamination. This alone destroys their usefulness as glutathione precursors, for which role they must be bioactive.

To maintain bioactivity, great care and specific techniques are required in the extraction of whey proteins from milk, and the process must be carefully monitored to assure success. Commercial whey products vary in their protein content from as little as 20% protein to more than 90%. Much more important is the extent to which GSH precursors are denatured (broken down). Some retain some bioactivity. Most have none.

Bioactive whey proteins

Bioactive whey proteins contain high levels of non-denatured protein and are also called undenatured whey proteins. In scientific terms, they preserve the original bioactivity of the thermolabile[13] components, as well as the physical structure of the proteins, guaranteeing maximum GSH-promoting activity.

Reliable reports of the GSH-sustaining effect of dietary whey proteins first emereged from research at Montreal's McGill University in the early 1980s. Dr. Gustavo Bounous and Dr. Patricia Kongshavn were studying protein supplementation when they stumbled upon the bioactive potential of whey protein. Investigating this protein's effect on the immune system at length, their published results stirred excitement. As a result, scientific teams around the world were encouraged to test the whey protein's GSH-enhancing qualities on a wide variety of diseases. This team went on to develop a method of production that maximized bioactivity of the isolated protein.

This protein was subsequently patented for its immuno-sustaining and GSH-enhancing effects. It is extracted from milk raised without antibiotics and refined to 90% purity. This particular whey protein extract has received a patent for its method of use, and has also been granted a USA patent as

13 Readily deactivated by heat.

a chemotherapeutic agent—the first natural supplement to receive such recognition.

Bounous's bioactive whey protein is backed up by phase I, II and III clinical trials that include research into infectious disease (HIV/AIDS, hepatitis, Lyme disease, bacterial infections), cancer therapy, pulmonary disease, chronic fatigue syndrome and other disorders associated with high oxidative stress and low glutathione activity. It has been sold in Europe and the Orient by pharmaceutical distributors. In North America this all-natural product is available without prescription. Some governmental agencies and insurance companies will reimburse patients with a physician's prescription.

Undenatured, bioactive whey protein is a natural extract of milk and an ideal way to raise and sustain GSH levels—safe, dependable and effective.

Co-Factors for GSH Production

Selenium

Selenium is a trace element that functions principally as an antioxidant, but plays roles in protein synthesis and other metabolic processes. It also acts synergistically (hand-in-hand) with other antioxidants—particularly vitamin E. Its clinical applications have aroused attention, and we expect to see an increase in the number of clinical trials using this mineral.

Plants absorb sodium selenite[14] and convert it into organic seleno-methionine. When we eat these plants the seleno-methionine is either used to make protein or converted once again, this time into seleno-cysteine. The cysteine portion of this molecule contributes to GSH production. The selenium portion is an essential component of the critically important enzyme glutathione peroxidase.

Browsing through a list of selenium research and clinical trials, one is reminded of similar research and clinical trials on GSH. Both deal with the same broad spectrum of disease, clinical symptoms and outcomes. Selenium has been linked with heart disease and atherosclerosis, cancer treatment and prevention, liver and pancreatic function, detoxification of heavy metals, immune support, male infertility, AIDS, Crohn's disease, pancreatitis, cystic fibrosis and multiple sclerosis—it reads like a table of contents for this book on GSH.

Most scientists agree that selenium principally fights these diseases by raising levels of glutathione peroxidase—the major metabolically active form of selenium.

A study sponsored by the National Cancer Institute (USA) caused quite a stir when it didn't go as expected. Based on favorable reports about selenium being cancer-preventive, the institute initiated a study on skin cancer. Patients were given either selenium or a placebo, and over eight years were monitored for any recurrence of their skin lesions. With no evidence that selenium protects against skin cancer recurrences, initial results caused disappointment. However, researchers continued crunching the data and found that their test group suffered significantly lower rates of other cancers—including lung, colon and prostate cancers (see Chapters 12, 13 and 20). These unexpected findings rolled over into a host of new studies, some still in progress.

Selenium is found abundantly in foods grown in selenium-rich soil and from the meat and dairy products of animals raised on those plants. The suggested daily intake is 40 to 70 micrograms (mcg)—an amount found in normal diets and not usually requiring supplementation.

Be careful! Too much selenium is known to be toxic, and some individuals suffer ill effects at doses as low as 250 mcg/day. At 1,000 mcg/day, many symptoms appear. Selenium is usually sold in doses ranging

---

14 An inorganic compound in the soil

from 25 to 200 mcg. It may be a natural food supplement, but it still must be approached with caution. People in good health with a reasonable diet generally do not need to take more than 25 to 50 mcg/day.

Vitamins B_1, B_2

The water-soluble vitamins B_1 (thiamine) and B_2 (riboflavin) were two of the first vitamins discovered back in the 1920s and 30s. They each perform several important functions in our body. Vitamin B_1 is essential for carbohydrate metabolism and energy production. It also helps conversion of fatty acids into steroid hormones. Vitamin B_2 is just as involved in energy production and hormone regulation. It also helps combine individual amino acids into larger proteins—glutathione being one of them.

Vitamins B_1 and B_2 maintain glutathione and its related enzymes in their active forms, enabling GSH to function optimally. They are integral constituents of coenzymes that produce glutathione reductase and NADPH – essential for recycling oxidized (inactive) glutathione (GSSG) back to reduced glutathione (GSH)—its active form.

The currently recommended daily intake of these two vitamins is 1 to 2 milligrams. Most clinicians believe that these values are far too low and it's just a matter of time before they are raised. Doses of 50 to 150 mg are not uncommon and many feel that the optimum level lies between 25 and 300 mg/day. It is apparently not toxic – these higher doses have revealed no adverse effects. Nutritionists at times prescribe 500 mg/day for some conditions, but for most near-normal states 10 to 50 mg/day should suffice.

Vitamins B6, B_{12}, & Folic acid (B^9)

Like their cousins B_1 and B_2, vitamins B_6(pyridoxine) and B_{12} (cobalamin) are also water soluble. Both play an indirect but important role in glutathione metabolism. Vitamin B_6 is one of the most widely used vitamins in our body and contributes to over sixty enzyme systems. It is crucial for the metabolism and function of many amino acids and essential fatty acids, so most of our tissues depend on it. Vitamin B_{12} acts as a coenzyme in the production and regulation of red blood cells, myelin and other neurological tissues. It is prone to depletion in various diseases including malabsorption[15], alcoholism, pernicious anemia and the complications of strict vegetarianism.

Folic acid (Vitamin B_9) – also known as folate or folacin – takes part in a number of various processes, including DNA synthesis and neurotransmission.[16] It works together with vitamin B_{12} in amino acid metabolism and protein synthesis. Its role has also been highlighted in cardiovascular disease, since it lowers elevated homocysteine levels—a serious risk factor. In the presence of folate (B_9), cysteine is more likely to participate in the production of glutathione rather than homocysteine.

North American recommended daily dietary allowances for vitamins B_6, B_{12} and folate (B_9) are 0.5 to 2 mg, 1 to 2 mcg, and 150 to 250 mcg respectively. Some nutritionists may recommend as much as 50 to 500 mg of vitamin B_6, 100 to 500 mcg of vitamin B_{12}, and 400 to 2,000 mcg of folic acid. Vitamin B_{12} has negligible toxicity but vitamin B_6 can be neurotoxic[17] at higher doses. Folic acid (B_9) is relatively safe unless taken alone by someone deficient in certain B-vitamins, particularly B_{12}. Under normal circumstances we recommend a maximum 10 to 50 mg of B_6, 10 to 50 mcg of B_{12}, and 400 mcg of folic acid (B_9) per day.

Vitamin C

The water-soluble vitamin C has various names, including ascorbate and ascorbic acid. It has been a focus for antioxidant research longer than any other antioxidant. Linus Pauling, the foremost researcher in vitamin C, is considered by many to be the grandfa-

---

15 Decreased ability to digest and/or absorb nutrients from food
16 The process by which neurons exchange information
17 Damaging to the nervous system

ther of free radical biology. He blazed the trail along which this and many other books have evolved. Thousands of articles have been written about vitamin C and research is still going strong. Yet, even after all this time, the topic of vitamin C in health and disease is still fraught with controversy.

The classic use of vitamin C is against scurvy.[18] More recently, it has been studied in cancer, anti-aging, cardiovascular disorders, emotional or physical stress, and of course in immunology and infectious disease. It is an antioxidant but performs many other functions in our body. It is involved in bone, cartilage and soft tissue repair; support of various biologic systems including the recycling of B-vitamins, folic acid and other antioxidants; iron storage and a list of other life-sustaining functions too long and involved to discuss in this book. It is is intimately involved in the GSH-driven glutathione-transhydrogenase enzyme system which keeps GSH, vitamin C, vitamin E and other antioxidants in a reduced (non-oxidized) state.

Many studies have demonstrated that vitamin C supports healthy glutathione levels and activity. Johnston, Meyer and Srilakshmi at Arizona State University conducted a double blind study comparing the GSH levels of three groups—one fed a low-vitamin C diet, another a diet with 500 mg/day of vitamin C, and a third receiving 2,000 mg/day. Those taking the vitamin had significantly higher GSH red blood cell counts than the low-vitamin C group. There was little difference in glutathione level between those who took 500 mg/day and those who took 2000 mg.

The converse is equally true. Vitamin C is much less effective and rapidly depleted whenever there's not enough glutathione to go around, because the two work together. A vitamin C molecule mops up a free radical, effectively neutralizing it. However, it now has its hands full. It (and its toxic prisoner) can be ejected from the cell and eliminated from the body, or it can hand off the captive radical to a recycling agent—in this case, glutathione. GSH and GSH enzymes accept the free radical from the vitamin C complex, freeing it up to get back to work. This cycle drives antioxidant function in our bodies (see Figure 6 in Chapter 1).

Mendiratta, May and Qu of Vanderbilt University in Nashville described a persuasive study demonstrating this interdependence of glutathione and vitamin C in human plasma and red blood cells. When GSH was intentionally depleted from plasma using the chemical diamide, vitamin C was either lost or remained functionally impaired in its oxidized state (dehydro-ascorbate). Glutathione enabled its transformation back into the functional form, ascorbate.

Despite decades of research, there is little agreement over the appropriate dosage of vitamin C. Both the American and Canadian recommended daily allowances of vitamin are in the range of 30 to 60 mg/day, but many scientists and nutritionists feel that this figure is too low. Advocates of megadosing with vitamin C are not averse to taking 10, 20, or 30 thousand mg/day.

It is well documented that supplies of vitamin C beyond a certain threshold are eliminated from the body, often along with cramps and diarrhea. Some researchers feel that vitamin C is potentially harmful at high doses. It may serve as a pro-oxidant, and it strongly competes with other antioxidants—occasionally impairing their function. Flagg and her team at Emory University in Atlanta showed that high levels of vitamin C intake corresponded to lowered GSH levels.

If glutathione levels are adequate, there is no reason to supplement more than 200 to 1,000 mg/day of vitamin C.

Vitamin E

The fat-soluble vitamin E is America's second most popular supplement after vitamin C. Given the wealth of information and positive clinical studies done on this vitamin, its popularity will probably continue to

---

[18] A wasting disease resulting from a lack of vitamin C.

grow—and so it should. Some authors have suggested that if all North Americans took enough vitamin E supplements, health-care costs could be reduced by billions of dollars.

Studies have shown the benefits of vitamin E in cancer prevention and therapy, cardiovascular disease, diseases of aging, wound healing, neurodegenerative disease and many other states of health. Besides its clearly defined role as an antioxidant, it also works in the detoxification of many compounds and in the immune system.

Like vitamin C, vitamin E has an important role in the GSH-driven glutathione-transhydrogenase enzyme system which keeps GSH, vitamin C, vitamin E and other antioxidants in their reduced (non-oxidized) state (see Figure 3 in Chapter 1). Studies with GSH and vitamin E resemble those with GSH and vitamin C because these antioxidants depend on each other for proper function and recycling. The synergistic effect of vitamin E and glutathione can be attributed to vitamin E's ability to assist GSH with antioxidation, and to its direct modulation of glutathione-related enzymes.

Vitamin E comes in several forms, natural and synthetic. This vitamin is actually a set of substances, the most active being alpha, beta, delta, and gamma-tocopherols. The most prevalent natural form of tocopherol is D-alpha-tocopherol, which is more potent and bioavailable[19] than the synthetic DL-alpha-tocopherol.

The daily recommended allowance ranges from 25 to 50 IU (international units); however, studies hint that most of us would benefit from much higher doses. Popular regimens range from 100 to 1200 IU/day. With adequate GSH levels, it is unlikely that one needs more than 400 IU/day. At excessive levels, vitamin E is toxic and can provoke gastrointestinal, cardiovascular and neurological side-effects.

Other micronutrients

A deficiency of magnesium can impair the enzyme gamma glutamyl transpeptidase (GGT), important in GSH synthesis.

Vanadium is a trace element that depends on glutathione to remain in a reduced (non-oxidized) state and to increase its bioavailability. Under certain conditions, vanadium recycles GSH. However, in high concentrations it is toxic and may deplete GSH.

Deficiency of zinc is also detrimental to the glutathione metabolism, resulting in reduced GSH concentration—particularly in red blood cells. Zinc in high levels carries a certain toxicity and may reduce GSH.

Nrf2 activators, epigenetics, sulforaphane

The past few decades of genetic research have opened up doors that were once sealed. Now we have the ability to read the actual DNA code that determines what makes us who we uniquely are. A better understanding of how DNA works has revealed that our genetic information is not necessarily "fixed" in hard-wired code that dictates how we turn out. DNA carries some reprogrammable "software" that's influenced by environmental factors, including diet. This phenomenon is called "Epigenetics," which is Latin for, "Over and above the genes."

Epigenetic "switches" have been identified that can "turn on (activate)" or "turn off (deactivate)" pieces of DNA coding, ultimately influencing how the DNA expresses itself. One dramatic example of this epigenetic environmental switch was described after Montreal's famous "ice storm" in 1998, when electric power was lost for weeks, causing great stress among the city's inhabitants. A retrospective study of the mothers who were pregnant in that period revealed that their

[19] A substance's ability to enter the circulation when introduced into the body and to have an active effect.

offspring had a much higher incidence of neurological disorders, including attention deficit disorder and autism.

Some genes are more affected than others by epigenetic switching. One is the Nrf2 gene. When "activated," it upregulates (adds force to) natural antioxidant production in the cell. Glutathione, being the cell's "master antioxidant" is greatly influenced by Nrf2 activation.

One of the first Nrf2 activators to be described was discovered on plants of the Brassica family—including broccoli. This discovery finally explained the positive effects of broccoli on health, including cancer suppression. Your grandmother was right all along when she made you eat your broccoli!

The most powerful substance identified in broccoli was a molecule called "sulphoraphane." Sulforaphane can now be isolated from the vegetable, and it remains bioavailable when eaten. Scientists from Johns Hopkins University described its anticancer benefits as early as 1992. Since then, a flood of articles have been written on this previously unknown organic molecule.

Much research has been done linking sulforaphane to glutathione. In the late 1990's cell culture studies showed how sulforaphane induced cells to increase their GSH activity. In the early 2000's several researchers had moved on to human studies, and showed how sulforaphane enhanced glutathione production. By 2011, scientists were examining the potential of sulforaphane-glutathione modulation not only in cancer therapy, but also in treating neurological conditions, including Alzheimer's disease, Parkinson's disease and age-related cognitive decline. More recently, human clinical trials are commonly reported in the literature. Back in the cradle of sulforaphane's discovery—Johns Hopkins University—neuropsychiatrists have described how sulforaphane augments glutathione and influences brain chemistry in human subjects. They suggest this field should be pursued in addressing psychiatric illnesses.

Conclusion

For our bodies to sustain healthy glutathione levels, the limiting factor in our daily intake of food is usually the amino acid cysteine. It must be in a form that can survive the trip from our mouths to our cells. Unfortunately, simply eating either glutathione—or its precursor, the free amino acid cysteine—does not supply the cell with the raw materials it needs to manufacture glutathione.

Several drugs and natural products do this efficiently. NAC (N-acetyl-cysteine) is a powerful drug commonly used in critical care medicine, toxicology, and pulmonary medicine. It has been the most researched of all the GSH-promoting modalities, and newer clinical applications are being developed all the time.

Some natural products exert positive effects by supporting or directly raising glutathione levels. Undenatured whey protein isolates are an exciting development, especially those with bonded cysteine (cystine). The discovery of epigenetic triggers such as Nrf2 activators like sulforaphane has broadened our ability to raise and sustain glutathione.

RAISING GSH LEVELS

REFERENCES

Aebi S, Assereto R, Lauterburg BH. *High-dose intravenous glutathione in man. Pharmacokinetics & effects on cyst(e)ine in plasma & urine.* Eur J Clin Invest 21(1):103-10, 1991

Allen J. *Inhaled glutathione for the prevention of air pollution-related health effects: a brief review.* Altern Ther Health Med 14(3):42-4, 2008

Allen J, Bradley RD. *Effects of oral glutathione supplementation on systemic oxidative stress biomarkers in human volunteers.* J Altern Complement Med 17(9):827-33, 2011

ALMASIO P, BORTOLINI M, PAGLIARO L, ET AL. *Role of s-adenosyl methionine in the treatment of intrahepatic cholestasis.* Drugs 40: (S3): 111-123, 1990

AMMON HP, MELIEN MC, VERPOHL EJ. *Pharmacokinetics of intravenously administered glutathione in the rat.* J Pharm Pharmacol 38(10):721-5, 1986

ANDERSON ME. *GSH & GSH delivery compounds.* Advances in Pharmacol. 38:65-78, 1997

ANDERSON ME, LEVY EJ, MEISTER A. *Preparation & use of glutathione monoesters.* Methods Enzymol. 234: 492-499, 1994

ANDERSON M, POWRIE F, PURI R, MEISTER A. *Glutathione monoethyl ester: Preparation, uptake by tissues, & conversion to glutathione.* Archives Biochemistry & Biophysiology 239:538-48, 1985

ANONYMOUS, RECORD SUPPLIED BY PUBLISHER. *Monograph: Alpha-lipoic acid.* Altern. Med. Rev. 3: 308-311, 1998

ASK M, MAPELLI V, HÖCK H, OLSSON L, BETTIGA M. *Engineering glutathione biosynthesis of Saccharomyces cerevisiae increases robustness to inhibitors in pretreated lignocellulosic materials.* Microb Cell Fact 12:87, 2013

BAGNATO GF ET AL. *Effect of inhaled glutathione on airway response to 'Fog' challenge in asthmatic patients.* Respiration 66(6):518-21, 1999

BALANSKY RB, D'AGOSTINI F, ZANACCHI P, DE FLORA S. *Protection by N-acetylcysteine of the histopathological & cytogenical damage produced by exposure of rats to cigarette smoke.* Cancer Lett. 64: 123-131, 1992

BARLOW-WALDEN LR, REITER RJ, ABE M, ET AL. *Melatonin stimulates brain glutathione peroxidase activity.* Neurochem. Int. 26: 497-502, 1995

BASOGLU M, YILIRGAN I, AKCAY F, ET AL. *Glutathione & nitric oxide concentrations in glutamine-infused rabbits with intestinal ischemia/reperfusion.* Eur. J. Clin. Chem. Clin. Biochem. 35: 415-419, 1997

BAST H, HAENEN GR. *Interplay between lipoic acid & glutathione in the protection against microsomal lipid peroxidation.* Biochem. Biophys. Acta. 963: 558-561, 1988

BAST H, HAENEN GR. *Regulation of lipid peroxidation by glutathione & lipoic acid : involvement of liver microsomal vitamin E free radical reductase.* Adv. Exp. Med. Biol. 264: 111-116, 1990

BAUR A, HARRER T, PEUKERT M, ET AL. *Alpha-lipoic acid is an effective inhibitor of human immuno-deficiency virus (HIV-1) replication.* Klin. Wochenschr. 69: 722-724, 1991

BIEWENGA GP, HAENEN GR, BAST. *The pharmacology of the antioxidant lipoic acid.* Gen. Pharmacol. 29: 315-331, 1997

BIRNBAUM S, WINITZ M, GREENSTEIN J. *Quantitative nutritional studies with water soluble, chemically defined diets. III - Individual amino acids as sources of "non-essential" nitrogen.* Archives Biochemistry & Biophysics 72:428-36, 1957

BISHAYEE A, CHATTERJEE M. *Selective enhancement of glutathione S-transferase activity in liver & extrahepatic tissues of rat following oral administration of vanadate.* Acta. Physiol. Pharmacol. Bulg. 19: 83-89, 1993

BISHAYEE A, CHATTERJEE M. *Time course effects of vanadium supplement on cytosolic reduced glutathione level & glutathione S-transferase.* Biol. Trace Elem. Res. 48: 275-285, 1995

BISHOP C, HUDSON VM, HILTON SC, WILDE C. *A pilot study of the effect of inhaled buffered reduced glutathione on the clinical status of patients with cystic fibrosis.* Chest 127(1):308-17, 2005

BJORKMAN L, LANGWORTH S, LIND B, ET AL. *Activity of antioxidative enzymes in erythrocytes & concentration of selenium in plasma related to mercury exposure.* J. Trace Elem. Electrolytes Health Dis. 7: 157-164, 1993

BONGERS V, DE JONG J, STEEN I, ET AL. *Antioxidant-related parameters in patients treated for cancer chemoprevention with N-acetylcysteine.* Eur. J. Cancer 31A:921-923, 1995

BOROK Z, BUHL R, GRIMES GJ ET AL. *Effect of glutathione aerosol on oxidant-antioxidant imbalance in idiopathic pulmonary fibrosis.* Lancet 338(8761):215-6, 1991

BOUNOUS G, GOLD P. *The biological activity of undenatured whey proteins: The role of glutathione.* Clinical Investigative Medicine 14:296-309, 1991

BOUNOUS G, KONGSHAVN P. *Influence of dietary whey proteins on the immune system of mice.* Journal of Nutrition 112:1747-55, 1982

BOUNOUS G, LETOURNEAU L, KONGSHAVN P. *Influence of dietary protein type on the immune system of mice.* Journal of Nutrition 113:1415-21, 1983 Bounous G, Batist G, Gold P. Immuno-enhancing property of dietary whey protein in mice: Role of glutathione. Clinical Investigative Medicine 12:154-61, 1989

BOUNOUS, DR. GUSTAVO BOUNOUS G, SHENOUDA N, KONGSHAVN P, OSMOND D. *Mechanism of altered B-cell response induced by changes in dietary protein type in mice.* Journal of Nutrition 115:1409-17, 1985

BRAY T, TAYLOR C. *Enhancement of tissue glutathione for antioxidant & immune functions in malnutrition.* Biochemistry Pharmacology 47:2113-23, 1994

BUHL R, VOGELMEIER C, CRITENDEN M ET AL. *Augmentation of glutathione in the fluid lining the epithelium of the lower respiratory tract by directly administering glutathione aerosol.* Proc Natl Acad Sci U S A 87(11):4063-7, 1990

Buonocore D, Grosini M, Giardina S et al. *Bioavailability Study of an Innovative Orobuccal Formulation of Glutathione.* Oxid Med Cell Longev 2016:3286365, 2016

Busse E, Zimmer G, Schopohl B, Kornhuber B. *Influence of alpha-lipoic acid on intracellular glutathione in vitro & in vivo.* Arzneimittelforschung 42: 829-831, 1992

Campos R, Garrido A, Guerra R, Valenzuela A. *Silybin dihemisuccinate protects against glutathione depletion & lipid peroxidation induced by acetaminophen on rat liver.* Planta Med. 55: 417-419, 1989

Cao Y, Feng Z, Hoos A, Klimberg VS. *Glutamine enhances gut glutathione production.* J. Parenter. Enteral Nutr. 22: 224-227, 1998

Chen JL, Xie L, Cai JJ, Yang CS, Duan XH. *Enzymatic synthesis of glutathione using engineered Saccharomyces cerevisiae.* Biotechnol Lett 35(8):1259-64, 2013

Clark LC, Combs GF Jr, Turnbull BW, et al. *Effects of selenium supplementation for cancer prevention in patients with carcinoma of the skin. A randomized controlled trial. Nutritional Prevention of Cancer Study Group.* JAMA 276: 1957-1963, 1996

Clark LC, Dalkin B, Krongrad A, et al. *Decreased incidence of prostate cancer with selenium supplementation : results of a double-blind cancer prevention trial.* Br. J. Urol. 81: 730-734, 1998

Clark LC, Hixson LJ, Combs GF Jr, et al. *Plasma selenium concentration predicts the prevalence of colorectal adenomatous polyps.* Cancer Epidemiol. Biomarkers Prev. 2: 41-46, 1993

Combs GF Jr, Clark LC, Turnbull BW. *Reduction of cancer risk with an oral supplement of selenium.* Biomed. Environ. Sci. 10: 227-234, 1997

Conaway CC, Jiao D, Kelloff GJ, et al. *Chemopreventive potential of fumaric acid, N-acetylcysteine, N-(4-hydroxyphenyl) retinamide & beta-carotene for tobacco-nitrosamine-induced lung tumors in A/J mice.* Cancer Lett. 124: 85-93, 1998

Constantinescu A, Pick U, Handelman et al. *Reduction & transport of lipoic acid by human erythrocytes.* Biochem. Pharmacol. 17: 253-261, 1995

Costagliola C, Menzione M. *Effect of vitamin E on the oxidative state of glutathione in plasma.* Clin. Physiol. Biochem. 8: 140-143, 1990

D'Agostini F, Bagnasco M, Giunciuglio D, et al. *Inhibition by N-acetylcysteine of doxorubicin-induced clastogenicity & alopecia, & prevention of primary tumors & micrometastasis in mice.* Int. J. Oncol. 13: 217-224, 1998

Davreux CJ, Soric I, Natens AB, et al. *N-acetylcysteine attenuates acute lung injury in the rat.* Shock 8: 432-438, 1997

Denno R, Rounds JD, Faris R, et al. *Glutamine-enriched total parenteral nutrition enhance plasma GSH in the resting state.* J. Surg. Res. 15: 35-38, 1996

Dickenson A. *Benefits of nutritional supplements.* Council for Responsible Nutrition. 1-68, 1998

Droge W. *Cysteine & glutathione deficiency in AIDS patients: a rationale for the treatment with N-acetyl-cysteine.* Pharmacology 46: 61-65, 1993

Dworkin BM. *Selenium deficiency in HIV infection & the acquired immunodeficiency syndrome (AIDS).* Chem. Biol. Interact. 91: 181-186, 1994

Ferreira de Oliveira JM, Costa M, Pedrosa T, Pinto P et al. *Sulforaphane induces oxidative stress & death by p53-independent mechanism: implication of impaired glutathione recycling.* PLoS One 9(3):e92980, 2014

Flagg EW, Coates RJ, Eley JW, et al. *Dietary glutathione intake in humans & the relationship between intake & plasma total glutathione level.* Nutrition & Cancer 21: 33-46, 1994

Floreani M, Skaper SD, Facci L, et al. *Melatonin maintains glutathione homeostasis in kainic acid-exposed rat brain tissues.* FASEB J 11: 1309-1315, 1997

Garcia-Gimenez JL, Roma-Mateo C, Pérez-Machado G, Peiró-Chova L, Pallardo FV. *Role of GSH in regulation of epigenetic mechanisms in disease.* Free Radic Biol Med 112:36-48, 2017

Griese M et al. *Improvement of alveolar glutathione & lung function but not oxidative state in cystic fibrosis.* Am J Respir Crit Care Med 169(7):822-8, 2004

Guerrero-Beltrán CE, Calderón-Oliver M, Pedraza-Chaverri J, Chirino YI. *Protective effect of sulforaphane against oxidative stress: recent advances.* Exp Toxicol Pathol 64(5):503-8, 2012

Guilford FT. *Commentary to "Randomized controlled trial of oral glutathione supplementation on body stores of glutathione".* Eur J Nutr 54(5):859-60, 2015

Gregus Z, Stein AF, Varga F, Klassen CD. *Effect of lipoic acid on biliary excretion of glutathione & metals.* Toxicol. Appl. Pharmacol. 114: 88-96, 1992

Han D, Handelman G, Marcocci L, et al. *Lipoic acid increases de novo synthesis of cellular glutathione by improving cysteine utilization.* Biofactors 6: 321-338, 1997

Han D, Tritschler HJ, Packer L. *Alpha-lipoic acid increases intracellular glutathione in a human T-lymphocyte Jurkat cell line.* Biochem. Biophys. Res. Commun. 207: 258-264, 1995

Hara M, Abe M, Suzuki T, Reiter RJ. *Tissue changes in glutathione metabolism & lipid peroxidation induced by swimming are partially prevented by melatonin.* Pharmacol. Toxicol. 78: 308-312, 1996

Hara KY, Aoki N, Kobayashi J et al. *Improvement of oxidized glutathione fermentation by thiol redox metabolism engineering in Saccharomyces cerevisiae. Appl Microbiol Biotechnol 99(22):9771-8, 2015*

HARTL D, STAROSTA V, MAIER K ET AL. *Inhaled glutathione decreases PGE2 & increases lymphocytes in cystic fibrosis lungs.* Free Radic Biol Med 39(4):463-72, 2005

HARWARD TR, COE D, SOUBA WW, ET AL. *Glutamine preserves gut GSH levels during intestinal ischemia/reperfusion.* J. Surg. Res. 56: 351-355, 1994

HEALTH CANADA. *Nutrition recommendations: The report of the Scientific Review Committee.* Health Canada, 1990

HIRAI R, NAKAI S, KIKUISHI H, KAWAI K. *Evaluation of the immunological enhancement activities of Immunocal.* Otsuka Pharm Co. Dec. 13, 1990

HOLDINESS MR. *Clinical pharmacokinetics of N-acetylcysteine.* Clin. Pharmacokinet. 20: 123-134, 1991

HOLROYD KJ, BUHL R, BOROK Z ET AL. *Correction of glutathione deficiency in the lower respiratory tract of HIV seropositive individuals by glutathione aerosol treatment.* Thorax 48(10):985-9, 1993

HOLYNSKA-IWAN I ET AL. *The application of N-acetylcysteine in optimization of specific pharmacological therapies.* Pol Merkur Lekarski 43(255):140-144, 2017

HONG RW, ROUNDS JD, HELTON WS, ET AL. *Glutamine preserves liver glutathione after lethal hepatic injury.* Ann. Surg. 215: 114-119, 1992

HYBERTSON BM, GAO B, BOSE SK, MCCORD JM. *Oxidative stress in health & disease:* the therapeutic potential of Nrf2 activation. Mol Aspects Med 32(4-6):234-46, 2011

INSTITUTE OF MEDICINE, FOOD & NUTRITION BOARD. *Public policy news—Translating the science behind the dietary reference intakes.* J. American Diet. Assoc. 98: 756, 1998

IP C. *Comparative effects of antioxidants on enzymes involved in glutathione metabolism.* Life Sci. 34: 2501-2506, 1984

JACOB C, MARET W, VALLEE BL. *Selenium redox biochemistry of zinc-sulfur coordination sites in proteins & enzymes.* Proc. Natl. Acad. Sci. USA. 96: 1910-1914, 1999

JAIN A, MADSEN DC, AULD P, ET AL. *L-2-Oxothiazolidine-4-carboxylate, a cysteine precursor, stimulates growth & normalizes tissue glutathione concentrations in rats fed a sulfur amino acid-deficient diet.* J. Nutr. 125: 851-856, 1995

JIANG LJ, MARET W, VALLEE BL. *The glutathione redox couple modulates zinc transfer from metallothionein to zinc-depleted sorbitol dehydrogenase.* Proc. Natl. Acad. Sci. USA. 95: 3483-3488, 1998

JOHNSTON CS, MEYER CG, SRILAKSHMI JC. *Vitamin C elevates red blood cell glutathione in healthy adults.* Amer. J. Clin. Nutr. 58: 103-105, 1993

KALAYJIAN RC, SKOWRON G, EMGUSHOV RT, ET AL. *A phase I/II trial of intravenous L-2-oxothiazolidine-4-carboxylic acid (procysteine) in asymptomatic HIV-infected subjects.* J. Acq. Immune Def. Syndr. 7: 369-374, 1994

KALEBIC T, KINTER A, POLI G, ET AL. *Suppression of human immunodeficiency virus expression in chronically infected monocyte cells by glutathione, glutathione ester, & N-acetylcysteine.* Proc. Natl. Acad. Sci. USA. 88: 986-990, 1991

KAPLOWITZ N, AW T, OOKHTENS M. *The regulation of hepatic glutathione.* Ann Revue Pharmacology & Toxicology 25:715-44, 1985

KELLY GS. *Clinical applications of N-acetylcysteine.* Altern. Med. Rev. 3: 114-127, 1998

KERN JK, GEIER DA, ADAMS JB, GARVER CR ET AL. *A clinical trial of glutathione supplementation in autism spectrum disorders.* Med Sci Monit 17(12):CR677-82, 2011

KIRIYAMA K, HARA KY, KONDO A. *Oxidized glutathione fermentation using Saccharomyces cerevisiae engineered for glutathione metabolism.* Appl Microbiol Biotechnol 97(16):7399-404, 2013

KLATZ R. *Grow young with HGH [ISBN 0-06-098434-1].* Harper Perennial. 1997

KLIMBERG VS, MCCLELLAN JL. CLAUDE H. ORGAN JR. *Hon. Lectureship: Glutamine, cancer, & its therapy.* American J. Surg. 172: 418-424, 1996

KOCH S, LEIS A, STOKIC D, KHAWLI F ET AL. *Side effects of IV N-acetylcysteine.* American Journal Respirology & Critical Care Medicine 149:A321, 1994

KOTLER M, RODRIGUEZ C, SAINZ RM, ET AL. *Melatonin increases gene expression for antioxidant enzymes in rat brain cortex.* J. Pineal Research 24: 83-89, 1998

LASH LH, JONES DP. *Distribution of oxidized & reduced forms of glutathione & cysteine in rat plasma. Arch Biochem Biophys 240(2):583-92, 1985*

LEDERMAN MM, GEORGER D, DANDO S, ET AL. *L-2-Oxothiazolidine 4-carboxylic acid (procysteine) inhibits expression of HIV & expression of the interleukin-2 receptor alpha chain.* J. Acq. Immune Def. Syndr. 8: 107-115, 1995

LEVY EJ, ANDERSON ME, MEISTER A. *Transport of glutathione diethyl ester into human cells.* Proc. Natl. Acad. Sci. U.S.A. 90: 9171-9175, 1993

LEVY EJ, ANDERSON ME, MEISTER A. *Preparation & properties of glutathione diethyl ester & related derivatives.* Methods Enzymol. 234: 499-505, 1994

LI Y, WEI G, CHEN J. *Glutathione:* a review on biotechnological production. Appl Microbiol Biotechnol 66(3):233-42, 2004

LIEBERMAN S, BRUNING N. *The Real Vitamin & Mineral Book. Second Ed.* Avery Pub., NY, 1997

Lockitch G. *Selenium: clinical significance & analytical concepts.* Crit. Rev. Clin. Lab. Sci. 27: 483-541, 1989

Lomaestro B, Malone M. *Glutathione in health & disease: Pharmacotherapeutic Issues.* Annals of Pharmacotherapy 29:1263-73, 1995

Look MP, Rockstroh JK, Rao GS, et al. *Serum selenium, plasma glutathione (GSH) & erythrocyte glutathione peroxidase (GSH-Px)-levels in asymptomatic versus symptomatic human immunodeficiency virus-1 (HIV-1)-infection.* Eur. J. Clin. Nutr. 51: 266-272, 1997

Maheo K, Morel F et al. *Inhibition of cytochromes P-450 & induction of glutathione S-transferases by sulforaphane in primary human & rat hepatocytes.* Cancer Res 57(17):3649-52, 1997

Marrades RM, Roca J, Barbera JA et al. *Nebulized glutathione induces bronchoconstriction in patients with mild asthma.* Am J Respir Crit Care Med 156(2 Pt 1):425-30, 1997

Mant T, Tempowski J, Volans G, Talbot J. *Adverse reactions to acetylcysteine & effects of overdose.* British Medical Journal 2 89:217-19, 1984

May JM, Mendiratta S, Hill KE, Burk RF. *Reduction of dehydroascorbate to ascorbate by the selenoenzyme thioreoxin reductase.* J. Biol. Chem. 272: 22607-22610, 1997

Meister A, Anderson ME. *Glutathione.* Ann Revue Biochemistry 52:711-60, 1983

Meister A. *New aspects of glutathione biochemistry & transport, selective alteration of glutathione metabolism.* Nutrition Revue 42:397-410, 1984

Mendiratta S, Qu ZC, May JM. *Erythrocyte ascorbate recycling: antioxidant effects in blood.* Free Radic. Biol. Med. 24: 789-797, 1998

Miguez MP, Anundi I, Sainz-Pardo LA, Lindros KO. *Hepatoprotective mechanism of silymarin: no evidence for involvement of cytochrome P450 2E1.* Chem. Biol. Interact. 91: 51-63, 1994

Mischley LK, Vespignani MF, Finnell JS. *Safety survey of intranasal glutathione.* J Altern Complement Med 19(5):459-63, 2013

Mischley LK, Leverenz JB, Lau RC et al. *A randomized, double-blind phase I/II study of intranasal glutathione in Parkinson's disease.* Mov Disord 30(12):1696-701, 2015

Mischley LK, Conley KE, Shankland EG et al. *Central nervous system uptake of intranasal glutathione in Parkinson's disease.* NPJ Parkinsons Dis 2:16002, 2016

Mischley LK, Lau RC, Shankland EG et al. *Phase IIb Study of Intranasal Glutathione in Parkinson's Disease.* J Parkinsons Dis 7(2):289-299, 2017

Misso NL, Powers KA, Gillon RL, et al. *Reduced platelet glutathione peroxidase activity & serum selenium concentration in atopic asthmatic patients.* Clin. Exp. Allergy 26: 838-847, 1996

Mizuno K, Kume T, Muto C et al. *Glutathione biosynthesis via activation of the nuclear factor E2-related factor 2 (Nrf2)—antioxidant-response element (ARE) pathway is essential for neuroprotective effects of sulforaphane & 6 (methylsulfinyl) hexyl isothiocyanate.* J Pharmacol Sci 115(3):320-8, 2011

Muzes G, Deak G, Lang I, et al. *Effect of silymarin (Legalon) therapy on the antioxidant defense mechanism & lipid peroxidation in alcoholic liver disease.* Orv. Hetil. 131: 863-866, 1990

Nath KA, Salahudeen AK. *Autoxidation of cysteine generates hydrogen peroxide: cytotoxicity & attenuation by pyruvate.* American J. Physiol. 262 (2 Pt 2): F306-F314, 1993

Nishiuch Y, Sasaki M, Nakayasu, et al. *Cytotoxicity of cysteine in culture media.* In Vitro 12: 635, 1976

Olney JW, Ho OL, Rhee V. *Cytotoxic effect of acid & sulphur containing amino acids on the infant mouse central nervous system.* Brain Res. 14: 61-76, 1971

O'Riordain MG, De Beaux A, Fearon KC. *Effect of glutamine on immune function in the surgical patient.* Nutrition 12(11-12 Suppl):S82-S84, 1996

Pablos MI, Agapito MP, Gutierrez R, et al. *Melatonin stimulates the activity of the detoxifying enzyme glutathione peroxidase in several tissues of chicks.* J. Pineal Research 19: 111-115, 1995

Pablos MI, Chuang J, Reiter RJ, et al. *Time course of the melatonin-induced increase in glutathione peroxidase activity in chick tissues.* Biol. Signals 4: 325-330, 1995

Packer L, Tritschler HJ, Wessel K. *Neuroprotection by the metabolic antioxidant alpha-lipoic acid.* Free Radic. Biol. Med. 22: 359-378, 1997

Packer L, Witt EH, Tritschler HJ. *Alpha-lipoic acid as a biologic antioxidant.* Free Radic. Biol. Med. 19: 227-250, 1995

Porta P, Aebi S, Summer K, et al. *L-2-Oxothiazolidine-4-carboxylic acid, a cysteine prodrug: Pharmacokinetics & effects on thiols in plasma & lymphocytes in human.* J. Pharmacol. Exp. Ther. 257: 331-334, 1991

Prousky J. The treatment of pulmonary diseases & respiratory-related conditions with inhaled (nebulized or aerosolized) glutathione. *Evid Based Complement Alternat Med 5(1):27-35, 2008*

Puri R, Meister A. *Transport of glutathione, as gamma-glutamylcysteinylglycyl ester, into liver & kidney.* Proceedings of the National Academy of Science USA 80:5258-60. 1983

Qian W, Fu Y, Cai C. *Engineering a high-yield glutathione strain of Hansenula polymorpha using ion beam implantation.* Prep Biochem Biotechnol 43(6):577-85, 2013

Redman C, Scott JA, Baines AT, et al. *Inhibitory effect of selenomethionine on growth of three selected human tumor cell lines.* Cancer Lett. 125: 103-110, 1998

Reiter RJ, Tang L, Garcia JJ, Munoz-Hoyos A. *Pharmacological actions of melatonin in oxygen radical pathophysiology.* Life Sci. 60: 2255-2271, 1997

Reiter RJ, Tang L, Cabrera J, et al. *The oxidant/antioxidant network: role of melatonin.* Biol. Signals Recept. 8: 56-63, 1999

Riedl MA, Saxon A, Diaz-Sanchez D. *Oral sulforaphane increases Phase II antioxidant enzymes in human upper airway.* Clin Immunol 130(3):244-51, 2009

Richie JP Jr, Nichenametla S, Neidig W et al. *Randomized controlled trial of oral glutathione supplementation on body stores of glutathione.* Eur J Nutr 52(2):251-63, 2015

Roederer M, Staal FJ, Ela SW, Herzenberg LA, Herzenberg LA. *N-acetylcysteine: potential for AIDS therapy.* Pharmacology 46: 121-129, 1993

Roum JH, Borok Z, McElvaney NG et al. *Glutathione aerosol suppresses lung epithelial surface inflammatory cell-derived oxidants in cystic fibrosis.* J Appl Physiol 87(1):438-43, 1985

Rouse K, Nwokedi E, Woodliff JE, Epstein J, Klimberg JS. *Glutamine enhances selectivity of chemotherapy through changes in glutathione metabolism.* Ann. Surg. 221: 420-426, 1995

Saez G, Thornally PJ, Hill HAO, et al. *The production of free radicals during the oxidation of cysteine & their effects on isolated rat hepatocytes.* Biochem Biophys Acta 719:24-31, 1982

Santana-Martinez RA, Galván-Arzate S, Hernandez-Pando R et al. *Sulforaphane reduces the alterations induced by quinolinic acid: modulation of glutathione levels.* Neuroscience 272:188-98, 2014

Sasaki K, Hara KY et al. *Nanofiltration concentration of extracellular glutathione produced by engineered Saccharomyces cerevisiae.* J Biosci Bioeng 121(1):96-100, 2016

Sedlak TW, Nucifora LG, Koga M et al. *Sulforaphane Augments Glutathione & Influences Brain Metabolites in Human Subjects:* A Clinical Pilot Study. Mol Neuropsychiatry3(4):214-222. 2018

Selhub J, Jacques PF, Bostom HG, D'Agostino RB, Wilson PWF, Belanger AJ, O'Leary DH, Wolf PA, Schaefer EJ, Rosenberg IH. *Association between plasma homocysteine concentrations & extracranial carotid-artery stenosis.* The New England Journal of Medicine 332:286-291, 1995

Shear NH, Malkiewicz IM, Klein D, et al. *Acetaminophen-induced toxicity to human epidermoid cell line A431 & hepatoblastoma cell line Hep G2, in vitro, is diminished by silymarin.* Skin Pharmacol. 8: 279-291, 1995

Shug AL, Madsen DC. *Protection of the ischemic rat heart by procysteine & amino acids.* J. Nutr. Biochem. 5: 356-359, 1994

Sinha R, Sinha I, Calcagnotto A et al. *Oral supplementation with liposomal glutathione elevates body stores of glutathione & markers of immune function. Eur J Clin Nutr doi:1038/ejcn.2017.132, 2017*

Souba WW. *Glutamine & cancer.* Ann. Surg. 218: 715-728, 1993

Stadtman TC. *Specific occurrence of selenium in enzymes & amino acid tRNAs.* FASEB J. 1: 375-379, 1987

Stone J, Hinks LJ, Beasly R, et al. *Reduced selenium status of patients with asthma.* Clin. Sci. 77: 495-500, 1989

Sunitha K, Hemshekhar M, Thushara RM et al. *N-Acetylcysteine amide: a derivative to fulfill the promises of N-Acetylcysteine.* Free Radic Res 47(5):357-67, 2013

Testa B, Mesolella M, Testa D et al. *Glutathione in the upper respiratory tract.* Ann Otol Rhinol Laryngol 104(2):117-9, 1995

Vale JA, Buckley BM. *Asthma associated with N-acetyl cysteine infusion & paracetamol poisoning.* British Medical Journal 287:1223, 1983

Vale JA, Wheeler DC. *Anaphylactoid reactions to N-acetyl cysteine.* Lancet 2(8305):988, 1982

Valenzuela A, Aspillaga M, Vial S, Guerra R. *Selectivity of silymarin on the increase of the glutathione content in different tissues of the rat.* Planta Med. 55: 420-422, 1989

Valenzuela A, Garrido A. *Biochemical bases of pharmacological action of flavonoid silymarin & of its structural isomer silibinin.* Biol. Res. 27: 105-112, 1994

Van Zandwijk N. *N-acetylcysteine for lung cancer prevention.* Chest 107: 1437-1441, 1995

Walton NG, Mann TAN, Shwa KM. *Anaphylactoid reactions to N-acetyl cysteine.* Lancet 2(8155):1298, 1979

Wang D, Wang C, Wu H, Li Z, Ye Q. *Glutathione production by recombinant Escherichia coli expressing bifunctional glutathione synthetase. J Ind Microbiol Biotechnol 43(1):45-53, 2016*

Wang C, Zhang J, Wu H, Li Z, Ye Q. *Heterologous gshF gene expression in various vector systems in Escherichia coli for enhanced glutathione production.* J Biotechnol 2014:63-8, 2015

Wendel A, Cikryt P. *The level & half-life of glutathione in human plasma.* FEBS Lett 120(2):209-11, 1980

Witschi A, Reddy S, Stofer B, Lauterberg B. *Systemic availability of oral glutathione.* European Journal of Clinical Pharmacology 43:667-9, 1992

Yoshida S, Kaibara A, Yamasaki K, et al. *Effect of glutamine supplementation on protein metabolism & glutathione in tumor-bearing rats.* J. Parenter. Enteral Nutrition 19: 492-497, 1995

Zarka MH, Bridge WJ. *Oral administration of y-glutamylcysteine increases intracellular glutathione levels above homeostasis in a randomized human trial pilot study. Redox Biol 11:631-636, 2017*

Zembron-Lacny A, Slowinska-Lisowska M et al. *Modulatory effect of N-acetylcysteine on pro-antioxidant status & haematological response in healthy men.* J Physiol Biochem 66(1):15-21, 2010

Zhang J, Quan C, Wang C et ael. *Systematic manipulation of glutathione metabolism in Escherichia coli for improved glutathione production.* Microb Cell Fact 15:38, 2016

Zhang Y, Talalay P, Cho CG, Posner GH. *A major inducer of anticarcinogenic protective enzymes from broccoli: isolation & elucidation of structure.* Proc Nath Acad Sci USA 89(6):2399-403, 1992

Zhang Y, Callaway EC. *High cellular accumulation of sulphoraphane, a dietary anticarcinogen, followed by rapid transporter-mediated export as a glutathione conjugate.* Biochem J 364(Pt 1):301-7, 2002

PART TWO

GLUTATHIONE IN SICKNESS

[CHAPTERS 5 TO 34]

The chapters of Part Two describe glutathione's activity in a wide variety of diseases and show how it plays specific roles in pathologies related to oxidative stress, toxicology and immune dysfunction.

5

Cancer

FEW WORDS STRIKE as much fear and loathing in a doctor's office as 'cancer.' More than one hundred types are known, of varying levels of aggression. Many are treatable or even curable. Still, cancer is the second greatest cause of death in North America, after cardiovascular disease. One third of Americans will eventually die of some form of cancer. It must be emphasized that many cancers can be prevented through the threefold regimen of diet, avoidance of carcinogens and reinforced bodily defenses.

The most common cancers are of the prostate (for men) and breast (for women), followed by lung and colorectal cancers. Next is bladder cancer for men, uterine cancer for women, lymphoma for men and ovarian cancer for women. See Figure 11.

Carcinogenesis

Healthy cells have a built-in mechanism that only allows cellular replication for three purposes: normal growth, healing of injured tissue and replacement of cells lost in normal metabolism. But cells can lose their ability to regulate growth, replicating uncontrollably and eventually forming a clump of cancerous tissue. This tumor can grow sufficiently to crowd out normal tissue, sometimes releasing diseased cells that spread the cancer into other parts of the body by the process of metastasis. Symptoms develop when the growth begins to interfere with bodily functions or deplete energy resources.

It is not clear precisely how and why these cells lose their self-regulation, although many possible causes have been singled out. Certain environmental carcinogens will predictably initiate cancerous growth, including a variety of chemicals and high radiation levels. Other factors are less predictable. Differences in our genetic makeup or immune systems apparently protect some people better than others. We also know that susceptibility to certain cancers is sometimes inherited from the family or racial gene pool, but the triggering factors are still unknown.

Apart from genetic factors, we can identify the following causal factors: the pollution of cigarette smoke, fossil fuel exhaust, heavy metals, pesticides and others; the ionizing radiation of X-rays, nuclear waste, ultraviolet

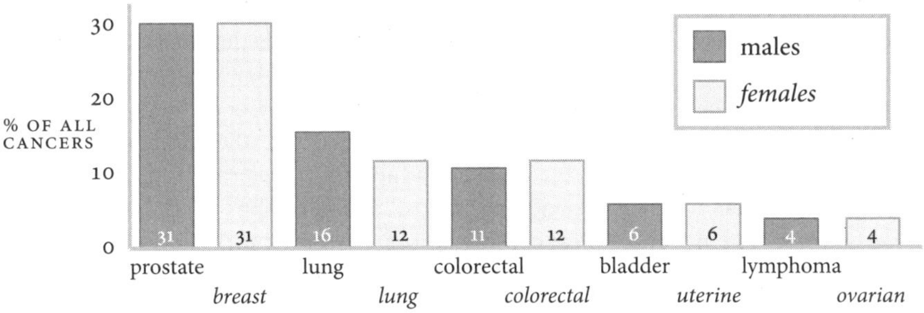

FIGURE 12: *Relative incidence of various types of cancer*

(UV) radiation from the sun intensified by a depleted ozone layer; poor diet is an important factor; finally, certain viruses can contribute to the development of cancer: AIDS, hepatitis C, Epstein-Barr disease and papilloma (see Figure 12).

The American Cancer Society makes the following suggestions to minimize the risk of cancer: maintain appropriate body weight, eat a varied diet including daily fruits and vegetables, eat more high-fiber foods (whole grains, cereals, legumes, etc.), cut down on total fat intake and limit consumption of alcoholic beverages and salt-cured, smoked and nitrate-preserved foods (see Figure 9).

Cancer starts with a mutation in the genetic code of the cell—a reprogramming of developmental patterns that results in uncontrolled growth. A combination of genetic and environmental factors, including diet, may contribute to this aberrant replication. One theory suggests that when free radicals form in the cell nucleus, its DNA code may be damaged. Another theory suggests that factors such as poor diet and cigarette smoke compromise the immune system and weaken bodily defenses which might otherwise destroy a newly cancerous cell at the outset, when it is still vulnerable. Regardless of theory, we owe it to ourselves to pay attention to all possible factors, and take advantage of any way to minimize the danger of cancer. One of these is by maintaining GSH levels.

GSH and cancer

Hundreds of medical articles describe the role of GSH in preventing and treating cancer. They fall into three main groups: 1) prevention, including detoxification of carcinogens, antioxidation and heightened immune response; 2) therapeutic possibilities, such as anti-tumor methodologies and the treatment and prevention of malnutrition and wasting, and 3) a special role for GSH in chemotherapy and radiotherapy that enhances the effectiveness of these arduous treatments while minimizing their side-effects (see Table 13).

Cancer prevention

As early as 1996, an article in the European Journal of Cancer actually suggested that free radicals be listed as an important class of carcinogens. Because of its great capacity as the cell's major antioxidant (see Chapter 1) GSH can soak up oxyradicals and other free radicals as they form in the cell. This prevents subsequent damage to various parts of the cell, particularly to the DNA in its nucleus. GSH has the additional benefit of enhancing the effect of other antioxidants such as vitamin C, vitamin E and selenium. This further strengthens the body's ability to destroy free radicals. To top it off, GSH also plays an important role in the synthesis and repair of DNA.

There is no doubt that a well-functioning glutathione enzyme system wards off cancer. This is clearly illustrated by a study published in the Journal of the National Cancer Institute. It focused on people deficient in the enzyme glutathione-S tranferase-mu-1 (GSTM1). GSTM1 is an important antioxidant that also detoxifies common bladder cancer carcinogens such as tobacco smoke. Approximately one person in two inherits two defective copies of the GSTM1 gene, impairing the function of this enzyme. It was found that 25% of all bladder cancers occurred in people missing this enzyme. Heavy smokers missing this gene were six times more likely to develop bladder cancer.

There is a link between the loss of glutathione activity and the development of prostate cancer. Another glutathione enzyme, glutathione-S-transferase-pi-1 (GSTP1) almost always disappears in both cancerous and pre-cancerous prostate lesions. Prostate cancer seems to begin with the inactivation of this glutathione enzyme. Many studies have made the connection between GSTP1 loss

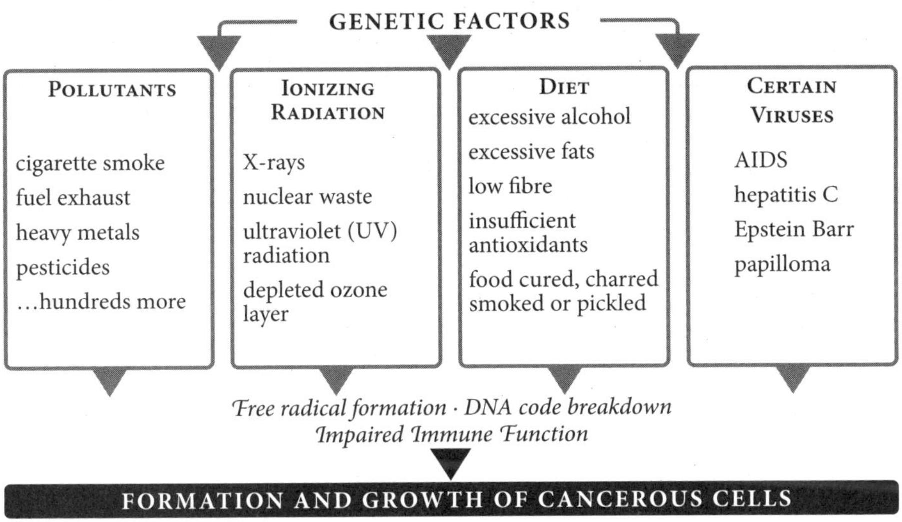

FIGURE 13: Factors leading to the development of cancer

and malignant transformation of prostatic tissues. Similar studies have linked GSH-defective genes to breast and lung cancer as well, especially in smokers. Several scientists have suggested that people should be screened for these genetic or enzymatic defects as a way to determine their risk level.

GSH also plays a specific role in detoxifying numerous well-known environmental carcinogens and mutagens. These cancer-causing substances are conjugated or neutralized by GSH and rendered into a form the body can eliminate. The role of GSH in detoxification simply can't be overstated. Since the liver is the body's principal detoxifying organ it is not surprising that it carries the highest concentrations of GSH in the body.

The Chemoprevention Branch of the National Cancer Institute (USA) has for the last few decades have been developing drugs to diminish the incidence of this dreaded disease. Substances that raise GSH levels, such as NAC and the selenium derivative selenomethionine (see Chapter 4), are on their short list of useful therapies. One of the major successes of their research efforts is their statistical demonstration that selenium protects against prostate cancer (see Chapter 4). Other studies have identified selenium as protecting against colon, rectal and lung cancers as well as colonic polyps. Balansky, Conaway, Witschi, and other American and European researchers have successfully shown that NAC can slow the growth of cancers induced by toxins including urethane, nitrosamines, doxorubicin, ethylnitrosourea and other cancer-causing agents.

NAC apparently protects against the carcinogenic properties of cigarette smoke. N. Van Zandwijk from the Cancer Institute of the Netherlands writes, "NAC has emerged as a most promising cancer chemopreven-

CANCER PREVENTION	THERAPEUTIC POSSIBILITIES	INTERACTION/TREATMENT OF SIDE-EFFECTS
Detoxification of carcinogens	Anti-tumor characteristics	Chemotherapy
Antioxidation	Treatment/ prevention of malnutrition, wasting	Radiotherapy
Heightened immune response		

TABLE 13: Potential roles of GSH in cancer

Maintain appropriate body weight	Cut down on total fat intake
Eat a varied diet	Limit consumption of alcoholic beverages
Include a variety of fruits and vegetables in your daily diet	Limit salt-cured, smoked and nitrite-preserved foods
Eat more high fiber foods (whole grains, cereals, legumes, etc.)	American Cancer Society guidelines, diet & nutrition

TABLE 14: American Cancer Society guidelines, diet & nutrition

tive agent." S. De Flora summarized a very large chemoprevention trial sponsored by Project Euroscan and described the many positive effects of NAC as a cancer prevention agent. It reviewed potential uses against lung, breast, bowel, and skin cancers, and the actual mechanisms by which NAC and GSH exert these protective effects.

One of glutathione's effects upon the immune system is to control and balance the growth of T-cell lymphocytes (a type of white blood cell), thereby strengthening the immune response. Immuno-depressed individuals are often more prone to cancer, a good example being Karposi's sarcoma, a cancer found mostly in AIDS patients. Cancer specialists have recently developed a strategy called immunotherapy—an attempt to optimize the body's natural defenses against the cancer. Immuno-therapy consists of tools to stimulate the immune system. A Japanese team from Kyoto University showed that adding NAC to cytokines—a class of immunotherapeutic agents—stimulated immune cells and their biochemical products. They suggest that this may be an effective complement for the treatment of primary liver cancer.

Other anti-cancer substances produced naturally by the immune system are TNF (tumor necrosis factor) and IL-2 (interleukin 2). Glaxo Wellcome Research and Development scientists showed that NAC acts against tumors by elevating TNF. In the laboratory NAC halted tumor growth in more than one third of mice injected with cancer cells. C.Y. Yim and J.B. Hibbs at the University of Utah had similar success in suppressing tumor growth by using NAC to stimulate IL-2 (a promoter of white blood cell activity) in lymphokine killer cells, a type of T-cell lymphocyte.

Therapeutic possibilities

Surgical removal of cancer is only feasible if the tumor is not widespread and is accessible. Radiation and/or chemical therapy can help, but both inflict great damage on normal as well as cancerous cells. A cornerstone of recent research has been the search for ways to limit the damage to normal cells by such anti-cancer treatments.

Chemotherapy is a controlled poisoning of the patient based on the idea that rapidly growing cancer cells are more sensitive to the poison than are normal cells. Many but not all chemo-therapeutic agents produce particularly unpleasant side effects. Radiation therapy works in a similar way. The cancerous area is targeted and bombarded with radiation. The tumor is theoretically more sensitive to the radiation than the surrounding healthy tissue, but this treatment can also produce severe side-effects.

Recent experiments show that the GSH content of both normal and cancerous cells makes them more or less susceptible to damage. High GSH levels clearly help protect cells from chemotherapy, low levels make them vulnerable. It would be ideal if GSH levels were high in normal cells and low in tumorous cells, but many human cancer cells have particularly high GSH levels. Cancer is the only known condition under which the otherwise tightly regulated GSH levels are exceeded. It is characteristic of cancer cells to bypass normal regulatory controls.

Tumor cells high in GSH often show resistance to chemotherapy, so there has been some effort to reduce GSH levels in cancerous cells with GSH-depleting drugs like BSO. The trouble is, BSO reduces GSH levels in healthy cells too, magnifying the already intolerable side-effects of chemotherapy. So this approach is impractical.

Nevertheless, there may be a way to diminish GSH in cancer cells alone. Paradoxically, the precursors that raise glutathione levels in normal cells trigger the opposite reaction in cancerous cells. Overstimulation of GSH in cancer cells shuts down glutathione production in a process called negative feedback inhibition, making them more susceptible to destruction. Meanwhile, normal tissue uses the precursors to make glutathione, leaving it with better defenses.

This paradox was described as early as 1986 by Russo's team in the journal Cancer Research. When the GSH-promoting drug OTZ was added to human lung cancer cells, their glutathione level did not increase even though GSH levels in surrounding normal cells did. McGill University researchers Sylvain Baruchel, Gerry Batist and their team in Montreal showed that OTZ could deplete GSH in breast cancer cells while enhancing it in normal cells. This team later worked with Dr. Gustavo Bounous and published similar results in the journal Cancer Research, using a specially-prepared cysteine-rich whey protein isolate (CRWPI) to provide dietary GSH precursors.

The same diet was studied on patients with metastatic carcinoma—cancer that is spreading through the body. They were fed a CRWPI (glutathione precursor) for six months. Although it did not cure the cancer, a significant proportion showed either tumor regression or stabilization. Most also experienced the advantage of normalized hemoglobin and white blood cell counts. The same researchers showed that elevated GSH levels may enhance the anti-cancer action of certain chemotherapeutic agents.

Another Canadian team—this one from the University of Saskatchewan—conducted trials on patients with advanced progressive cancer. They were given toxic doses of acetaminophen as chemotherapy, plus NAC to raise glutathione levels. They hoped that NAC would raise GSH in normal cells only, and their results bear them out. More than half the patients showed either improvement or stabilization.

Nevertheless, cancer specialists are still concerned that elevating GSH non-selectively might in certain cases diminish the advantages of chemotherapy. I addressed this question in a review entitled "Therapeutic Potential of Glutathione Augmentation in Cancer Patients Receiving Chemotherapy or Radiotherapy" published in the Journal of Nutritional Oncology, 2016. In it I report that attempts to raise glutathione in human subjects have not been shown to interfere with treatment. Only in-vitro (test-tube) studies to increase GSH demonstrated negative effects. Nevertheless, I strongly suggest that this approach be discussed with the treating physician before trying.

Additional studies have investigated the effects of nutritional proteins on cancer-causing chemicals in animals. Researchers doing similar experiments in Canada and Australia

aflatoxin B1	dimethylnitrosamine
n-acetyl-2-aminofluorine	ethyl methane sulfonate
benzanthracene	n-methyl-4-aminoazobenzine
benzapyrene	7-methyl-benzanthracene
benzidine	3-methyl-cholanthracene
dimethylhydrazine	1-nitropyrene

TABLE 15: Some important environmental carcinogens & mutagens

subjected rodents to the powerful carcinogen dimethylhydrazine—which causes colonic cancer similar to humans—and fed them a variety of proteins. Animals fed on undenatured whey protein concentrate showed fewer tumors and a reduced tumor load. The scientists found that this protein offered "considerable protection to the host," more so than any other protein.

It is accepted as a fact of life that the incidence and mortality rates of cancer increase with age. Certain cancers may in fact be considered diseases of aging, especially cancer of the prostate gland (see Chapter 23). Specific changes of aging render patients more susceptible to cancer. They also have less protection against oxidative damage, and diminished immune response (see Chapter 6). The protective effect of GSH diminishes with age. We generally lose from 20 to 40% of GSH after age 65.

A recent study convincingly showed that normal levels of androgens (male sex hormones) in older men lead to decreased GSH levels in the prostate gland. Anti-androgen therapy—also known as chemical castration—is a common treatment for prostate cancer. However, androgens act as oxidative stressors and can upset the prooxidant-antioxidant balance. Lowered GSH levels lead to loss of antioxidant function and may contribute to prostatic carcinogenesis.

The prostate specific antigen (PSA) blood test is used to screen for prostate cancer and to track the progress of men suffering from this cancer. Higher PSA levels usually indicate disease progression, while falling levels show the success of treatment. Studies following PSA levels in patients taking GSH-promoting substances are in progress. GSH therapy has minimal toxic potential and one hopes it will become a standard treatment.

Prevention/treatment of side-effects

Chemotherapy and radiotherapy lead to huge increases in free radical formation and a build-up of toxic metabolites. If the problem is not addressed, the side effects grow worse. Numerous studies have shown that when patients eat well—especially when their diets include vitamins and supplements—their tolerance of these unpleasant therapies improves. Patients with higher intracellular GSH levels experience far fewer chemotherapeutic side effects and cells with higher levels of GSH carry more protection against radiation damage, thereby lessening the side effects of radiotherapy.

Radiotherapists studying the protective role of GSH have correlated higher pretreatment glutathione levels with fewer subsequent radiation burns. Pre-treatment or simultaneous treatment with products that raise and maintain GSH levels enables patients to better tolerate therapy. Chapter 2 explains GSH and radiation toxicity at greater length.

Women with cancer were treated at the University of California (San Diego) with the standard chemotherapy cisplatin and supplemented with intravenous glutathione. This enabled them to take higher doses of chemotherapy while experiencing fewer side-effects. A similar but much larger study was carried out at the Western General Hospital in Edinburgh, Scotland. Over 150 patients being treated for ovarian cancer with cisplatin and glutathione were monitored for side effects, quality of life and outcome, and compared to another group receiving no glutathione. The first group showed statistically less depression, vomiting, hair loss, shortness of breath and neurotoxicity. Their mental concentration and kidney function improved measurably and there was a distinct trend toward better outcome.

The hair loss that often results from chemotherapy may not be life-threatening but it can be extremely disheartening, especially at this time when patients don't need additional stress. Hair loss may also suggest damage inflicted on other cells that regenerate quickly, like those lining the intestine. The researcher Jimenez at the University of Miami and others have demonstrated that NAC can protect from the baldness caused by common chemotherapy agents like cyclophosphamide.

Evidence suggests that glutathione-enhancing strategies may increase the efficiency of certain chemotherapy agents, including Adriamycin, cyclophosphamide, cisplatin and others. Before beginning any GSH-enhancing therapy patients must talk to their treating physician. It is possible that non-specific glutathione elevation might interfere with the anti-cancer treatment. This risk diminishes after the course of chemotherapy and/or radiotherapy is complete.

Malnutrition/wasting/recovery from treatment

Anti-cancer treatment is often accompanied by loss of weight, appetite, energy and strength. Good nutrition is critical and should include appropriate dietary supplements. The cancer itself, the anti-cancer treatment and the resulting state of nutritional compromise all decrease intracellular GSH levels. This greatly weakens antioxidant and immune defenses, rendering patients more susceptible to other diseases and opportunistic infections. Well-known German immunologist and researcher Wulf Droge has studied weight and muscle loss in cancer, AIDS, sepsis and other diseases. He has noted the similarities among them and points to a common cause—GSH depletion. He and others have gone on to test the possibility that glutathione-enhancing therapy may slow or halt this process of degeneration.

Increased GSH synthesis depends on the intake of cysteine-containing foods. Rich sources of this GSH-precursor are very hard to come by and often are not well tolerated by the patient. Cysteine is available as a free amino acid and may be taken, but it has toxic qualities and is not recommended. The drugs NAC and OTC (see Chapter 4) can raise GSH levels but their effects are short-lived. These pharmaceutical drugs also have little nutritional value. Whey proteins have excellent nutritional value but usually lack GSH-precursors. The ideal source of dietary cysteine should be natural, nutritional, bioactive and undenatured.

In 2007 a multi-centered, double-blinded, placebo controlled clinical trial was published by a team headed up by world-eminent researchers Drs. Richard Tozer and Wulf Droge. The objective of the study was to see if a specially-prepared whey protein isolate (CRWPI) could improve quality-of-life variables in cancer patients receiving chemotherapy. Not only were these outcomes improved, but they demonstrated a statistically significant improvement in preventing and even reversing the severe weight loss (cachexia) normally seen in these patients. A secondary finding related to survival was that, after one year, 50% of the placebo group were deceased while 80% of the treatment group were alive.

A Canadian team led by Dr. Franco Carli has been on the forefront of a new strategy termed "Prehabilitation". Prehabilitation differs from "rehabilitation." Prehabilitation takes place before, rather than after, an intervention like surgery or chemotherapy. Prior to surgery for colorectal cancer, patients underwent a month of psychological counseling and nutrition using a CRWPI (glutathione precursor) versus a placebo group. The CRWPI group experienced meaningful improvements in muscular strength and endurance.

Case Histories

Quebecer Ivy-Marie is a very active thirty-seven year-old breast cancer survivor. After undergoing her initial surgery, the pathologist's report suggested she undergo a dozen sessions of chemotherapy and radiotherapy. She experienced many side-effects, including profound weakness and fatigue – a new experience for her. After ten sessions of therapy and many visits to her doctor to treat side-effects, she was put on 30 gm/day of a whey protein concentrate. Her strength and sense of well-being improved within a week and she tolerated her last two sessions of chemotherapy with few side-effects. She is back to her usual routine, and remains disease-free.

Complaining of abdominal pain, Louisa from Alberta was 54 when she found out she had ovarian cancer. While awaiting surgery, she fell ill with a persistent cough and malaise which turned out to be a metastasis (spreading cancer) which had traveled to her lung. She ultimately needed pelvic surgery to relieve her discomfort, but decided not to undergo treatment for her lung metastasis. She started taking a specifically prepared bioactive whey-protein and multivitamins daily and noticed a great improvement after several weeks. Four months later, repeat chest x-rays showed no increase in tumor size. Nine months later the radiographs revealed a decrease in tumor size. Louise continued to enjoy tending to her family and household.

Conclusion

There are many types of cancer, and perhaps hundreds of potential causes, but most cases are accompanied by poor antioxidant defenses. To make matters worse, most anti-cancer therapies place an enormous burden on the body and may deplete whatever natural defenses remain. Cancer sufferers must place themselves in the best possible medical hands, but must also take special care of their nutrition. Patients are heavily dosed with pharmaceutical drugs and suffer from poor appetite and low energy, especially while undergoing chemical or radiation therapy. A natural source of energy that can also reinforce antioxidant defenses may make all the difference for people undergoing this distressing disease and its noxious treatment. Undenatured, bioactive whey proteins such as CRWPI (cysteine-rich whey protein isolate) are an ideal way to increase GSH levels and simultaneously address protein requirements. Elevated glutathione replenishes antioxidant defenses, contributes to synthesis and repair of DNA and helps detoxify numerous carcinogens and mutagens.

CANCER

REFERENCES

AMES BN. *Understanding causes of aging & cancer.* Microbiologia 11: 305-308, 1995

BALANSKY RB, D'AGOSTINI F, ZANACCHI P, ET AL. *Protection by n-acetylcysteine of the histopathological & cytogenetic damage produced by exposure of rats to cigarette smoke.* Cancer Lett. 64: 123-131, 1992

BALANSKY RM, DE FLORA S. *Chemoprevention by n-acetylcysteine of urethane-induced clastogenicity & lung tumors in mice.* Int. J. Cancer 77: 302-305, 1998

BALTRUSKEVICIENCE E, ET AL. *Changes of reduced glutathione & glutathione S-transferase levels in colorectal cancer patients undergoing treatment.* Tumori 25: 2017.

BARUCHEL S, VIAU G. *In vitro selective modulation of cellular GSH by a humanized native milk protein isolate in normal cells & rat mammary carcinoma model.* Anticancer Res. 16: 1095-1100, 1996

BARUCHEL S, VIAU G, OLIVIER R, BOUNOUS G, WAINBERG M. *Nutriceutical modulation of GSH with a humanized native milk serum protein isolate, Immunocal: application in aids & cancer.* In: Oxidative Stress in Cancer, aids, & Neurodegenerative Diseases. Editors L. Montagnier, R. Olivier, C. Pasquier. Institute Pasteur. Pub. Marcel Dekker Inc. 1996

BARTA O, BARTA VD, CRISMAN MV, AKERS RM. *Inhibition of blastogenesis by whey.* American J. Vet. Res. 52: 247-253, 1991

BELL DA, TAYLOR JA, PAULSON DF, ET AL. *Genetic risk & carcinogen exposure: a common inherited defect of the carcinogen-metabolism gene glutathione S-transferase M1 (GSTM1) that increases susceptibility to bladder cancer.* J. Natl. Cancer Inst. 85: 1159-1164, 1993

BENHAR M, SHYTAJ IL, STAMLER JS, SAVARINIO A. *Dual targeting of the thioredoxin & glutathione systems in cancer & HIV.* J Clin Invest. 126(5);1630-1639, 2016.

BEUTLER E, GELBART T. *Plasma glutathione in health & in patients with malignant disease.* Journal of Laboratory & Clinical Medicine 105: 581-584, 1985

Bhattathiri VN, Sreelekha TT, Sebastian P, et al. *Influence of plasma GSH level on acute radiation mucositis of the oral cavity.* Int. J. Radiat. Oncol. Biol. Phys. 29: 383-386, 1994

Bongers V, de Jong J, Steen I, et al. *Antioxidant-related parameters in patients treated for cancer chemoprevention with n-acetylcysteine.* Eur. J. Cancer 31: 921-923, 1995

Boone CW, Kelloff GJ. *Biomarker end-points in cancer chemoprevention trials.* IARC Sci. Publ. 142: 273-280, 1997

Bounous G, Batist G, Gold P. *Whey proteins in cancer prevention.* Cancer Letters 57:91-94, 1991

Bounous G, Papenburg R, Kongshavn P, Gold P, Fleiszer D. *Dietary Whey protein inhibits the development of dimethyl-hydrazine induced malignancy.* Clinical & Investigative Medicine 11:213-217, 1988

Bourtourault M, Buleon R, Samperez S, et al. *Effect of proteins from bovine milk serum on the multiplication of human cancerous cells.* C. R. Seances Soc. Biol. Fil. 185: 319-323, 1991

Bray TM, Taylor CG. *Enhancement of tissue GSH for antioxidant & immune functions in malnutrition.* Biochemical Pharmacology 47:2113-2123, 1994

Brigelius-FloheR, Kipp A. *Glutathione peroxidases in different stages of carcinogenesis.* Biochem Biophys Acta. 1790(11):1555-1568, 2009.

Burt RW. *Cohorts with familial disposition for colon cancers in chemoprevention trials.* Journal of Cellular Biochemistry – Supplement 25: 131-135, 1996

Cai Q, Wang Z, et al. *Association between glutathione S-transferases & M1 & T1 gene polymorphisms & prostate cancer risk: a systematic review & meta-analysis.* Tumour Biol 35(1);247-256, 2014.

Cheng SB, Liu HT, Chen SY, Lin PT, Lai CY, Huang YC. *Changes of oxidative stress, glutathione, & its dependent antioxidant enzyme activities in patients with hepatocellular carcinoma before & after tumor resection.* PLoS One. 12(1):e0170016, 2017.

Cheng SH, Tseng YM, Wu SH, Tsai SM, Tsai LY. *Selective effects of whey protein concentrate on glutathione levels & apoptosis in rats with mammary tumors.* Food Chem Toxicol. 107: 440-448, 2017.

Clark LC, Combs GF Jr, Turnbull BW, et al. *Effects of selenium supplementation for cancer prevention in patients with carcinoma of the skin. A randomized controlled trial.* Nutritional Prevention of Cancer Study Group. JAMA 277: 1520, 1997

Clark LC, Dalkin B, Krongrad A, et al. *Decreased incidence of prostate cancer with selenium supplementation: results of a double-blind cancer prevention trial.* Br. J. Urol. 81: 730-734, 1998

Clark LC, Hixson LJ, Combs GF Jr, et al. *Plasma selenium concentration predicts the prevalence of colorectal adenomatous polyps.* Cancer Epidemiol. Biomarkers Prev. 2: 41-46, 1993

Combs GF Jr, Clark LC, Turnbull BW. *Reduction of cancer mortality & incidence by selenium supplementation.* Med. Klin. 92 (Suppl 3): 42-45, 1997

Conaway CC, Jiao D, Kelloff GJ, et al. *Chemopreventive potential of fumaric acid, n-acetylcysteine, N-(4-hydroxyphenyl) retinamide & beta-carotene for tobacco-nitrosamine-induced lung tumors in A/J mice.* Cancer Lett. 124: 85-93, 1998

D'Agostini F, Bagnasco M, Giunciuglio D, et al. *Inhibition by oral n-acetylcysteine of doxorubicin-induced clastogenicity & alopecia, & prevention of primary tumors & lung micrometastases in mice.* Int. J. Oncol. 13: 217-224, 1998

De Flora S, et al. *Antioxidant activity & other mechanisms of thiols involved in chemoprevention of mutation & cancer.* The American Journal of Medicine 91:3c-122s–3c-130s, 1991

De Flora S, Cesarone CF, Balansky RM, et al. *Chemopreventive properties & mechanisms of N-Acetylcysteine. The experimental background.* J. Cell Biochem. Suppl. 22: 33-41, 1995

Delneste Y, Jeannin P, Potier L, et al. *N-acetyl-L-cysteine exhibits antitumoral activity by increasing tumor necrosis factor alpha-dependent T-cell cytotoxicity.* Blood 90: 1124-1132, 1997

Deutz NE, et al. *Muscle protein synthesis in cancer patients can be stimulated with a specially formulated medical food.* Clin Nutr 30(6):759-768, 2011.

Di Pietro G, Magno LA, Rios-Santos F. *Glutathione S-transferases: & overview in cancer research.* Expert Opin Drug Metab Toxicol. 6(2);153-170, 2010.

Dreher D, Junod AF. *Role of oxygen free radicals in cancer development.* Eur. J. Cancer 32: 30-38, 1996

Droge W, Gross A, Hack V, Kinscherf R, Schykowski M, Bockstette M, Mihm S, Galter D. *Role of cysteine & GSH in hiv infection & cancer cachexia: Therapeutic intervention with n-acetylcysteine.* Advances in Pharmacology 38: 581-600, 1997.

Falconer W, Ducruet T, Karabadjian A, Bounous G, Molson J, Droge W. *Cysteine-rich protein reverses weight loss in lung cancer patients receiving chemotherapy or radiotherapy.* Antioxidants & Redox Signaling, (in press), 2008

Franco R, Cidlowski JA. *Apoptosis & glutathione: beyond an antioxidant.* Cell Death Differ. 16(10);1303-1314, 2009.

Gamcsik MP, Kasibhatia MS, Teeter SD, Colvin OM. *Glutathione levels in human tumors.* Biomarkers. 17(8); 671-691, 2012.

Gillis C, Loiselle SE, Fiore JF Jr, Awatsthi R, Wykes L, Liberman AS, Stein B, Charlebois P, Carli F. *Prehabilitation with whey protein supple-*

mentation on preoperative functional exercise capacity in patients undergoing colorectal resection for cancer: A pilot double-blinded randomized placebo-controlled trial. J Acad Nutr Diet. 116(5):802-812, 2016.

Guengerich FP, Their R, Persmark M, et al. *Conjugation of carcinogens by theta class glutathione s-transferases: mechanisms & relevance to variations in human risk.* Pharmacogenetics 5 Spec. No: S103-107, 1995

Gutman J. *Therapeutic potential of glutathione augmentation in cancer patients receiving chemotherapy or radiotherapy.* Journal of Nutritional Oncology 1 (1): 40-44, 2016.

Harries LW, Stubbins MJ, Forman D, et al. *Identification of genetic polymorphisms at the glutathione S-transferase Pi locus & association with susceptibility to bladder, testicular & prostate cancer.* Carcinogenesis 18: 641-644, 1997

Heckbert SR, Weiss NS, Hornung SK, et al. *Glutathione S-transferase & epoxide hydrolase activity in human leukocytes in relation to risk of lung cancer & other smoking-related cancers.* J. Natl. Cancer Inst. 84: 414-422, 1992

Hietanen E, Bartsch H, Bereziat JC, et al. *Diet & oxidative stress in breast, colon & prostate cancer patients: a case-control study.* Eur. J. Clin. Nutr. 48: 575-586, 1994

Hu XY, Huang XY, Ma J, Zuo Y, Lou NB, Lai SL, Su DK. *GSTT1 & GSTM1 polymorphisms predict treatment outcome for breast cancer: a systemic review & meta-analysis.* Tumour Biol 37(1);151-162, 2016.

Izzotti A, Orlando M, Gasparini L, et al. *In vitro inhibition by n-acetylcysteine of oxidative DNA modifications detected by 32P postlabeling.* Free Radic. Res. 28: 165-178, 1998

Jimenez JJ, Huang HS, Yunis AA. *Treatment with ImuVert/n-acetylcysteine protects rats from cyclophosphamide/cytarabine-induced alopecia.* Cancer Invest. 10: 271-276, 1992

Kennedy RS, Konok JP, Bounous G, Baruchel S, Lee TDG. *The use of a whey protein concentrate in the treatment of patients with metastatic carcinoma: A phase I-II clinical study.* Anticancer Research 15:2643-2650, 1995

Ketterer B, Harris JM, Talaska G, et al. *The human glutathione S-transferase supergene family, its polymorphism, & its effects on susceptibility to lung cancer.* Environmental Health Perspectives 98: 87-94, 1992

Kobrinsky NL, Hartfield D, Horner H, et al. *Treatment of advanced malignancies with high-dose acetaminophen & n-acetylcysteine rescue.* Cancer Invest. 14: 202-210, 1996

Liu D, Sun L, Tong J, Chen X, Li H, Zhang Q. *Prognostic significance of glutathione peroxidase 2 in gastric carcinoma.* Tumour Biol. 39(6):1010428317701443, 2017.

Lenton KJ, Therriault H, Fulop T, et al. *Glutathione & ascorbate are negatively correlated with oxidative DNA damage in human lymphocytes.* Carcinogenesis 20: 607-613, 1999

Lubos E, Loscaizo J, Handy DE. *Glutathione peroxidase-1 in health & disease: from molecular mechanisms to therapeutic opportunities.* Antiox Redox Signal. 15(7);1957-1997, 2011.

Luo W, Kinsey M, Schiffman JD, Lessnick SL. *Glutathione s-transferases in pediatric cancer.* Front Oncol. 1:39, 2011.

Marchewka Z, Piwowar A, Ruzik S, Dlugosz A. *Glutathione S-transferases class Pi & Mi & their significance in oncology.* Postepy Hig Dosw (online). 19:71(0):541-550, 2017.

McIntosh GH, Regester GO, LeLeu RK, Royle PJ, Smithers GW. *Dairy proteins protect against dimethyl-hydrazine induced intestinal cancers in rats.* Journal of Nutrition 125:809-816, 1995

Milla P, Airoldi M, Weber G, Drescher A, Jaehde U, Cattel L. *Administration of reduced glutathione in FOLFOX4 adjuvant treatment for colorectal cancer: effect on oxaliplatin pharmacokinetics, Pt-DNA adduct formation, & neurotoxicity.* Anticancer Drugs. 20(5):396-402, 2009.

Mohandas J, Marshall JJ, Duggin GG, et al. *Low activities of glutathione-related enzymes as factors in the genesis of urinary bladder cancer.* Cancer Res. 44: 5086-5091, 1984

Moslehi A, et al. *N-acetyl cysteine for prevention of oral mucositis in hematopoietic SCT: a double-blind, randomized, placebo-controlled trial.* Bone Marrow Transplant. 49(6): 818-823, 2014.

Mulders TMT, Keizer HJ, Breimer DD, Mulder GJ. *In Vivo characterization & modulation of the glutathion/glutathione S-transferase system in cancer patients.* Drug Metab. Rev. 27: 191-229, 1995

Nakanishi Y, Matsuki H, Takayama K, et al. *Glutathione derivatives enhance Adriamycin cytotoxicity in a human lung adenocarcinoma cell line.* Anticancer Res. 17: 2129-2134, 1997

O'Dwyer PJ, Hamilton TC, Yao KS, Tew KD, Ozols RF. *Modulation of GSH & related enzymes in reversal of resistance to anticancer drugs.* Hematology/Oncology Clinics of North America 9(2):383-396, 1995

Ortega AL, Mena S, Estrela JM. *GSH in cancer cell death.* Cancers (Basel). 3(1);1285-1310, 2011.

Parodi, PW. *A role for milk proteins & their peptides in cancer prevention.* Curr Pharm Des. 13(8):813-828, 2007.

Papenburg R, Bounous G, Fleiszer D, Gold P. *Dietary milk proteins inhibit the development of dimethyl-hydrazine induced malignancy.* Tumor Biology 11:129-136, 1990

Plaxe S, Freddo J, Kim S, et al. *Phase I trial*

of cisplatin in combination with glutathione. Gynecologic Oncology 55: 82-86, 1994

Redman C, Scott JA, Baines AT, et al. *Inhibitory effect of selenomethionine on the growth of three selected human tumor cell lines.* Cancer Lett. 125: 103-110, 1998

Richie JP Jr. *The role of GSH in aging & cancer.* Experimental Gerontology 27:615-626, 1992

Ripple MO, Henry WF, Rago RP, Wilding G. *Prooxidant-antioxidant shift induced by androgen treatment of human prostate carcinoma cells.* Journal of the National Cancer Institute 89:40-48. 1997

Ross RK, Jones PA, Yu MC. *Bladder cancer epidemiology & pathogenesis.* Seminars in Oncology. 23: 536-545, 1996

Ross DA, Kish P, Muraszko KM, et al. *Effect of dietary vitamin A or NAC on ethylnitrosourea-induced rat gliomas.* J. Neurooncol. 40: 29-38, 1998

Rotstein JB, Slaga TJ. *Effect of exogenous glutathione on tumor progression in the murine skin multistage carcinogenesis model.* Carcinogenesis 9: 1547-1551, 1988

Russo A, DeGraff W, Friedman N, et al. *Selective modulation of glutathione levels in human normal versus tumor cells & subsequent differential response to chemotherapy drugs.* Cancer Res. 46: 2845-2848, 1986

Schroder CP, Godwin AK, O'Dwyer PJ, Tew KD, Hamilton TC, Ozois RF. *GSH & drug resistance.* Cancer Investigation 14:158-168, 1996

Schwartz JL, Shklar G. *Glutathione inhibits experimental oral carcinogenesis, p53 expression, & angiogenesis.* Nutrition & Cancer 26: 229-236, 1996

Shklar G, Schwartz J, Trickler D, Cheverie SR. *The effectiveness of a mixture of beta-carotene, alpha-tocopherol, GSH, & ascorbic acid for cancer prevention.* Nutrition & Cancer 20:145-151, 1993

Singh DK, Lippman SM. *Cancer chemoprevention. Part 1: Retinoids & carotenoids & other classic antioxidants.* Oncology (Huntingt.) 12: 1643-1653, 1657-1660, 1998

Singh DK, Lippman SM. *Cancer chemoprevention. Part 2: hormones, nonclassic antioxidant natural agents, NSAIDs, & other agents.* Oncology (Huntingt.) 12: 1787-1800, 1998

Smyth JF, Bowman A, Perren T, Wilkinson P, Prescott RJ, Quinn KJ, Tedeschi M. *GSH reduces the toxicity & improves the quality of life of women diagnosed with ovarian cancer treated with cisplatin: results of a double blind, randomized trial.* Annals of Oncology 8:569-573, 1997

Tozer RG, Tai P, Falconer W, Ducruet T, Karabadjian A, Bounous G, Molson J, Droge W. *Cysteine-rich protein reverses weight loss in lung cancer patients receiving chemotherapy or radiotherapy.* Antioxidants & Redox Signaling 10(2): 395-402, 2008

Trickler D, Shklar G, Schwartz J. *Inhibition of oral carcinogenesis by glutathione.* Nutr. Cancer 20: 139-144, 1993

Tsuchiya T et al. *Oral administration of the amino acids cysteine & theanine attenuates the adverse events of S-1 adjuvant chemotherapy in gastrointestinal cancer patients.* Int J Clin Oncol. 21(6);1085-1090, 2016.

Tsuyuki S, Yamauchi A, Nakamura H, et al. *Possible availability of NAC as an adjunct to cytokine therapy for hepatocellular carcinoma.* Clin. Immunol. Immunopathol. 88: 192-198, 1998

van Zandwijk N. *N-acetylcysteine for lung cancer prevention.* Chest 107: 1437-1441, 1995

van Zandwijk N. *N-acetylcysteine (NAC) & glutathione (GSH): antioxidant & chemopreventive properties, with special reference to lung cancer.* J. Cell Biochem. Suppl. 22: 24-32, 1995

Vos O, Roos-Verhey WS. *Endogenous versus exogenous thiols in radioprotection.* Pharmacological Therapeutics 39:169-177, 1988

Wang T, Chen X, Schecter RL, Baruchel S, Alaoui-Jamali M, Melnychuk D, Batist G. *Modulation of GSH by a cysteine pro-drug enhances in vivo tumor response.* Journal of Pharmacology & Experimental Therapeutics 276:1169-1173, 1996

Weisburger JH. *Nutritional approach to cancer prevention with emphasis on vitamins, antioxidants & carotinoids.* American Journal of Clinical Nutrition 53:226s-237s, 1991

White EL, Ross LJ, Steele VE, et al. *Screening of potential cancer preventing chemicals as antioxidants in an in vitro assay.* Anticancer Res. 18: 769-773, 1998

Witschi H, Espiritu I, Yu M, et al. *The effects of phenethyl isothiocyanate, n-acetylcysteine & green tea on tobacco smoke-induced lung tumors in strain A/J mice.* Carcinogenesis 19: 1789-1794, 1998

Wu JH, Batist G. *Glutathione & glutathione analogues; therapeutic potentials.* Biochem Biophys Acta. 1830(5);3350-3353, 2013.

Yim CY, Hibbs JB Jr, McGregor JR, et al. *Use of n-acetylcysteine to increase intracellular glutathione during the induction of antitumor responses by IL-2. J.* Immunol. 152: 5796-5805, 1994

Zhang ZJ, Hao K, Shi R, Zhao G, Jiang GX, Song Y, Xu X, Ma J. Am J *Glutathione S-Transferase M1 (GSTM1) & Glutathione S-Transferase T1 (GSTT1) Null Polymorphisms, Smoking, & Their Interaction in Oral Cancer: A HuGE Review & Meta-Analysis* Epidemiol 173(8):847-857, 2011.

6

Aging

The rules for aging are definitely being broken. In 1900 a North American's life expectancy was 49 years. By year 2018 it was 82 in Canada, 80 in the USA, and 78 in Mexico. With scientific and medical advances a new breed of physician has emerged—the longevity specialist. Doctors may now write certified board exams to obtain their specialty in anti-aging. Dr. Ronald Klatz, founder and president of the American Academy of Anti-Aging Medicine (A4M), representing over 26,000 members worldwide in 2017, states, "These health professionals believe aging is not inevitable.... In less than thirty years from now when millions of baby boomers start reaching the century mark, we will look back on the medical science of today as though it were the dark ages."

Duke University demographer James Vaupel says, "There is no evidence that human life expectancy is anywhere close to its ultimate limit." Many believe that 100-120 years is an obtainable goal. See Figure 13.

Twentieth century improvements in sanitation, occupational health and lifestyle as well as advances in antibiotics, vaccines and medical care have helped to extend the human life span. Twenty-first century science is furthering knowledge of neuroscience, genetics, epigenetics and individualized medical treatment. This will undoubtedly accelerate our abilities to extend the life span.

We all want to maintain health during our senior years. A practical knowledge of GSH can help us ensure they bring a good quality of life. More than 15% of North Americans

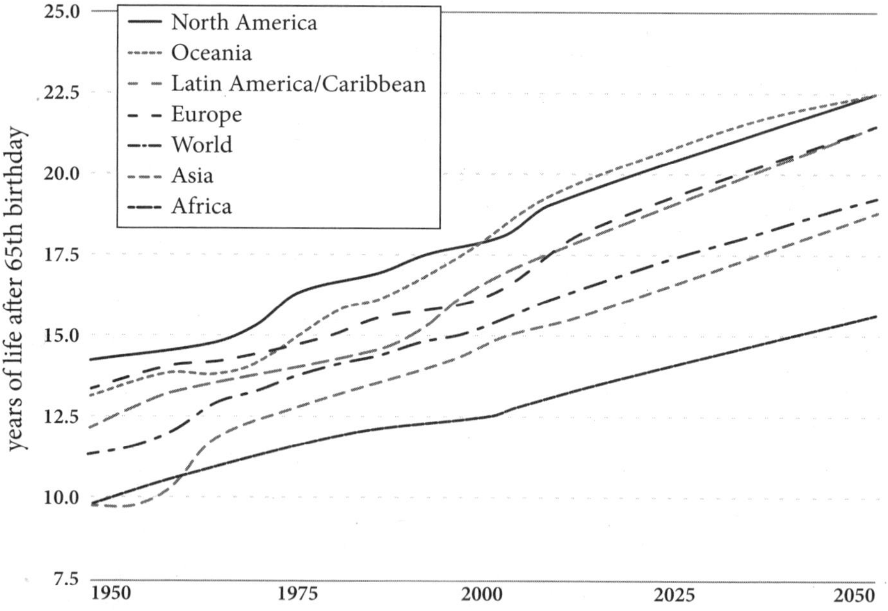

Figure 14: Worldwide Increase in life expectancy, 1950 - 2050

Disease	Chapter	Disease	Chapter
Heart disease	7	Parkinson's Disease	25
Stroke	32	Prostate disease	20
Certain types of cancer	5	Macular degeneration	17
Rheumatoid arthritis	3	Cataracts	17
Alzheimer's Disease	26	Immune deficiency	2, 3

TABLE 16: Diseases of aging discussed in this book

are over 65 and occupy a growing proportion of the population as baby boomers age. Most will suffer from heart disease, stroke, certain cancers, arthritis, Alzheimer's Disease, Parkinson's Disease, cataracts and other debilitating diseases (see Table 16). Oxidative stress is common to all these diseases, and the free-radical theory of aging based on oxidative damage underlies most anti-aging treatments.

GSH & Aging

In a 2015 review on anti-aging, authors Homma and Fuji state "Glutathione is now entering a new era of therapeutic application. Decreased GSH levels are associated with the common features of aging as well as of a wide range of pathological conditions, including neurodegenerative disorders."

The GSH antioxidant system is the body's powerhouse for diffusing and disposing of free radicals that threaten cell, tissue and organ damage, thus slowing the approach of aging. John T. Pinto of Sloan Kettering Cancer Center in New York proclaims GSH "The master antioxidant." Jean Carper in her bestseller Stop Aging Now! underlines the same point: "You must get your levels of GSH up if you want to keep your youth and live longer. High blood levels of GSH predict good health as you age and a long life. Low levels predict early disease and death."

These scientific opinions result from convincing research and experimentation. Age-specific decreases in GSH are seen in all tissues, including those of liver, kidney, lung, heart, spleen and the brain. Laboratory studies on the role of GSH in aging show GSH deficiency in all creatures, from mosquitoes and houseflies to rats and mice (see Table 17).

Similar findings in humans indicate that elderly subjects bear increased risk of disease and impairment. Blood-GSH concentrations in younger people (20-40 years) are 20 to 40% higher than in those aged 60-80 years.

A study with elderly people suggests that elevated GSH levels provide a physical, psychological and sociological advantage over those with lower levels. Researchers Mara Julius and Calvin Lang measured glutathione concentrations in community-based individuals over 60 years of age, mapping these values to a) health, b) number of illnesses, and c) risk factors for chronic disease (tobacco, alcohol, cholesterol, blood pressure and obesity). Higher glutathione levels corresponded to lessened effects of aging and better general health. Those with 20% higher levels experience about one-third the rate of arthritis, high blood pressure, heart disease, circulatory difficulties and other maladies.

Dr. Lang looked at glutathione levels in other age groups too: 20-40, 40-60, 60-80 and 80-100 years. The youngest group had acceptable levels but 14% of 40-60 year olds and 53% of 60-80 year olds had critically low

liver	29%	kidney	22%	spleen	22%
lung	39%	heart	27%	brain	33%

TABLE 17: GSH decrease in older mice (Richie JP Jr., 1992)

levels. Interestingly, only 24% of the oldest group had low levels. Perhaps that's how they reached such a ripe old age in the first place.

In Italy, G. Paolisso and M.R. Tagliamonte went one step further, comparing adults under age 50 with those over 50. Both the GSH and antioxidant function were compromised in the older group. However, those over 100 years of age had higher GSH levels than the over-50 group. Again, this may explain their unusual longevity.

Several researchers over the years have shown that life span can be extended by restricting diet and maintaining low body weight. No satisfactory explanation has emerged for this phenomenon, but some scientists have demonstrated that glutathione levels rise in these longer-living individuals. They suggest that glutathione may be involved in a molecular mechanism that contributes to longevity.

Nuttal and his British team published a revealing study in The Lancet, comparing GSH levels in individuals of different ages and states of health. The highest levels of GSH were found in the healthy young, then in the healthy elderly. The lowest levels were found in sick, elderly patients. The results showed that GSH levels fall, a) as we age, and b) as we become ill. The more severe the illness, the more evident the decrease.

Back in the laboratory, scientists are trying to find out whether elevated GSH levels actually extend the lifespan. Aging expert John Richie Jr. thinks that glutathione deficiency may be a biochemical cause of the aging process. In some of his experiments MgTC—a GSH-promoting drug similar to OTC—was fed to mosquitoes. GSH levels were found to be 50 to 100% higher, and life span was increased by almost 40%. In another experiment, Diane Birt at the University of Nebraska fed hamsters the whey-protein concentrate lactalbumin—a GSH-precursor. These animals also lived longer.

Interestingly, control hamsters on a diet including either, a) mixture of casein and cysteine, or b) methionine did not benefit. In fact high cysteine loads proved harmful, making the point that both cysteine and methionine (sometimes considered glutathione precursors) don't work well. The bioactivity of these amino acids changes when they are constituents of a larger protein, as opposed to acting as free amino acids.

Using yet another product, Dr. Gustavo Bounous and other researchers at McGill University were able to demonstrate the anti-aging effect of elevated GSH levels. Mice fed a specially-developed whey protein isolate were compared to mice on a standard diet. Not only were their tissue GSH levels found to be higher, the whey-fed mice had an average life span of 27 months (corresponding to a human age of 80 years) whereas the mice on the control diet averaged 21 months (human equivalent of 55 years). This is an increase of 30%. Further experiments using both cysteine and caseine (another milk protein) neither increased longevity nor raised GSH levels.

This doesn't apply only to mice. In humans too, glutathione deficiency resulting from poor cellular synthesis of GSH can be corrected. A 2011 article in the American journal of Clinical Nutrition documented the progress of elderly subjects whose diet was supplemented with glutathione precursors. Normal glutathione levels (as compared to a younger population) were restored in just two weeks.

This is especially important for elderly vegetarians. A review study by McCarty and DiNicolantonio stresses the need for glutathione precursors for elderly subjects who follow a plant-based diet or who commonly have a suboptimal protein intake.

Aging & detoxification

As we age, GSH levels fall and we become increasingly susceptible to the toxic accumulation of many drugs and pollutants. This is highly significant considering the widespread use of prescription drugs among the elderly. Older people have enough health challenges without this additional threat. Renowned aging researchers T.S. Chen, J.P. Ritchie and C.A. Lang have suggested that lower GSH levels in aging livers diminish the body's ability to counteract poisons, including toxic levels of acetaminophen.

Aging & exercise

Increased physical activity as a way of life is clearly associated with longevity and improved health. There are many reasons, and some researchers have focused on the role of antioxidants and GSH. Allessio and Blasi at Miami University's Department of Physical Education summed it up, saying that exercise can elevate antioxidant enzymes (and their cofactors), and that antioxidant levels are inversely related to mortality.

In a series of reports on glutathione levels among the elderly, German researchers Kretzschmar and Muller suggest that exercise compensates for age-related decline, and that the resultant increase in GSH levels can protect against many of the diseases common to older people. In Israel, Reznick and Witt went further, suggesting that raised antioxidant function enables aging people to tolerate more exercise without the ill-effects of over-training.

This approach was confirmed by Nyberg and his team when they measured glutathione levels in the muscle tissue of both young and old individuals, focusing on ways to preserve them. The message is unequivocal: exercise or grow old faster.

In Chapter 23 on glutathione and athletic performance, read how glutathione levels increase with exercise and how this wards off some of the down sides of too much exercise. It has been suggested on several occasions that physical activity promotes longevity by increasing glutathione levels.

Immunity, Aging and GSH

It's well known that the immune system declines with age. This helps explain the increased incidence of cancer and other diseases—especially the infections typically found among older people. Fidelius and Tsan from the Veterans Administration Research Service have directly tied low GSH levels to this increased susceptibility and were able to shift the immune response up and down by raising and depleting glutathione levels respectively.

As the immune system ages, T-cell lymphocytes (see Chapter 3) undergo the most significant changes, leaving us less prepared to fight viruses, bacteria and other threats. The same T-cell decline has also been identified in some autoimmune diseases, including rheumatoid arthritis (RA) and systemic lupus erythematosus (SLE).

Separate study groups have enhanced the immune response of aging laboratory animals using GSH or GSH-promoting drugs like OTC (ornithine decarboxylase) or 2ME (2-mercapto-ethanol), and the same tests were migrated into human studies. Tufts University researchers Drs. Simin Meydani & Dayang Wu showed that adding GSH to the white blood cells of elderly people brought their immune activity to levels typical of much younger individuals. The same team of leading researchers in aging and immunology carried out an in-vivo study in human patients, feeding them supplements known to raise GSH levels. These tests had equally positive benefits for the immune response. These studies all point to the same conclusion: increased oxidative stress and/or lower consumption of antioxidants contribute to the decline of white-blood cell function and weakened immune response in the aged.

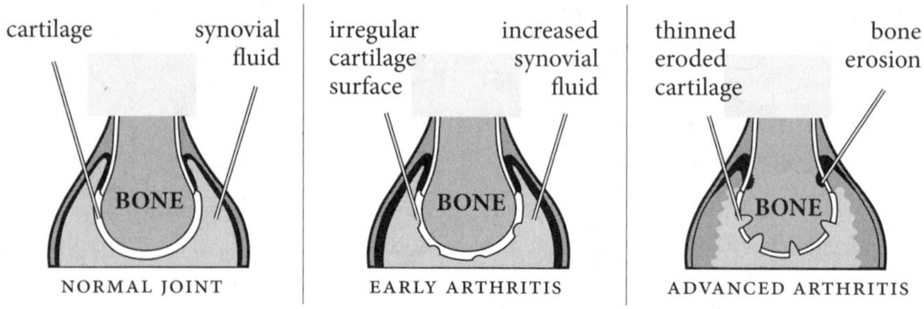

FIGURE 15: Progression of rheumatoid arthritis

Rheumatoid arthritis

Rheumatoid arthritis (RA) is a common chronic inflammatory joint disease that gets worse with age (see Figure 14). Although its exact cause is unknown, several factors have been identified. Strong evidence shows that many of the changes in RA-affected joints result from oxidation and free radical damage. Some researchers have also implicated poor T-cell activity and overactive B-cells. Scientists have also demonstrated that the GSH content of T-cells in rheumatoid joints is much lower than in nearby T-cells of the same patients.

GSH modulation seems to play a role in the progression or remission of RA. A team of rheumatologists from Leiden University Medical Center in the Netherlands used NAC to raise glutathione in these tissues, and noted reduced inflammation at a cellular level.

Conclusion

There's little doubt that oxidative damage to cells worsens the decline of aging and its diseases. We know that those who live to a hundred or more have unusually high levels of glutathione. We also know how destructive oxyradicals are. Given that GSH is a powerful antioxidant, there's every reason to connect longevity to GSH. At the very least, it should improve immune defenses and quality of life at a time when many people experience one health problem after another.

The extension of the life span of mice by 30 to 50% suggests that GSH may reduce the wear and tear of aging on overall health. Quite apart from the process of aging, good health in general is associated with high GSH levels. Also, GSH helps the liver deal with the toxic effects of medications that are commonly used by the elderly. It may also improve the value of exercise by energizing the GSH system and contributing to better overall health and well-being.

GSH can enhance the immune response at a time when it generally starts to decline. It can ward off diseases of aging and improve T-cell function—a critical part of the immune system. Finally, the aging of brains due to glutathione deficiency has been a topic of great focus and will be important in anti-aging medicines of the future.

AGING

REFERENCES

ALESSIO HM, BLASI ER. *Physical activity as a natural antioxidant booster & its effect on a healthy life span.* Res. Q. Exerc. Sport. 68:292-302, 1997

BENZI G, PASTORIS O, MARZATICO F, VILLA RF. *Age-related effect induced by oxidative stress on the cerebral glutathione system.* Neurochem. Res. 14:473-481, 1989

BIANCO RA, ZIEGLER TR, CARLSON BA, CHENG PY, PARK Y, COTSONIS GA, ACCARDI CJ, JONES DP. *Diurnal variation in glutathione & cysteine redox states in human plasma. Am J Clin Nutr. 86(4); 1016-1023, 2007.*

Birt DF, Schuldt GH, Salmasi S. *Survival of hamsters fed graded levels of two protein sources.* Lab. Animal Sci. 32:363-366, 1982

Boccatonda A, Tripaldi R, Davi G, Santilli F. *Oxidative Stress Modulation Through Habitual Physical Activity.* Curr Pharm Des 22(24):3648-80, 2016

Bounous G, Gervais F, Amer V, Batist G, Gold P. *The influence of dietary whey protein on tissue GSH & the diseases of aging.* Clin. & Investig. Med. 12: 343-349, 1989

Carper J. *Stop Aging Now!* Harper Collins Publishers, New York, NY 1995

Chen TS, Richie JP Jr, Lang CA. *The effects of aging on glutathione & cysteine levels in different regions of the mouse brain.* Proc. Soc. Exp. Biol. Med. 190:399-402, 1989

Chen TS, Richie JP Jr, Lang CA. *Life span profiles of glutathione & acetaminophen detoxification.* Drug Metab. Dispos. 18:882-887, 1990

Currais A, Maher P. *Functional consequences of age-dependent changes in glutathione status in the brain.* Antioxid Redox Signal. 19(8):813-22, 2013

Currais A, Maher P. *Functional consequences of age-dependent changes in glutathione status in the brain. Antioxid Redox Signal 19(8):813-22, 2013*

Eshkoor SA. et al. *Association of GSTM1 & GSTT1 with ageing in auto repair shop workers.* Genet Mol Res 11(2):1486-96, 2012

Fidelus RK, Tsan MF. *GSH & lymphocyte activation: a function of aging & autoimmune disease.* Immunology 61:503-508, 1987

Fletcher RH, Fletcher SW. *GSH & Aging: Ideas & evidence.* Lancet 344:1379-1380, 1994

Furukawa T, Meydani SN, Blumberg JB. *Reversal of age associated decline in immune responsiveness by dietary GSH supplementation in mice.* Mechanisms of Aging & Development 38:107-117, 1987

Galiniak S, Bartosz G, Sadowska-Bartosz I. *Glutathione is the main endogenous inhibitor of protein glycation.* Gen Physiol Biophys 36(2):175-185, 2017

Gemma C, Vila J, Bachstetter A, Bickford PC. *Oxidative Stress & the Aging Brain: From Theory to Prevention.* In: Riddle DR, editor: Brain Aging: Models, Methods, & Mechanisms. Boca Raton (FL): CRC Press/Taylor & Francis; 2007. Chapter 15.

Gringhuis SI, Leow A, Papendrecht-Van Der Voort EA, et al. *Displacement of linker for activation of T cells from the plasma membrane due to redox balance alterations results in hyporesponsiveness of synovial fluid T lymphocytes in rheumatoid arthritis.* . Immunol. 164:2170-2179, 2000

Gutteridge JM. *Aging & free radicals.* Med. Lab. Sci. 49:313-318, 1992

Guttmann RP. *Redox regulation of cysteine-dependent enzymes.* J Anim Sci 88(4):1297-306, 2010

Han C, Someya S. *Maintaining good hearing: calorie restriction, Sirt3, & glutathione.* Exp Gerontol 48(10):1091-5, 2013

Harman D. *Free radicals in aging.* Mol. Cell. Biochem. 84:155-161, 1988

Harman D. *Free radical theory of aging.* Mutat. Res. 275:257-266, 1992

Hazelton GA, Lang CA. *Glutathione contents of tissues in the aging mouse.* Biochem. J. 188:25-30, 1980

Hazelton GA, Lang CA. *Glutathione peroxidase & reductase activities in the aging mouse.* Mech. Aging Dev. 29:71-81, 1985

Homma T, Fujii J. *Application of Glutathione as Anti-Oxidative & Anti-Aging Drugs.* Curr Drug Metab 16(7):560-71, 2015

Ji, LL. *Antioxidant enzyme response to exercising & aging.* Med. Sci. Sports Exerc. 25:225-231, 1993

Julius M, Lang CA, Gleiberman L, et al. *GSH & morbidity in a community based sample of elderly.* Journal of Clinical Epidemiology 47: 1021-1026, 1994

Khanna SC, Garg SK, Sharma SP. *Antioxidant-influenced alterations in glutathione reductase activity in different age groups of male mice.* Gerontology 38:9-12, 1992

Klatz R. *Grow young with HGH [ISBN 0-06-098434-1].* Harper Perennial. 1997

Knight JA. *Free radicals: their history & current status in aging & disease.* Ann. Clin. Lab. Sci. 28:331-346, 1998

Kretzschmar M, Muller D. *Aging, training & exercise.* A review of effects on plasma glutathione & lipid peroxides. Sports Med. 15:196-209, 1993

Kretzschmar M, Muller D, Hubscher J, et al. *nfluence of aging, training & acute physical exercise on plasma glutathione & lipid peroxides in man.* nt. J. Sports Med. 12, 218-222, 1991

Kumar H. et al. *The role of free radicals in the aging brain & Parkinson's Disease: convergence & parallelism.* Int J Mol Sci 13(8):10478-504, 2012

Lang CA, Naryshkin S, Schneider DL, Mills BJ, Lindeman RD. *Low blood GSH in healthy aging adults.* Journal of Laboratory & Clinical Medicine 120:720-725, 1992

Lang CA, Wu WK, Chen T, Mills BJ. *Blood glutathione: a biochemical index of life span enhancement in the diet restricted Lobund-Wistar rat.* Prog. Clin. Biol. Res. 287:241-246, 1989

Mari M. et al. *Mitochondrial glutathione, a key survival antioxidant.* Antioxid Redox Signal

11(11):2685-700, 2009

McCarty ME, DiNicolantonio JJ. *An increased need for dietary cysteine in support of glutathione synthesis may underlie the increased risk for mortality associated with low protein intake in the elderly.* Age (Dordr) 37(5):96, 2015

Maurice MM, Van der Voort EAM, Vilet AI, Tak PP, Breedveld FC, Verweij CL. *Chronic oxidative stress in rheumatoid arthritis: Implications for T-cell function. Oxidative Stress in Cancer, AIDS & Neurodegenerative Diseases.* Institute Pasteur. Editors Montagnier L, Olivier R, Pasquier C. Marcel Dekker, 1998.

Mazzetti AP, Fiorile MC, Primavera A, Lo Bello M. *Glutathione transferases & neurodegenerative diseases.* Neurochem Int 82:10-8, 2015

Merry P, Winyard PG, Morris CJ, Grootveld M, Blake DR. *Oxygen-free radicals, inflammation, & synovitis: the current status.* Annals of Rheumatic Disease 48:864-870, 1989

Meydani SN, Wu D, Santos MS, Hayek MG. *Antioxidants & immune response in aged persons: overview of present evidence.* American Journal of Clinical Nutrition 62(s):1462-1476, 1995

Michelet F, Gueguen R, Leroy P, et al. *Blood & plasma glutathione measured in healthy subjects by HPLC: relation to sex, aging, biological variables, & life habits.* Clin. Chem. 41:1509-1517, 1995

Nohi H. *Involvement of free radicals in aging: a consequence or cause of senescence.* Br. Med. Bull. 49:653-667, 1993

Nutall SL, Martin U, Sinclair AJ, Kendall MJ. *Glutathione in sickness & in health.* Lancet 351: 645-646, 1998

Nguyen D. et al. *Impaired mitocondrial fatty acid oxidation & insulin resistance in aging: novel protective role of glutathione.* Aging cell 12(3):415-25, 2013

Nyberg M, Mortensen SP, Cabo H, Gómez-Cabrera MC, Viña J, Hellsten Y. *Roles of sedentary aging & lifelong physical activity in Exchange of glutathione across exercising human skeletal muscle.* Free Radic Biol Med 73:166-73, 2014

Paolisso G, Tagliamonte MR, Rizzo MR, et al. *Oxidative stress & advancing age: results in healthy centenarians. American Geriatric Soc. 46:833-838, 1998*

Peng C. et al. *Biology of ageing & role of dietary antioxidants.* Biomed Res Int 2014:831841, 2014

Poot M. *Oxidants & antioxidants in proliferative senescence.* Mutat. Res. 256:177-189, 1991

Presnell CE. et al. *Computational insights into the role of glutathione in oxidative stress.* Curr Neurovasc Res 10(2):185-94, 2013

Remacle J, Michiels C, Raes M. *The importance of antioxidant enzymes in cellular aging & degeneration.* EXS. 62:99-108, 1992

Reznick AZ, Witt EH, Silbermann M, Packer L. *The threshold of age in exercise & antioxidants action.* EXS. 62:423-427, 1992

Richie JP Jr. *Correction of a GSH deficiency in the aging mosquito increases its longevity.* Proc. of the Society for Experimental Biology & Medicine 184:113-117, 1987

Richie JP Jr. *The role of GSH in aging & cancer.* Experimental Gerontology 27:615-626, 1992

Salminen LE, Paul RH. *Oxidative stress & genetic markers of suboptimal antioxidant defense in the aging brain: a theoretical review.* Rev Neurosci 25(6):805-19, 2014

Salmon M, Gaston JSH. *The role of T-cell lymphocytes in rheumatoid arthritis.* British Medical Bulletin 51:332-345, 1995

Sekhar RV. et al. *Deficient synthesis of glutathione underlies oxidative stress in aging & can be corrected by dietary cysteine & glycine supplementation.* Am J Clin Nutr 94(3):847-53, 2011

Soysal P. et al. *Oxidative stress & frailty: A systematic review & synthesis of the best evidence.* Maturitas 99:66-72, 2017

Vina J, Sastre J, Anton V, et al. *Effect of aging on glutathione metabolism.* Protection by antioxidants. EXS. 62:136-144, 1992

Wu D, Meydani SN, Sastre J, Hayek M, Meydani M. *In vitro GSH supplementation enhances interleukin-2 production & mitogenic response of peripheral blood mononuclear cells from young & old subjects.* Journal of Nutrition 124: 655-663, 1994

7

Cardiovascular Disease

"CARDIOVASCULAR" refers to the heart (cardia) and the vessels (vascula) that circulate blood throughout your body. This chapter discusses heart disease, stroke, cholesterol, and hypertension (high blood pressure). Before we look at the differences between these problems, let's consider the primary process underlying most of them—arteriosclerosis.

Arteriosclerosis

Heart disease and stroke are the principal cause of death in North America. Both result from arteriosclerosis—also called atherosclerosis or hardening of the arteries. This is such a common disease in the developed world that for a time it was considered a normal part of the aging process. Nowadays, overwhelming evidence links it closely to diet and lifestyle issues such as smoking and lack of exercise, suggesting that this major cause of mortality and morbidity is preventable, and that its progress may be slowed or even reversed.

Although more common in older people, the early stages of this disease are sometimes found in children, and people in their thirties may suffer significant damage too.

The consequences of arteriosclerosis are serious—heart failure, heart attack, stroke, kidney failure, high blood pressure, impaired circulation and other ailments. Additional contributing factors aggravate this condition and must be managed throughout life to ensure health and longevity (see Table 18).

Figure 15 shows the three layers of an artery wall—a tough epithelium, a thick muscular mesothelium and the endothelium—a delicate lining especially prone to damage.

FIBER	A high-fiber diet is critical. Include a variety of fruits, vegetables and grains.
FAT	Eat high-fat foods only occasionally. These include fried food, junk food, meat products, butter, lard, margarine and rich dairy products.
COOKING OIL	Use pure, cold-pressed olive oil or unrefined canola oil. Heating oil increases its damaging effects.
FAMILY HISTORY	If your family has a history of cardiovascular disease, see your doctor for regular checkups.
STRESS	Reduce stress levels and use relaxation techniques.
EXERCISE	Take regular, moderate exercise, at least three times weekly for 30-45 minutes.
BLOOD PRESSURE	Monitor and maintain normal blood pressure.
TOBACCO	Avoid smoking and second-hand smoke. This is a powerful source of oxidation.
WEIGHT	Maintain an appropriate body weight.

TABLE 18: How to avoid arteriosclerosis

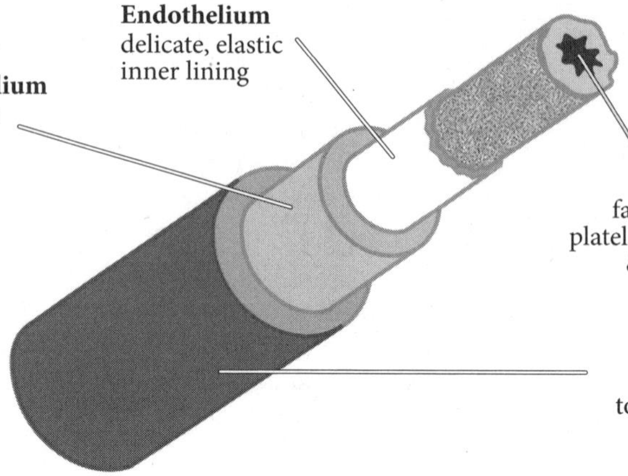

Figure 16: To understand how GSH helps prevent and treat this disease, we must first understand how arteriosclerosis develops

Thin streaks of fatty deposits are liable to accumulate on this lining. In a healthy artery, this process is combated in several ways, including our natural antioxidant defenses. In arteries damaged or affected by aggravating factors such as high blood pressure, stress or cigarette smoking these fatty deposits have an opportunity to accumulate. Trying to contain this damage, the body lays down platelets, calcium and scar tissue, complicating the issue further. Plaque thickens and makes the area stickier than usual, enabling additional lipids to accumulate. Eventually, the artery becomes clogged enough to inhibit blood flow and deprive organs and muscles of oxygen.

Heart disease

Poor circulation may affect all organ systems, including the brain, kidneys, eyes and extremities, but the major burden it causes on the medical system is through heart disease.

When blood flow through the coronary arteries and into the heart is obstructed (ischemia), a heart attack results. Inadequate blood flow also triggers the pain of angina when the heart suffers from a lack of oxygen. Furthermore, a heart with insufficient blood flow weakens, leading to possible 'heart failure.' On top of that, blocked and hardened arteries cause high blood pressure, compromising heart function even more.

Physicians treat this downward spiral with medications to lower blood pressure, thin the blood, decrease cholesterol, strengthen heart muscle contractions and improve blood flow through the arteries. Surgery is occasionally performed to work around blockages. A coronary bypass grafts a vein to 'bypass' the blockage. A simpler procedure, angioplasty, squashes the plaque back against the artery wall, widening the passageway and allowing blood to flow more freely.

Stroke

A stroke results from an oxygen shortage in the brain caused by poor blood flow. All vital organs are prone to a similar kind of ischemia whenever the arteries feeding them become narrow and hard. Treatment begins with blood thinners and control of cholesterol, and may be followed by surgery to remove arterial plaque.

Impeded oxygen flow to brain tissue causes significant damage. To make things complicated, the reintroduction of oxygen (the life-saving process of reperfusion) causes more oxidative damage of cells. Neurologists from the University of California (San Francisco) showed how important glutathione was at such times by artificially lowering glutathione levels in the brains of animals, which then experienced a stroke. Compared with animals with normal glutathione levels, brain damage was significantly greater. Neurosurgeons at the same institution explored the spiraling stages of damage, demonstrating that glutathione depletion contributes to yet more narrowing of arteries, starving oxygen-starved brain cells of even more oxygen.

Cholesterol and plaque formation

The buildup of plaque (atherogenesis, Figure 16) is a long, slow and complex process that takes years to produce noticeable symptoms. However, we know that certain types of fatty substances (lipids) are more dangerous than others. LDL[1] (bad cholesterol) leads to plaque formation, while HDL[2] (good cholesterol) prevents it. Other factors add to the danger of these lipids—especially oxidative stress.

Oxidation is a chemical reaction that makes fat rancid. When that happens to the fats in our bloodstream, the chemical change causes fatty deposits to stick to the inside of artery walls. Meanwhile, the free radicals left over from oxidation do further damage, causing lipid peroxidation that leads to hardening of the arteries.

Other factors contribute to this process. Cigarette smoke releases huge amounts of free radicals into the blood stream, explaining why more smokers die of cardiovascular disease than of lung cancer. For similar reasons, diabetics are prone to the complications of vascular damage.

Researchers have focused on many aspects of cardiovascular atherogenesis, from the biochemical changes that result in lipid peroxidation to concerns about the associated inflammatory response, platelet function and cardiac muscle aging. A whole field of free-radical biology has arisen, leading to a clearer understanding of oxidative stress and its role in cardiac disease. Thousands of articles have examined the role of antioxidants in arteriosclerosis. The great promise first held for antioxidants in preventing heart disease was likely overblown, but antioxidant therapy nevertheless plays an important, well-established role.

An important article published by a combined team of Canadian and Japanese heart researchers reviews the evidence for the role of oxidative stress in acute ischemic heart disease. They suggest using antioxidant therapy before procedures such as angioplasty, coronary bypass and thrombolysis (treatment to dissolve clots and improve flow) to minimize complications.

Without adequate protective mechanisms to combat free radical formation and lipid peroxidation, vascular systems are quickly overcome by atherosclerosis. Kendal's team at the University of Birmingham performed a randomized clinical trial of more than 2,000 patients with coronary artery disease. Those who took antioxidant supplements were at 47% less risk. Large-scale, well-defined clinical trials have not yet proven beyond doubt that antioxidants are essential, and yet a poll of cardiologists published in the American Journal of Cardiology showed that a full 44% of them take antioxidants themselves.

GSH and Arteriosclerosis

The principal antioxidant in our cells is glutathione. This applies to the endothelial cells of the arteries as well as red blood cells and platelets. University of British Columbia

1 low-density lipoproteins
2 high-density lipoproteins

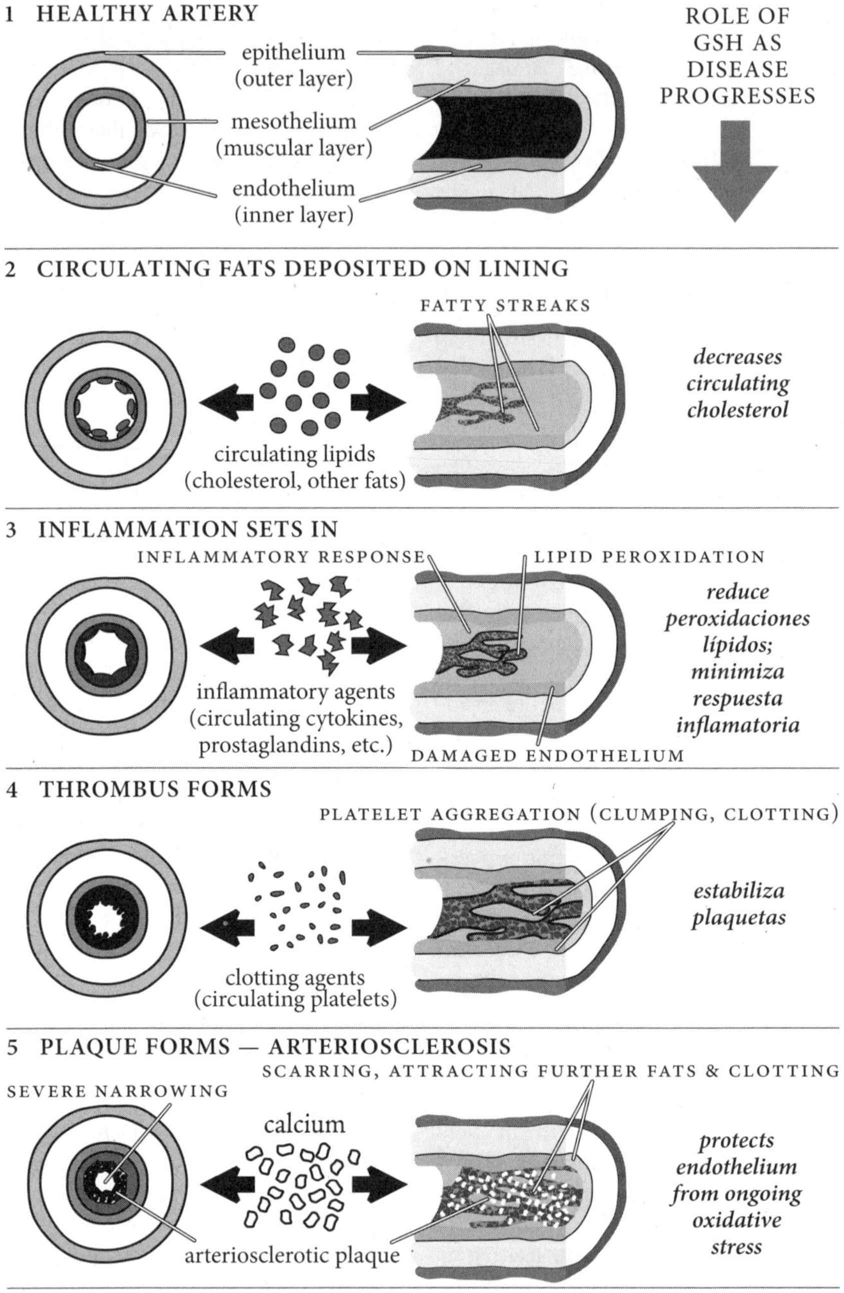

FIGURE 17: *Atherogenesis*

researchers led by Cheng correlated cholesterol levels, GSH levels and plaque formation in the aorta (the main artery coming out of the heart). Ji, Dillon & Wu published data indicating that age-related low GSH levels contribute to atherosclerosis. Although the importance of the antioxidant vitamins C and E are increasingly appreciated, neither one occurs "naturally" in the human body—they must first be ingested. GSH, on the other hand, does occur naturally. It is produced within our cells. GSH also serves to recycle other antioxidants into their functionally active form, doubling its importance.

To determine a person's risk of cardiovascular disease, doctors test for elevated levels of two "markers": lipoprotein-a (Lp[a]), and homocysteine. Gavish, Breslow and other researchers set out to see whether they could reduce Lp[a] levels by using the GSH-promoting drug NAC (N-acetylcysteine). They reported a 50-70% reduction in Lp[a] using 2 to 4 grams of NAC per day. Other researchers—using lower doses to minimize drug side-effects—have not as successfully reduced Lp[a], but have suggested that NAC may influence atherosclerosis in other ways. It appears that the resultant increase in GSH levels correspondingly reduces levels of LDL ('bad' cholesterol), and inhibits free radical formation by white blood cells.

The association between homocysteine and GSH metabolism is currently under investigation and will likely have important repercussions in the future. Stamler & Slivka in a lead review article discuss the roles of GSH, its interaction with homocysteine, and the protective effect of GSH on the vascular system. Like Gavish and Breslow, the Swedes Wiklund, Fager and their group were also able to bring about a lowering of homocysteine levels using NAC (N-acetylcysteine).

An article of great interest appeared in the Japan Heart Journal, describing a study by the Turkish researcher Usal. Taking 21 patients who had suffered heart attacks, he measured their red blood cell glutathione levels and compared them to 21 healthy individuals. He confirmed that the cardiac patients had suffered measurable glutathione depletion, and supported the suggestion that GSH is in greater demand at such times. The question arises—might low glutathione levels predict cardiac risk?

GSH as a measure of heart health

The role of oxidative stress in the onset and progression of arteriosclerosis (hardening and blockage of the arteries) has been described in minute detail—and yet there's always more to learn. Recently there's been more focus on the long-term consequences of adverse cardiovascular events. They are hard to trace because the links are broad and interdependent, involving such risk factors as high blood pressure, high cholesterol levels, metabolic syndrome, obesity and diabetes. What everyone suffering from these factors has in common is: high levels of oxidative stress and low glutathione levels. It's no coincidence that all are at higher risk of cardiovascular disease.

It has been suggested that if oxidized fats (cholesterol and other lipids) are a major factor in the development of cardiovascular disease, and if glutathione peroxidase decreases lipid oxidation, then higher levels of glutathione would be protective. This appears to be so.

At a basic level of inquiry, it seems that individuals with genetic errors in certain glutathione enzymes are at greater risk of heart attack. You can see in many other chapters in this book that abnormal glutathione genetics are linked to a plethora of health problems.

By examining glutathione levels in under-45 year olds with premature coronary artery disease (early heart disease), Musthafa and his team noted low GSH levels. Compared to a healthy group of similar ages, his patients were deficient in glutathione.

Looking at older populations, the Hisayama study suggested that low glutathione levels correlate not only with the risk of heart attack, but even more so with stroke. Emory University cardiologists determined that low GSH was an independent predictor of impaired coronary circulation and plaque breakdown.

Diabetics tend to experience increased cardiac problems associated with low GSH levels. Italian researchers found the arterial tissue of diabetics to be severely low in GSH. To combat this problem, a paper in the American Journal of Cardiovascular Drugs reviewed studies using NAC on diabetic-associated cardiovascular complications. Results were promising enough for them to suggest it as an active area of investigation.

One surgical procedure that has become routine in the past few decades is angioplasty, in which coronary vessels are pressed open to reestablish circulation. Polish cardiologist Pietruszyński and his team found that low or high glutathione levels predicted whether patients would have a major adverse event or not during this procedure. This suggests that glutathione correction prior to angioplasty may be advisable. A team from Italy showed similar evidence: following a heart attack, patients with low GSH levels were much more likely to suffer a second cardiac event.

A major 2016 paper appearing in the journal Circulation proposed that glutathione be measured as a biomarker predicting risk of death from heart disease. Other papers have suggested that raising glutathione could be an effective way to prevent heart attack (myocardial infarction), and even heart disease itself.

GSH and cholesterol

As we saw in Chapter 4, undenatured whey proteins can raise cellular GSH. High quality whey protein isolates may also contain unusually high levels of lactoferrin, an important protein known to prevent the oxidation of bad cholesterol. In addition, raised GSH levels have been shown to help eliminate cholesterol by raising the activity of the enzyme cholesterol hydroxylase.

Zhang and Beynen compared the ability of various proteins to reduce cholesterol in the blood and liver. Their results showed that whey proteins were more effective than any other milk protein, or any amino acid combination. They suggest the mechanism that reduces cholesterol levels works by inhibiting cholesterol synthesis in the liver.

Selenium plays one major active biological role in the body: as a co-factor in the formation of glutathione peroxidase. Also, it has been shown that high or low selenium levels are matched by high or low levels of HDL.[3] Using selenium supplementation in a double-blind study, Luoma's teams successfully improved HDL/LDL[4] ratios (proportion of 'good' to 'bad' cholesterol) in healthy subjects. In Italy Franceschini and Werba were able to do the same using NAC (N-acetylcysteine).

An international team of American, German, Norwegian and Korean scientists showed that patients with low glutathione were at greater risk of dying from a heart attack. They did this by establishing the direct connection between low glutathione peroxidase levels, low HDL levels and increased cardiovascular mortality.

GSH and reperfusion injury

When tissues are deprived of blood flow and oxygen for more than a few minutes, the body does several things to compensate. When supplies are reestablished, the tissues are said to be 'reperfused,' or reoxygenated. However, everything doesn't just go back to normal. While reperfusion is an immediate life-saver, the flow of freshly oxygenated blood may cause yet more damage to the affected tissues. This is called reperfusion injury. Reperfusion occurs not only after heart attack and stroke, but also after bypass surgery or when 'thrombolytic' drugs have been used to break down a clot. Doctors need to be prepared.

Cardiologists have discovered that even more damage occurs during reperfusion as oxyradicals and free radicals form. The immune system responds to the damage by increasing production of neutrophils[5]—the most common white blood cell and

---

[3] HDL: high-density lipoproteins; 'good' cholesterol
[4] LDL: low-density lipoproteins; "bad" cholesterol
[5] a type of white blood cell

the main ingredient of pus). Neutrophils penetrate interstitial[6] tissue, releasing even more reactive oxygen species and hydrolytic enzymes. Pharmacologists Kilgore and Luchesi from the University of Michigan long ago suggested that antioxidants should be administered during thromobolytic therapy. Doctors at the University of Brescia have shown significant glutathione depletion after cardiac ischemia, and that this depletion can be remedied by restoring GSH levels with N-acetylcysteine.

GSH and high blood pressure

Hypertension (high blood pressure) is an independent risk factor for cardiovascular disease. In other words, the higher the blood pressure, the greater the likelihood of heart attack, stroke or other circulatory problem. When no single cause is identified for a patient's high blood pressure, doctors refer to it as "essential hypertension." However, a closer look at glutathione levels may help to identify a potential cause in many of these patients.

Some individuals are born with abnormal GSH enzymes, a condition which can be identified through genetic testing. Such people are at significantly higher risk of cardiovascular problems, including hypertension. This fact alone points to glutathione's role in minimizing high blood pressure.

As for glutathione's biochemical role in the cascade of events leading to hypertension, a Polish team led by Robaczewska observed that as glutathione levels fall with age, there is a corresponding increase in blood pressure. This suggests that regulation of the glutathione metabolism might counteract age-dependent increases in blood pressure.

Since high blood pressure at any age goes along with low glutathione levels, some cardiology researchers have suggested that GSH be used as a marker for both diagnosis and outcome. In the Journal of Hypertension, a study of juvenile essential hypertension revealed that oxidative stress was significant even among these children and adolescents. At the other end of the age scale, a study appearing in Cardiovascular Toxicology revealed the very same association in elderly hypertension patients. Again, low GSH levels correlated with high blood pressure and difficulty controlling it.

Across the board, individuals with essential hypertension have low glutathione levels. Furthermore, when hypertension is adequately treated GSH levels often normalize, raising the "chicken or egg" question. Studies are underway into the potential role of the GSH-precursor NAC (N-acetylcysteine) as an adjunctive treatment for hypertension.

GSH and circulation

Many other vascular-protective effects of GSH have been demonstrated, beyond the scope of this book. These involve the role played by GSH in maintaining smooth muscle tone in vessel walls, as well as the delicate balance of immune and anti-inflammatory substances including prostaglandins, leukotrienes, thromboxanes and platelet factors. These are dealt with more fully in the references.

Conclusion

Glutathione has been shown to reduce the oxidation of fats (lipid peroxidation), decrease circulating cholesterol, minimize the inflammatory response around arteriosclerotic plaque, stabilize platelets, and protect the sensitive lining of the arteries (endothelium). These are all critical ways to combat hardening of the arteries.

---

[6] fluid-filled areas surrounding the cells of a particular tissue

Glutathione also decreases tissue damage caused by oxygen deprivation (ischemia), and the complications that follow as the tissues are reperfused with fresh blood (reperfusion injury). By measuring glutathione levels, we may be able to predict cardiac disease and its outcomes.

The term "essential hypertension" implies that no clear reason exists for the presence of high blood pressure, but this approach may be outdated. It can be argued that many cases are indeed explained by low GSH levels.

The huge impact of cardiovascular disease on modern society is largely preventable. While a reasonable diet and life-style is always the best strategy, there are many cases in which raising GSH may prevent or even treat this all-too prevalent illness.

CARDIOVASCULAR DISEASE

REFERENCES

Ambrosio G, Tritto I, Golino P. *Reactive oxygen metabolites & arterial thrombosis.* Cardiovasc. Research 34:445-452, 1997

Berenson GS, Srinivasan SR, Bao W, Newman WP III, Tracy RE, Wattigney WA. *Association between multiple, cardiovascular risk factors & atherosclerosis in children & young adults.* New England Journal of Medicine 338: 1650-1656, 1998

Balta N, Gatina R, Loan M, et al. *Activity of glutathione-s-transferase, gammaglutamiltransferase & catalase in the erythrocytic membrane in arterial hypertension.* Rom J Physiol. 36:237-251, 1999

Blankenberg S, Rupprecht HJ, Bickel C, et al. *Glutathione peroxidase 1 activity & cardiovascular events in patients with coronary artery disease.* New England Journal of Medicine 349: 1605-1613, 2003

Breslow JL, Azrolan N, Bostom A. *N-acetylcysteine & lipoprotein.* Lancet 339: 126-127, 1992

Buijsse B, Lee DH, Steffen L, et al. *Low serum glutathione peroxidase activity is associated with increased cardiovascular mortality in individuals with low HDLc's.* PLoS One 7: e38901, 2012

Ceconi C, Curello S, Cargnoni A, et al. *The role of glutathione status in the protection against ischaemic & reperfusion damage: effects of N-acetylcysteine.* J. Mol. Cell. Cardiol. 20: 5-13, 1988

Cheng KM, Aggrey SE, Nichols CR, Garnett ME, Godin DV. *Antioxidant enzymes & atherosclerosis in Japanese quail: Hereditability & genetic correlation estimates.* Canadian Journal of Cardiology 13:669-676, 1997

De Chiara B, Mafrici A, Campolo J, et al. *Low plasma glutathione levels after reperfused acute myocardial infarction are associated with late cardiac events.* Coron Artery Dis. 18: 77-82, 2007

Dhalla NS, Golfman L, Takeda S, et al. *Evidence for the role of oxidative stress in acute ischemic heart disease: A brief review.* Can. J. Cardiol. 15: 587-593, 1999

Dhawan SS, Eshtehardi P, McDaniel MC, et al. *The role of plasma aminothiols in the prediction of coronary microvascular dysfunction & plaque vulnerability.* Atherosclerosis 219: 266-272, 2011

Dludia PV, Dias SC, Obonye N, et al. *A Systematic Review on the Protective Effect of N-Acetyl Cysteine Against Diabetes-Associated Cardiovascular Complications. Am J Cardiovasc Drugs 18:283-298, 2018*

Du Y, Wang H, Fu X, et al. *GSTT1 null genotype contributes to coronary heart disease risk: a meta-analysis. Mol Bio Rep. 39: 8571-8579, 2012*

Eslami S, Sahebkar A. *Glutathione-S-transferase M1 & T1 null genotypes are associated with hypertension risk: a systematic review & meta-analysis of 12 studies.* Curr Hypertens Rep. 16: 432, 2014

Fan NC, Tsai CM, Hsu CN, et al. *N-acetylcysteine prevents hypertension via regulation of the ADMA-DDAH pathway in young spontaneously hypertensive rats.* Biomed Res Int. 2013: 696317, 2013

Francheschini G, Werba JP, Safa O, et al. *Dose-related increase of HDL-cholesterol levels after N-acetylcysteine in man.* Pharmacol. Res. 28: 213-218, 1993

Frei B. *Reactive oxygen species & antioxidant vitamins: Mechanisms of action.* American J. Med. 97(suppl 3A): 5S-13S, 1994

Gavish D, Breslow JL. *Lipoprotein[a] reduction by NAC.* The Lancet 337: 203-204, 1991

Gaziano JM. *Antioxidant vitamins & coronary artery disease risk.* The American Journal of Medicine 97: 3a 18S-3a-21S, 1994

Gaziano JM. *Randomized trials of dietary antioxidants in cardiovascular disease prevention & treatment.* J. Cardiovascular Risk 3: 368-371, 1996

Ge B, Song Y, Zhang Y, et al. *Glutathione S-transferase M1 (GSTM1) & T1 (GSTT1) null polymorphisms & the risk of hypertension: a meta-analysis.* PLoS One 5: 118897, 2015

Goutzourelas N, Orfanou M, Charizanis I,

ET AL. *GSH levels affect weight loss in individuals with metabolic syndrome & obesity following dietary therapy.* Exp Ther Med. 16:635-642, 2018

HALLIWELL B. *Current status review: Free radicals, reactive oxygen species, & human disease: a critical evaluation with special reference to atherosclerosis.* British Journal of Experimental Pathology 70:737-757, 1989

HANDY DE, LOSCALZO J. *Responses to reductive stress in the cardiovascular system.* Free Radic Biol Med. 109:114-124, 2017

HANSEN PR. *Lipoprotein (a) reduction by N-acetylcysteine.* Lancet 337: 672-673, 1991

HASSAN AS, HACKLEY JJ, JEFFERY EH. *Role of GSH in the regulation of hepatic cholesterol 7a-hydroxylase, the rate-limiting enzyme of bile acid biosynthesis.* Steroids, 44:373-380, 1984

HENNEKENS CH, GAZIANO JM. *Antioxidants & heart disease: Epidemiology & clinical evidence.* Clinical Cardiology 16: I.10-I.15, 1993

HESS ML, MANSON NH. *The oxygen free radical system & myocardial dysfunction.* Advances in Myocardiology 5:177-181, 1985

HILDEBRANDT W, SAUER R, BONATERRA G, ET AL. *Oral N-acetylcysteine reduces plasma homocysteine concentrations regardless of lipid or smoking status.* Am J Clin Nutr. 102:1014-1024, 2015

HO E, KARIMI GALOUGAHI K, LIU CC, ET AL. *Biological markers of oxidative stress:* Applications to cardiovascular research & practice. Redox Biol. 1:483-491, 2013

HODIS HN, MACK WJ, LABREE L, CASHIN-HEMPHILL L, SEVANIAN A, JOHNSON R, AZEN SP. *Serial coronary angiographic evidence that antioxidant vitamin intake reduces progression of coronary artery atherosclerosis.* Journal of the American Medical Association 273: 1849-1854, 1995

HOFFMAN RM, GAREWAL HS. *Antioxidants & the prevention of coronary heart disease.* Archives of Internal Medicine 155: 241-246, 1995

HOLTZMAN JL. *The role of low levels of the serum glutathione-dependent peroxidase & glutathione & high levels of serum homocysteine in the development of cardiovascular disease.* Clin Lab. 48: 129-130, 2002

IZAWA K, OKADA M, SUMITOMO K, ET AL. *Impaired glutathione redox system paradoxically suppresses angiotensin II-induced vascular remodeling.* PLoS One 9: 108115, 2014

JI LL, DILLON D, WU E. *Myocardial aging: antioxidant enzyme systems & related biochemical properties.* American Journal of Physiology 261:R386-R392, 1991

KASHIWAGI A, ASAHINA T, NISHIO Y, IKEBUCHI M, TANAKA Y, KIKKAWA R, SHIGETA Y. *Glycation, oxidative stress, & scavenger activity: glucose metabolism & radical scavenger dysfunction in endothelial cells.* Diabetes 45: S84-S86, 1996

KENDALL MJ, NUTTALL SL, MARTIN U. *Antioxidant therapy – a new therapeutic option for reducing mortality from coronary artery disease.* J. Clin. Pharm. Ther. 23: 323-325, 1998

KIDD PM. *Cell membranes, endothelia, & atherosclerosis - the importance of dietary fatty acid balance.* Alt. Medicine Reviews 1: 148-167, 1996

KIDD PM. *Glutathione: Systemic protectant against oxidative & free radical damage.* Alternative Medicine Review 2:155-176, 1997

KILGORE KS, LUCCHESI BR. *Reperfusion injury after myocardial infarction: The role of free radicals & the inflammatory response.* Clin. Biochem. 26: 359-370, 1993

KUBOW S, GOYETTE N, KERMASHA S, STEWART-PHILLIP J, KOSKI K. *Effects of dietary lipid & protein composition on serum lipids & tissue lipid peroxidation in the Syrian Hamster.* Inform 3:484, 1992

KUZUYA M, ANDO F, IGUCHI A, ET AL. *Glutathione peroxidase 1 Pro198Leu variant contributes to the metabolic syndrome in men in a large Japanese cohort.* Am J Clin Nutr. 87: 1939-1944, 2008

LAPENNA D, CIOFANI G, CALAFIORE AM, ET AL. *Impaired glutathione-related antioxidant defenses in the arterial tissue of diabetic patients.* Free Radic Biol Med. 124: 525-531, 2018

LEONCINI G, SIGNORELLO MG, PIANA A, CARRUBBA M, ARMANI U. *Hyperactivity & increased hydrogen peroxide formation in platelets of NIDDM patients.* Thrombosis Research 86: 153-160, 1997

LUOMA PV, SOTANIEMI EA, KORPELA H, KUMPULAINEN J. *Serum selenium, glutathione peroxidase activity & high-density lipoprotein cholesterol – effect of selenium supplementation.* Res. Commun. Chem. Pathol. Pharmacol. 46: 469-472, 1984

MACIEL SS, PEREIRA ADA C, SILVA GJ, ET AL. *Association between glutathione S-transferase polymorphisms & triglycerides & HDL-cholesterol.* Atherosclerosis. 206: 204-208, 2009

MANSEGO ML, BLESA S, GONZALES-ALBERT V, ET AL. *Discordant response of glutathione & thioredoxin systems in human hypertension?* Antioxid Redox Signal. 9: 507-514, 2007

MARTINEZ Y, LI X, LIU G, ET AL. *The role of methionine on metabolism, oxidative stress, & diseases.* Amino Acids. 49: 2091-2098, 2017

MEHTA J. *Intake of antioxidants among American cardiologists.* American J. Cardiol. 79: 1558-1560, 1997

MIURA K, ET AL. *Cysteine uptake & glutathione level in endothelial cells exposed to oxidative stress.* American Journal of Physiology 262: C50-C58, 1992

Mizui T, Kinouchi H, Chan PH. *Depletion of glutathione by buthionine sulfoximine enhances cerebral ischemic injury in rats.* Am. J. Physiol. 262:H313-H317, 1992

Muda P, Kampus P, Zilmer M, et al. *Homocysteine & red blood cell glutathione as indices for middle-aged untreated essential hypertension patients.* J Hypertens. 12: 2329-2333, 2003

Musthafa QA, Abdul Shukor MF, Ismail NAS, et al. *Oxidative status & reduced glutathione levels in premature coronary artery disease & coronary artery disease.* Free Radic Res. 51: 787-798, 2017

Ochi H, Morita I, Murota S. *Roles of GSH & glutathione peroxidase in the protection against endothelial cell injury induced by 15-hydroperoxyeicosatetraenoic acid.* Archives of Biochemistry & Biophysiology 294:407-411, 1992

O'Keefe JH, Lavie CJ, McCallister BD. *Insights into the pathogenesis & prevention of coronary artery disease.* Mayo Clinic Proceedings 70: 69-79, 1995

Oniki K, Hori M, Takata K, et al. *Association between glutathione S-transferase A1, M1 & T1 polymorphisms & hypertension.* Pharmacogenet Genomics 18: 275-277, 2008

Pastore A, Piemonte F. *Protein glutathionylation in cardiovascular diseases.* Int J Mol Sci. 14: 20845-20876, 2013

Pastori D, Pignatelli P, Farcomeni A, et al. *Aging-Related Decline of Glutathione Peroxidase 3 & Risk of Cardiovascular Events in Patients With Atrial Fibrillation.* J Am Heart Assoc. 5: e003682, 2016

Patel RS, Ghasemzadeh N, Eapen DJ, et al. *Novel Biomarker of Oxidative Stress Is Associated With Risk of Death in Patients With Coronary Artery Disease.* Circulation. 133: 361-369, 2016

Pietruszynski R, Markuszewski L, Masiarek K, et al. *Role of preprocedural glutathione concentrations in the prediction of major adverse cardiac events in patients with acute coronary syndrome treated with percutaneous coronary intervention.* Pol Arch Med Wewn 123: 228-237, 2013

Pignatelli P, Menichelli D, Pastori D, et al. *Oxidative stress & cardiovascular disease: new insights.* Kardiol Pol. 76: 713-722, 2018

Pimentel D, Haeussier DJ, Matsui R, et al. *Regulation of cell physiology & pathology by protein S-glutathionylation: lessons learned from the cardiovascular system.* Antioxid Redox Signal. 16: 524-542, 2012

Porter M, Pearson DJ, Suarez-Mendez VJ, Blann AD. *Plasma, platelet & erythrocyte glutathione peroxidases as risk factors in ischaemic heart disease in man.* Clin Sci (Lond). 83: 343-345, 1992

Rafiee L, Shokouh P, Roohafza H, et al. *Association of glutathione S-transferases M1 & T1 gene polymorphisms with the risk of metabolic syndrome in an Iranian population.* Adv Biomed Res. 5:63, 2016

Rimm EB, Stampfer MJ. *The role of antioxidants in preventive cardiology.* Curr. Opin. Cardiol. 12: 188-194, 1997

Robaczewska J, Kedziora-Kornatowska K, Kozakiewicz M, et al. *Role of glutathione metabolism & glutathione-related antioxidant defense systems in hypertension.* J Physiol Pharmacol. 67: 331-337, 2016

Rose AH, Hoffmann PR. *Selenoproteins & cardiovascular stress.* Thromb Haemost. 113: 494-504, 2015

Rush JW, Ford RJ. *Nitric oxide, oxidative stress & vascular endothelium in health & hypertension.* Clin Hemorheol Microcirc. 37: 185-192, 2007

Rybka J, Kupczyk D, Kedziora-Kornatowska K, et al. *Glutathione-related antioxidant defense system in elderly patients treated for hypertension.* Cardiovasc Toxicol. 11: 1-9, 2011

Scanu AM. *N-acetylcysteine & immunoreactivity of lipoprotein[a].* The Lancet 337: 1159, 1991

Schutte R, Schutte AE, Huisman HW, et al. *Blood glutathione & subclinical atherosclerosis in African men:* the SABPA Study. Am J Hypertens. 22: 1154-1159, 2009

Shimizu H, Kiyohara Y, Kato I, et al. *Relationship between plasma glutathione levels & cardiovascular disease in a defined population: the Hisayama study.* Stroke. 35: 2072-2077, 2004

Song Y, Shan Z, Luo C, et al. *Glutathione S-Transferase T1 (GSTT1) Null Polymorphism, Smoking, & Their Interaction in Coronary Heart Disease:* A Comprehensive Meta-Analysis. Heart Lung Circ. 26: 362-370, 2017

Spanidis Y, Mpesios A, Stagos D, et al. *Assessment of the redox status in patients with metabolic syndrome & type 2 diabetes reveals great variations.* Exp Ther Med. 11: 895-903, 2016

Stamler JS, Slivka A. *Biological chemistry of thiols in the vasculature & in vascular-related disease.* Nutrition Reviews 54:1-30, 1996

Stampfer MJ, Malinow MR. *Can lowering homocysteine levels reduce cardiovascular risk?* The New England Journal of Medicine 332:328-329, 1995

Truscelli G, Tanzilli G, Viceconte N, et al. *Glutathione sodium salt as a novel adjunctive treatment for acute myocardial infarction.* Med Hypotheses 102: 48-50, 2017

Turi S, Friedman A, Bereczki C, et al. *Oxidative stress in juvenile essential hypertension.* J Hypertens. 21: 145-152, 2003

Usal A, Acarturk E, Yuregir GT, et al. *Decreased glutathione levels in acute myocardial infarction.* Japan Heart J. 37: 177-182, 1996

VARADHARAJ S, KELLY OJ, KHAYAT RN, ET AL. *Role of Dietary Antioxidants in the Preservation of Vascular function & the Modulation of Health & Disease.* Front Cardiovasc Med. 4: 64, 2017

VAVROVA L, KODYDKOVA J, ZEMAN M, ET AL. *Altered activities of antioxidant enzymes in patients with metabolic syndrome.* Obes Facts. 6: 39-47, 2013

VIOLI F, LOFFREDO L, CARNEVALE R, ET AL. *Atherothrombosis & Oxidative Stress: Mechanisms & Management in Elderly.* Antioxid Redox Signal. 27: 1083-1124, 2017

WIKLUND O, FAGER G, ANDERSON A, ET AL. *N-acetylcysteine treatment lowers plasma homocysteine but not serum lipoprotein(a) levels.* Atherosclerosis 119: 99-106, 1996

ZHANG X, BEYNEN AC. *Lowering effect of dietary milk- whey protein v. casein on plasma & liver cholesterol concentrations in rats.* British Journal of Nutrition 70:139-146, 1993

ZHOU D, MAYBERG MR, LONDON S, GAJDUSEK C. *Reduction of intracellular glutathione levels produces sustained arterial narrowing.* Neurosurgery 39: 991-997, 1996

8

Diabetes

Diabetes mellitus or 'sugar diabetes' is the most common glandular condition in North America. It affects over 30 million people in the USA, representing about 10% of the population, many of whom have yet to be diagnosed. In Mexico, figures are more difficult to estimate, but most authorities believe both the incidence and the number of new cases are even higher.

Diabetics run an above-average risk of developing heart disease and stroke, the leading causes of death in North America. Given that most types of diabetes and its complications are related to lifestyle and environment, this is for the most part a preventable problem.

Diabetes mellitus is an insulin disorder that impairs the body's sugar metabolism. The important hormone insulin is responsible for the absorption of sugar into cells for on-demand energy and into the liver and fat cells for energy storage. There are two main types of diabetes mellitus.

Types of Diabetes

In Type 1 diabetes mellitus, insulin-producing cells in the pancreas are destroyed. This may be caused by toxins or an injury, but most commonly by an autoimmune phenomenon. With regular injections of insulin, the patient can lead a normal life. Without it, he or she may lapse into coma and die.

In Type 2 diabetes mellitus, pancreatic production of insulin is diminished, or the body gradually loses its ability to utilize it. This is by far the most common form of diabetes and is usually linked to bad eating habits, obesity and poor lifestyle.

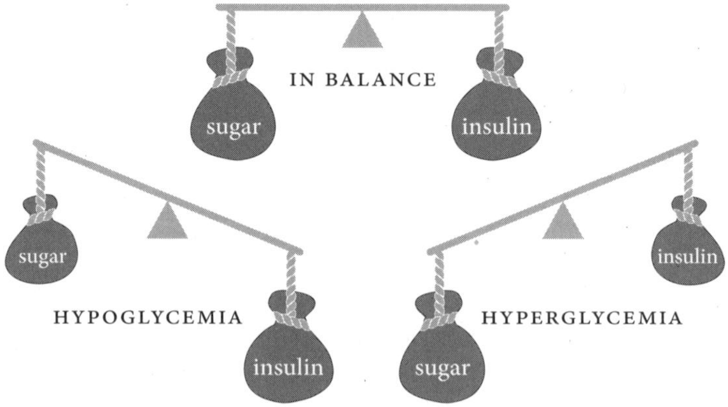

Figure 18: Levels of sugar in the blood must be balanced with levels of insulin

Living with diabetes

Both Type 1 and Type 2 diabetes are generally characterized by high blood sugar (hyperglycemia). However, blood sugar levels can plummet (hypoglycemia) in cases of overmedication or illness/stress during medication. Both extremes are potentially serious.

Hyperglycemia produces excessive thirst and urination, fatigue, weight loss, and dehydration. Occasionally, life-threatening illnesses (hyperosmolar coma or ketoacidosis) may result from excessive sugar levels. These are medical emergencies requiring immediate hospitalization.

Some diabetics take insulin injections or pills to lower sugar levels, and are susceptible to the complications of low blood sugar levels. This may happen because they take too much medication, skip a meal, increase energy expenditures, become sick or febrile, or suffer any sort of stress. This condition too must be treated immediately. Usually, a sweet drink or food will produce rapid results.

Apart from the emergencies resulting from such blood sugar imbalances, most diabetics fall ill from complications of diabetes itself. There are two: reduced ability to fight infection and damage to the circulatory system, including both small and large blood vessels. Such complications can cause symptomatic problems with the eyes, muscle, kidneys and bladder. They can also reduce energy levels, promote thirst, and cause tingling in the extremities. Cardiovascular plaque buildup is another result of diabetic complications.

Diabetic health complications

Diabetics are considered immune-compromised because they're prone to infections they can normally resist. Their immune systems may be overwhelmed by thrush (Candida) as well as other fungal infections of the skin and even the bloodstream. Bacterial infections are more common and their consequences are serious—gangrene (especially of the toes and foot) and sepsis. Diabetics with any sort of infection must always be treated immediately and aggressively.

Most illness and death in diabetics is due

Immune system support against infection
Decrease of oxidative stress from hyperglycemia
Decrease of platelet aggregation
Prevention of vascular complications including: Atherosclerosis (as well as heart disease & stroke) — Nephropathy (kidney damage) — Retinopathy (retinal damage) — Neuropathy (nerve damage)

TABLE 19: Possible help provided by elevated GSH levels

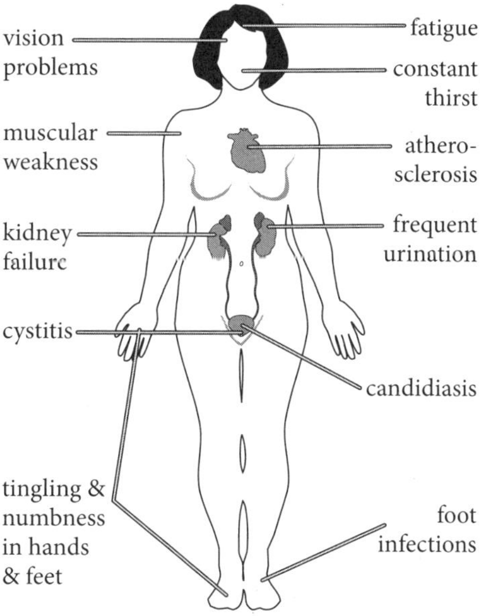

FIGURE 19: Living with Diabetes

to circulatory damage from heart disease, myocardial infarction, high blood pressure, atherosclerosis, stroke, renal failure, neuropathy, blindness and other effects of impaired blood circulation. Diabetic complications are the major cause of blindness in the USA. Diabetics are also more prone to cataracts and glaucoma (see Chapter 17).

Glutathione's role in diabetes

Although not primarily targeting blood glucose (sugar) levels, glutathione nevertheless plays a critical role in preventing long-term complications of diabetes. We have seen that it can prevent circulatory problems such as arteriosclerosis and stroke—the main causes of diabetic death (see Chapter 7). GSH also enhances the immune system. Many visits to the doctor or hospital would be avoided if diabetics were less prone to infection. Elevated GSH levels may help, as shown in Table 19.

Dozens of articles have been written to describe the high levels of oxidative stress, free radical damage and lowered GSH levels in both type 1 and type 2 diabetes. These descriptions show how this leads to long-term complications for diabetics. On the bright side, studies have correlated better glutathione status with improved outcomes, and several authors have suggested measuring glutathione levels as a way to mark progression of the disease.

There is strong circumstantial evidence for the importance of glutathione in diabetes. Some people suffer from genetic GSH abnormalities (polymorphisms), meaning they cannot make proper use of GSH. It appears their defective GSH genes render them prone to diabetes, and increase their risk of complications like diabetic retinopathy (eye disease), nephropathy (kidney disease), hyperlipidemia (cholesterol elevation), peripheral neuropathy (nerve damage), and morbid obesity.

Glutathione and blood sugar

Glutathione itself plays only a minor role in blood sugar control. However, researchers in the early 2000s who looked into diabetes and the body's use of cysteine (a vital glutathione precursor) correlated its availability with levels of insulin resistance.

Insulin in the blood of non-diabetics triggers healthy cells to absorb glucose (sugar), also circulating naturally in the blood. The cells of diabetics resist the influence of circulating insulin, putting them under a double threat: first, cells are starved of sugar; second, sugar accumulates in the blood to intolerable levels.

When insulin "resistance" is overcome at least to some degree, then more sugar is available to cells, and doesn't accumulate in circulating blood. Several good review articles detailing this approach are found in the references at the end of this chapter.

Glutathione and diabetic infection

Diabetics are, by definition, immune compromised. They have a higher rate of skin infection, bladder infection, pneumonia, gangrene, and other infectious complications than the non-diabetic population. The reasons for this are complex and varied. Not only does high sugar provide an excellent environment for bacterial growth, but because diabetics often have impaired circulation, this limits the flow of immune cells to fight a good battle. When researchers have examined more minute levels of immune impairment in diabetics, they have uncovered problems with specific types of white blood cells, specific immune signaling molecules and specific inflammatory agents. This opens the door to opportunistic infections from bacteria, fungi and other microbes.

Glutathione and diabetic cardiovascular disease

The major cause of complication and death in diabetes is from impaired circulation. Damaged microcirculation not only affects the eyes, kidneys and nerves of diabetic patients (see below), but also larger blood vessels, leading to heart attacks, stroke and other vascular catastrophes.

Damage to the arteries is complex, but two general statements can be made about diabetic circulation.

1) Vascular disease is closely tied to dangerous levels of circulating fat (such as cholesterol). When oxidized by free radicals, these fats (aka "lipids") become even more dangerous. This process is called "lipid peroxidation." The principal substance produced by the human body to prevent lipid peroxidation is the enzyme "glutathione peroxidase." Low glutathione leads to low glutathione peroxidase, freeing cholesterol and other lipids to do even more damage. For this reason, diabetics are placed on cholesterol-lowering medication earlier than non-diabetics.

2) The lining of the arteries (endothelium) is particularly sensitive to damage caused by the generalized inflammation of oxidative stress. This lining requires protection by higher-than-usual levels of glutathione. Without high GSH levels to keep it in check, oxidative damage may lead to swelling and plaque formation, platelet aggregation and organ damage.

Glutathione and diabetic neuropathy

Nerve damage ("neuropathy") commonly results from the restricted blood flow of poorly-controlled diabetes. This manifests from numbness or tingling in the hands and feet all the way to pure pain. Similarly, damage to digestive arteries causes digestive problems.

Diabetic neuropathy correlates with oxidative stress, free radical damage and low GSH levels. Studies show improvement in symptoms when GSH levels are restored.

Glutathione and diabetic kidney disease

In a similar process to diabetic neuropathy, both oxidative stress and microcirculatory damage lead to kidney disease. In the kidneys, another factor that comes into play are mitochondria—important structures in the cell responsible for energy production. Unfortunately, energy production requires high levels of oxygen and leads to oxidative stress. This impairs the kidney's bioenergetic processes and leads to kidney failure.

Nephrologists Sar, Saler & team have demonstrated the protective effects of NAC

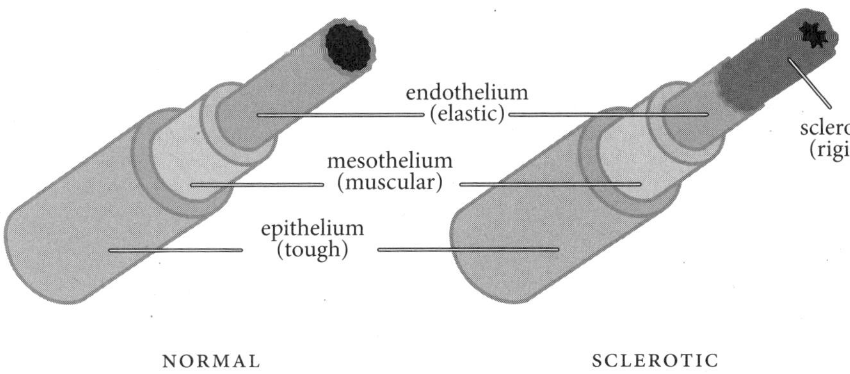

FIGURE 20: Blood vessels clogged by by-products of lipid peroxidation, leading to "sclerosis"

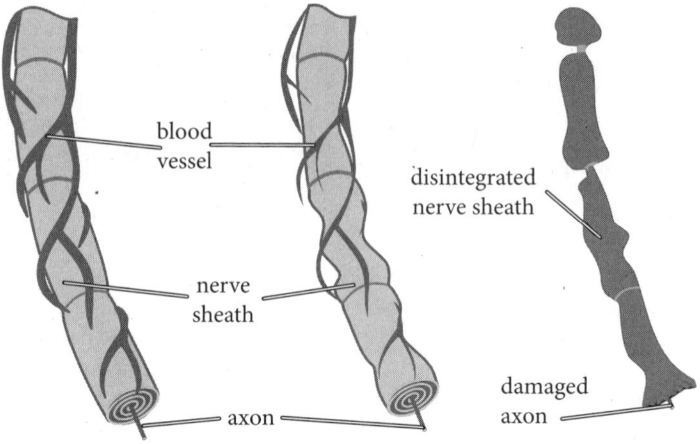

FIGURE 21: Progression of diabetic neuropathy

on the kidneys. Japanese researchers Osawa and Kato among others have demonstrated similar protective properties of GSH against kidney damage.

Glutathione and diabetic eye disease

Diabetic eye disease (retinopathy) results from damage to the visual receptors in the back lining of the eye—the "retina." Diabetic retinopathy is a preventable disease if diabetes is well controlled. The links between lowered glutathione levels and high oxidative stress are well documented. Although still in its early stages, intervention with NAC shows some promise in reducing the damage of diabetic retinopathy.

Case Study

DEANA WAS A MOTIVATED, POSITIVE ENTREPRENEUR who developed a wellness health center even though she suffered from serious diabetes. Increasingly fatigued, this 32 year-old Texan continued to run her center even after receiving and rejecting a kidney transplant, failing eyesight and dialysis treatments. Eventually she developed a chronic foot infection that required weekly debriding of dead tissue. Her doctor feared that amputation might prove necessary. She began taking high doses of CRWPI (a protein-based glutathione precursor) and her energy levels increased over several weeks. Kidney function tests and hemoglobin levels improved. Medication doses for her anemia and hypertension were decreased or eliminated. Peripheral circulation was better. Five months later the foot was healed. Deana has since married and continues to run her clinic.

Conclusion

Circulatory damage contributes substantially to diabetic complications, and GSH helps fight the oxidation that amplifies this damage. In fact, the blood and tissues of diabetics are marked by critically low GSH levels. These complications could be avoided or minimized by making diabetics less prone to infection. Elevated GSH levels may help to do just that (see Chapter 4).

DIABETES

REFERENCES

Asmat U, Abad K, Ismail K. *Diabetes mellitus & oxidative stress-A concise review.* Saudi Pharm J 24(5):547-553, 2016

Blouet C. et al. *Dietary cysteine alleviates sucrose-induced oxidative stress & insulin resistance. Free Radic Biol Med 42(7):1089-97, 2007*

Bravenboer B, Kappelle AC, Hamers FPT, Van Buren T, Erkelens DW, Gispen WH. *Potential use of glutathione for the prevention & treatment of diabetic neuropathy in the streptozotocin-induced diabetic rat.* Diabetologia 35:813-817, 1992

Carpi-Santos R. et al. *Early changes in system [Formula: see text] & glutathione in the retina of diabetic rats. Exp Eye Res 146:35-42, 2016*

Ceriello A, Curcio F, dello Russo P, Pegoraro I, Stel G, Amstad P, Cerutti P. *The defense against free radicals protects endothelial cells from hyperglycemia-induced plasminogen activator inhibitor 1 over-production.* Blood Coagulation & Fibrinolysis 6:133-137, 1995

Ceriello A, Giacomello R, Stel G, Motz E, Taboga C, Tonutti L, Pirisi M, Falleti E, Bartoli E. *Hyperglycemia-induced thrombin formation in diabetes. The possible role of oxidative stress.* Diabetes 44:924-928, 1995

Ceriello A, Motz E, Cavarape A, Lizzio S, Russo A, Quatraro A, Giugliano D. *Hyperglycemia counterbalances the antihypertensive effect of glutathione in diabetic patients: evidence linking hypertension & glycemia through the oxidative stress in diabetes mellitus.* Journal of Diabetes Complications 11:250-255, 1997

Ciuchi E, Odetti P, Prando R. *Relationship between glutathione & sorbitol concentrations in erythrocytes from diabetic patients.* Metabolism 45:611-613, 1996

Ciuchi E, Odetti P, Prando R. *The effect of acute glutathione treatment on sorbitol level in erythrocytes from diabetic patients.* Diabetes Metabolism 23:58-60, 1997

Curcio F, Ceriello A. *Decreased cultured endothelial cell proliferation in high glucose medium is reversed by antioxidants: new insights on the pathophysiological mechanisms of diabetic vascular complications.* In Vitro Cell Developmental Biology 28A: 787-790, 1992

Curcio F, Pegoraro I, dello Russo P, Falleti E, Perrella G, Ceriello A. *SOD & GSH inhibit the high glucose-induced oxidative damage & the PDGF increased secretion in cultured human endothelial cells.* Thrombolysis & Hemostasis: 74:969-973, 1995

Darmaun D, Smith SD, Sweeten S, Hartman BK, Welch S, Mauras N. *Poorly controlled type 1 diabetes is associated with altered GSH homeostasis in adolescents: apparent resistance to N-acetylcysteine supplementation.* Pediatr Diabetes 9(6):577-82, 2008

De Hann JB, Cooper ME. *Targeted antioxidant therapies in hyperglycemia-mediated endothelial dysfunction. Front Biosci 3:709-29, 2011*

Di Simplicio P, de Giorgio LA, Cardaioli E, Lecis R, Miceli M, Rossi R, Anichini R, Mian M, Seghieri G, Franconi F. *Glutathione, glutathione utilizing enzymes & thioltransferase in platelets of insulin-dependent diabetic patients: relation with platelet aggregation & with microangiographic complications.* European Journal of Clinical Investigation 25:665-669, 1995

Donnini D, Zambito AM, Perrella G, Ambesi-Impiombato FS, Curcio F. *Glucose may induce cell death through a free radical-mediated mechanism.* Biochem Biophys Research Communications 219:412-417, 1996

El-Bab MF, Zaki NS, Mojaddidi MA, Al-Barry M, El-Beshbishy HA. *Diabetic retinopathy is associated with oxidative stress & mitigation of gene expression of antioxidant enzymes.* Int J Gen Med 6:799-806, 2013

El Boghdady NA, Badr GA. *Evaluation of oxidative stress markers & vascular risk factors in patients with diabetic peripheral neuropathy.* Cell Biochem Funct 30(4):328-34, 2012

Gamage AM, Lee KO, Gan YH. *Effect of oral N-acetyl cysteine supplementation in type 2 diabetic patients on intracellular glutathione content & innate immune responses to Burkholderia pseudomallei.* Microbes Infect 16(8):661-71, 2014

Garcia-Fontana B. et al. *Relationship between Proinflammatory & Antioxidant Proteins with the Severity of Cardiovascular Disease in Type 2 Diabetes Mellitus. Int J Mol Sci 16(5):9469-83, 2015*

Gawlik K et al. *Markers of Antioxidant Defense in Patients with Type 2 Diabetes.* Oxid Med Cell Longev 2016:2352361, 2016

Gillani SW, Azeem E, Siddiqui A, Mian RI, Poh V. Sulaiman SA, Baig MR. *Oxidative Stress Correlates (OSC) in Diabetes Mellitus Patients. Curr Diabetes Rev 12(3):279-84, 2016*

González de Vega R, Fernández-Sánchez ML, Fernández JC, Alvarez-Menéndez FV, Sanz-Medel A. *Selenium levels & Glutathione peroxidase activity in the plasma of patients with type II diabetes mellitus. J Trace Elem Med Biol 37:44-49, 2016*

Goyal R, Singhai M, Faizy AF. *Glutathione*

peroxidase activity in obese & nonobese diabetic patients & role of hyperglycemia in oxidative stress. J Midlife Health 2(2):72-6, 2011

Hakki Kalkan I, Suher M. *The relationship between the level of glutathione, impairment of glucose metabolism & complications of diabetes mellitus.* Pak J Med Sci 29(4):938-42, 2013

Harmon JS. et al. *beta-Cell-specific overexpression of glutathione peroxidase preserves intranuclear MafA & reverses diabetes in db/db mice. Endocrinology 150(11):4855-62, 2009*

Hermers-Uliana C. et al. *Is L-glutathione more effective thaqn L-glutamine in preventing enteric diabetic neuropathy?* Dig Dis Sci 59(5):937-48, 2014

Hernandez Guerrero C. et al. *Glutathione peroxidase-1 pro200Leu polymorphism (RS1050450) is associated with morbid obesity independently of the presence of prediabetes or diabetes in women from Central Mexico.* Nutr Hosp 32(4):1516-25, 2015

Jain SK. *L-cysteine supplementation as an adjuvant therapy for type 2 diabetes. Can J Physiol Pharmacol 90(8):1061-4, 2012*

Jain SK, McVie R. *Effect of glycemic control, race & duration of diabetes on reduced glutathione content in erythrocytes of diabetic patients.* Metabolism 43:306-309, 1994

Jain SK, Micinski D, Huning L, Kahlon G, Bass PF, Levine SN. *Vitamin-D & L-cysteine levels correlate positively with GSH & negatively with insulin resistance levels in the blood of type 2 diabetic patients. Eur J Clin Nutr 68(10):1148-53, 2014*

Kakkar R, Mantha SV, Radhi J, Prasad K, Kalra J. *Antioxidant defense system in diabetic kidney: a time course study.* Life Science 60:667-679, 1997

Kamboj SS, Vasishta RK, Sandhir R. *N-acetylcysteine inhibits hyperglycemia-induced oxidative stress & apoptosis markers in diabetic neuropathy.* J Neurochem 112(1):77-91, 2010

Kashiwagi A, Asahina T, Nishio Y, Ikebuchi M, Tanaka Y, Kikkawa R, Shigeta Y. *Glycation, oxidative stress, & scavenger activity: glucose metabolism & radical scavenger dysfunction in endothelial cells.* Diabetes 45:S84-S86, 1996

Kasznicki J. et al. *Evaluation of oxidative stress markers in pathogenesis of diabetic neuropathy.* Mol Biol Rep 39(9):8669-78, 2012

Kornhauser C, Garcia-Ramirez JR, Wrobel K, Perez-Luque EL, Garay-Sevilla ME, Wrobel K. *Serum selenium & glutathione peroxidase concentrations in type 2 diabetes mellitus patients. Prim Care Diabetes 2(2):81-5, 2008.*

Kulkarni R, Acharya J, Ghaskadbi S, Goel P. *Oxidative stress as a covariate of recovery in diabetes therapy. Front Endocrinol (Lausanne) 5:89, 2014*

Kundu D, Mandal T, Nandi M, Osta M, Bandyopadhyay U, Ray D. *Oxidative stress in diabetic patients with retinopathy. Ann Afr Med 13(1):41-6, 2014*

Langman M. et al. *Investigating the causes for decreased levels of glutathione in individuals with type II diabetes. Plos One 10(3):e0118436, 2015*

Lash LH. *Mitochondrial Glutathione in Diabetic Nephropathy.* J Clin Med 4(7):1428-47, 2015

Lasram MM, Dhouib IB, Annabi A, El Fazaa S, Gharbi N. *A review on the possible molecular mechanism of action of N-acetylcysteine against insulin resistance & type-2 diabetes development. Clin Biochem 48(16-17):1200-8, 2015*

Lee DH, Jacobs DR Jr. *Hormesis & public health: can glutathione depletion & mitochondrial dysfunction due to very low-dose chronic exposure to persistent organic pollutants be mitigated?* J Epidemiol Community Health 69(3):294-300, 2015

Lei XG, Vatamaniuk MZ. *Two tales of antioxidant enzymes on β cells & diabetes. Antioxid Redox Signal 14(3):489-503, 2011*

Li S. et al. *Impacat of glutathione-HbA1c on HbA1c measurement in diabetes diagnosis via array isoelectric focusing, liquid chromatography, mass spectrometry & ELISA.* Talanta 115:323-8, 2013

Low PA, Nickander KK, Tritschler HJ. *The roles of oxidative stress & antioxidant treatment in experimental diabetic neuropathy.* Diabetes 46:S38-S42, 1997

Mastana SS, Kaur A, Hale R, Lindley MR. *Influence of glutathione S-transferase polymorphisms (GSTT1, GSTM1, GSTP1) on type-2 diabetes mellitus (T2D) risk in an endogamous population from north India.* Mol Biol Rep 40(12):7103-10, 2013

Mendez MM. et al. *Altered glutathione system is associated with the presence of distal symmetric peripheral polyneuropathy in type 2 diabetic.* J Diabetes Complications 29(7):923-7, 2015

Moasser E, Azarpira N, Shirazi B, Saadat M, Geramizadeh B. *Genetic polymorphisms of glutathione-s-transferase M1 & T1 genes with risk of diabetic retinopathy in Iranian population. Iran J Basic Med Sci 17(5):351-6*

Mohammedi K. et al. *Glutathione peroxidase-1 gene (GPX1) variants, oxidative stress & risk of kidney complications in people with type 1 diabetes.* Metabolism 65(2):12-9, 2016

Murakami K, Kondo T, Ohtsuka Y, Fujiwara Y, Shimanda M, Kawakami Y. *Impairment of glutathione metabolism in erythrocytes from patients with diabetes mellitus.* Metabolism 38:753-758, 1989

Orlewski J, Orlewska E. *Effects of genetic polymorphisms of glutathione S-transferase genes (GSTM1, GSTT1, GSTP1) on the risk of diabetic nephropathy: a meta-analysis. Pol Arch Med Wewn 125(9):649-58, 2015*

Osawa T, Kato Y. *Protective role of antioxidative food factors in oxidative stress caused by hyperglycemia.* Ann N Y Acad Sci 1043:440-51, 2005

Pinheiro DS. et al. *Evaluation of glutathione S-transferase GSTM1 & GSTT1 deletion polymorphisms on type-2 diabetes mellitus risk. PLoS One 8(10):e76262, 2013*

Pieme CA et al. *Relationship between hyperglycemia, antioxidant capacity & some enzymatic & non-enzymatic antioxidants in African patients with type 2 diabetes. BMC Res Notes 10(1):141, 2017*

Pittaluga M, Sgadari A, Dimauro I, Tavayyi B, Parisi P, Caporossi D. *Physical exercise & redox balance in type 2 diabetics: effects of moderate training on biomarkers of oxidative stress & DNA damage evaluated through comet assay. Oxid Med Cell Longev 2015:981242, 2015*

Reddy VS, Agrawal P, Sethi S, Gupta N, Garg R, Madaan H, Kumar V. *Associations of FPG, A1C & disease duration with protein markers of oxidative damage & antioxidative defense in type 2 diabetes & diabetic retinopathy.* Eye (Lond) 29(12):1585-93, 2015

Rodriguez-Carrizalez et al. *Oxidants, antioxidants & mitochondrial function in non-proliferative3 diabetic retinopathy.* J Diabetes 6(2):167-75, 2014

Rudich A, Kozlovsky N, Potashnik R, Bashan N. *Oxidant stress reduces insulin responsiveness in 3T3-L1 adipocytes.* American Journal of Physiology 272:E935-E940, 1997

Ruskovska T, Berniohr DA. *Oxidative stress & protein carbonylation in adipose tissue-implications for insulin resistance & diabetes mellitus. J Proteomics 92:323-34, 2013*

Saadat M. *Null genotypes of glutathione S-transferase M1 (GSTM1) & T1 (GSTT1) polymorphisms increased susceptibility to type 2 diabetes mellitus, a meta-analysis.* Gene 532(1):160-2, 2013

Sánchez-Gómez FJ, Espinosa Diez C, Dubey M, Dikshit M, Lamas S. *S-glutathionylation: relevance in diabetes & potential role as a biomarker. Biol Chem 394(10):1263-80, 2013*

Sar F, Saler T, Ecebay A, Saglam ZA, Ozturk S, Kazancioglu R. *The efficacy of n-acetlcysteine in preventing contrast-induced nephropathy in type 2 diabetic patients without nephropathy.* J Nephrol 23(4):478-82, 2010

Sedighi O, Markhlough A, Shorkrzadeh M, Hoorshad S. *Association between plasma selenium & glutathione peroxidase levels & severity of diabetic nephropathy in patients with type two diabetes mellitus.* Nephrourol Mon 6(5):e21355, 2014

Stoian A. et al. *Influence of GSTM1, GSTT1, & GSTP1 Polymorphisms on Type 2 Diabetes Mellitus & Diabetic Sensorimotor Peripheral Neuropathy Risk. Dis Markers 2015:638693, 2015*

Sun L, Zhang Y, Xiong Y. *GSTM1 & GSTT1 null genotype & diabetic retinopathy: a meta-analysis. Int J Clin Exp Med 8(2):1677-83, 2015*

Sundaram RK, Bhaskar A, Vijayalingam S, Viswanathan M, Mohan R, Shanmugasundaram KR. *Antioxidant status & lipid peroxidation in Type II diabetes mellitus with & without complications.* Clinical Science 90:255-260, 1996

Tan KS. et al. *GSH deficiency in type 2 diabetes impairs cytokine responses & control of intracellular bacteria. J Clin Invest 122(6):2289-300, 2012*

Tesauro M. et al. *The possible role of glutathione-S-transferase activity in diabetic nephropathy.* Int J Immunopathol Pharmacol 28(1):129-33, 2015

Thornalley PJ, McLellan AC, Lo TW, Benn J, Sonksen PH. *Negative association between erythrocyte reduced glutathione concentration & diabetic complications.* Clin Sci (Lond) 91(5):575-82, 1996

Tsai GY. et al. *Effect of N-acetylcysteine on the early expression of inflammatory markers in the retina & plasma of diabetic rats. Clin Exp Ophthalmol 37(2):223-31, 2009*

Tsai CJ, Hsieh CJ, Tung SC, Kuo MC, Shen FC. *Acute blood glucose fluctuations can decrease blood GSH & adiponectin levels in patients with type 2 diabetes.* Diabetes Res Clin Pract 98(2):257-63, 2012

Thornalley PJ, McLellan AC, Lo TW, Benn J, Sonksen PH. *Negative association between erythrocyte reduced glutathione concentration & diabetic complications.* Clinical Science 91:575-582, 1996

Vats P, Sagar N, Singh TP, Banerjee M. *Association of Superoxide dismutases (SOD1 & SOD2) & Glutathione peroxidase 1 (GPx1) gene polymorphisms with type 2 diabetes mellitus. Free Radic Res 49(1):17-24, 2015*

Vijayalingam S, Parthiban A, Shanmugasundaram KR, Mohan V. *Abnormal antioxidant status in impaired glucose tolerance & non-insulin-dependent diabetes mellitus.* Diabetic Medicine 13:715-719, 1996

Waggiallah H, Alzohairy M. *The effect of oxidative stress on human red cells glutathione peroxidase, GSH reductase level, & prevalence of anemia among diabetics.* N Am J Med Sci 3(7);344-7, 2011

Wright WS. et al. *Influence of glutathione on the electroretinogram in diabetic & non-diabetic rats.* Curr Eye Res 36(9):831-7, 2011

Yoshida K, Hirokawa J, Tagami S, Kawakami Y, Urata Y, Kondo T. *Weakened cellular scavenging activity against oxidative stress in diabetes mellitus: regulation of glutathione synthesis & efflux.* Diabetologia 38:201-210, 1995

Zhu Y, Zhang XL, Zhu BF, Ding YN. *Effect of antioxidant NAC on diabetic retinopathy & expression of VEGF & ICAM-1 from retinal blood vessels of diabetic rats.* Mol Biol Rep 39(4):3727-35, 2012

9

The Liver & Hepatitis

Hepatitis is an inflammation of the liver. The two main types in North America are alcoholic hepatitis (a type of toxic hepatitis) and infectious (viral) hepatitis, usually caused by virus types A, B or C. Other liver problems in this chapter include fatty liver (steatohepatitis), autoimmune hepatitis and other toxin-related liver damage.

Toxic hepatitis

Toxic hepatitis is a non-infectious condition caused by exposure to chemicals that damage the liver. The list of harmful agents is quite extensive, but simple alcohol abuse accounts for the vast majority of cases. Alcoholism tends to be a chronic disease, and this prolonged inflammation often leads to cirrhosis—replacement of healthy liver cells by scar tissue.

It's a surprise to many people that the second most common drug used in an intentional overdose or suicide attempts is acetaminophen (also called paracetamol and known under the trade names Tylenol, Atasol and others). The most common overdosed toxin in these patients is alcohol, but acetaminophen can actually be deadly in sufficient amounts. A large

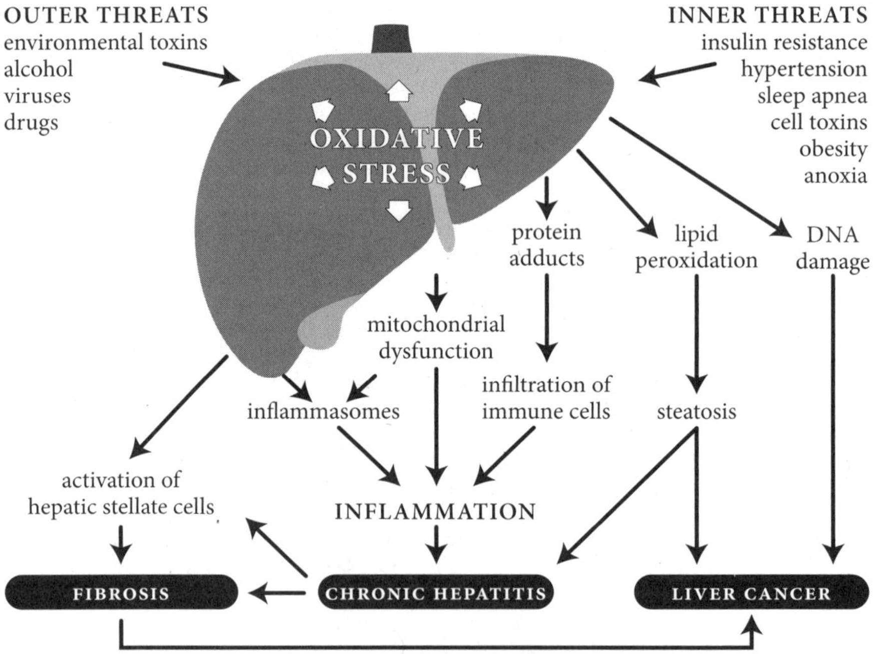

Figure 22: Toxins, disease and oxidative stress contribute to hepatitis and other liver ailments

bottle of extra-strength acetaminophen can potentially kill. Children's acetaminophen doses are intentionally distributed in very small bottles to prevent accidental overdose.

Acetaminophen damages the liver by producing unopposed oxidative stress and by depleting glutathione. Although conventional doctors are not necessarily well-versed in glutathione, they know one thing about it for sure—the drug NAC (a potent GSH precursor) is the antidote to acetaminophen overdose. This is the oldest and most widespread use of NAC in conventional medicine. Massive doses (up to 40 grams) are sometimes used to save a life.

NAC treatment has also been used to counter mushroom poisoning, sulfur mustard exposure, phosgene inhalation, paraquat ingestion, arsenic and other toxic exposures leading to liver damage.

Infectious hepatitis

Infectious hepatitis is the most common of all serious infectious diseases in North America. It is estimated that as many as a half million Americans per year contract the disease. Given the growing prevalence of a relatively newly-recognized hepatitis virus—Type C—this number is likely to increase. An accurate count is difficult because most cases of acute hepatitis go undiagnosed or unreported—the illness often feels no more serious than the flu. Other viruses and pathogens can cause hepatitis, but less frequently than hepatitis virus types A, B and C (see Table 20).

The course of the disease is variable. It can range from being entirely without symptoms to (in few cases) causing death. Most people with infectious hepatitis suffer a few weeks of a flu-like illness consisting of fatigue, aches and pains, mild fever, loss of appetite, abdominal pain, nausea and vomiting. More serious cases exhibit jaundice, dark colored urine, light colored stools, itching and altered mental states lapsing occasionally into coma. Most patients experience full recovery, but some progress to chronic hepatitis and sometimes cirrhosis.

The extent of liver inflammation determines how poorly the liver works. In hepatic dysfunction it cannot filter and eliminate toxins, help digestion, regulate the chemical composition of the blood, process and store nutrients, and perform other vital functions. The extent of dysfunction can be determined by liver function tests (LFT's), a measure of certain liver enzymes in the blood. LFT's are a sensitive indicator of the liver's health.

Treatment for acute hepatitis usually promotes a conservative regimen—lots of rest, good nutrition and plenty of fluids. Special care must be taken to avoid spreading the disease, which is highly contagious.

Chronic hepatitis

Some cases of toxic or infectious hepatitis decline further into chronic hepatitis. Chronic cases may be treated with steroids or interferon. In both cases, benefits need to be weighed against side-effects. In toxic hepatitis, the patient must be removed from the offending toxin. This is challenging when the cause is alcohol dependency.

Prevention

All forms of hepatitis can be prevented through sanitation and hygiene, as well as screening of blood products and vaccination. One should also beware of such toxins as alcohol and intravenous drugs and take special care to avoid contact with the bodily fluids of infected people.

	HEPATITIS A	HEPATITIS B	HEPATITIS C
transmission	Fecal contamination of water and food. Feces are infected from two to three weeks before until eight days after onset of jaundice.	Contaminated blood transfusions, sexual exchange of bodily fluids, needle-sharing. Transmission possible from mother to unborn child.	Shared hypodermic needles, unprotected sex and pre-1992 blood transfusions. Transmission possible from mother to unborn child.
symptoms	Flu-like symptoms such as fatigue, stomach and intestinal pain, appetite loss, nausea, diarrhea, darkened urine and jaundice. Occasionally symptom-free.	Jaundice, fatigue, abdominal pain, joint pain, loss of appetite, nausea and vomiting. May lead to liver cirrhosis or cancer. Most infected people do not develop chronic infection. Occasionally symptom-free.	Usually without acute symptoms. Fatigue, abdominal and joint pain, loss of appetite, jaundice, nausea and vomiting. Can cause chronic liver damage including cirrhosis and cancer.
traditional treatment	Bed rest, increased fluid intake, Vaccines available. Immunization with immunoglobulin.	Interferon reduces chances of recurrence and is effective in 30-40% of cases. Vaccines available.	Interferon. If not effective, Rebetron, a combination of interferon and ribavirin. No vaccine.
infections per year	Up to 200,000	From 150,000 to 300,000	From 150,000 to 300,000

TABLE 20: Three types of hepatitis

GSH in the liver

Hepatologists (liver specialists) know that GSH plays a critical role in the liver—it is that organ's most abundant antioxidant enzyme. We've already noted that GSH concentrations are higher in the liver than any other organ. This is because it functions as a substrate for key detoxification processes in the liver (see Chapter 2).

Phase I liver detoxification transforms toxins into a water-soluble form suitable for disposal. GSH appears in Phase II, when it neutralizes or conjugates these products, helping the body remove them through the gut or kidneys. If either of these two detoxification phases is impaired, toxins accumulate in the body and lead to disease.

Medical science has long known that GSH deficiency invariably accompanies liver damage. When hepatitis results from acute overdoses of hepatotoxic pharmaceutical drugs such as acetaminophen (Tylenol, Atasol, etc.), the GSH-enhancing drug NAC (N-acetylcysteine) is used to raise GSH levels rapidly. This eliminates the toxic breakdown products of the overdose. If the GSH deficiency is not addressed, the illness is compounded and falls into a downward spiral.

The liver produces less GSH when overcome by alcoholic cirrhosis, sicknesses due to exposure to hydrocarbons and other toxins, viral hepatitis, fatty livers and even aging individuals. Ongoing research aims to raise GSH levels in an attempt to support liver function in patients with these ailments. This approach is even being explored in the treatment of fulminant (acute) hepatic failure.

GSH and alcoholic hepatitis

Alcoholic liver disease is the leading cause of death from liver disease in the world. Alcoholic patients with lower GSH levels are more prone to liver damage. This has prompted researchers to try to treat alcoholic liver disease by raising GSH levels, and both clinical symptoms and liver function test results have improved with this method.

Several natural products that raise glutathione have been used in attempts to aid alcoholic hepatitis. They include silymarin, milk thistle, SAMe (S-adenosyl-methionine), curcumin and whey protein. The pharmaceutical drug NAC (N-acetylcysteine) (common in the treatment of acetaminophen overdose) has also shown promise in treating alcoholic hepatitis.

GSH in the treatment of viral hepatitis

Weiss and his team at the Max Planck Institute demonstrated the antiviral properties of NAC in human tissue cultures. Watanabe found that undenatured whey protein, a natural GSH precursor, was effective in improving liver function abnormalities and immunological parameters in hepatitis B patients. Improvements continued even after treatment ended, reflecting the long-term benefits of this approach.

Treatment options for chronic hepatitis C sufferers are far from ideal. Barbaro's team in Italy eloquently described the systemic depletion of GSH in hepatitis C patients, suggesting how this deficiency could account for their resistance to interferon therapy. Beloqui's team confirmed their hypothesis in a controlled study of hepatitis C positive individuals. By successfully raising one group's GSH levels with NAC therapy, they showed that interferon therapy was enhanced.

Watanabe and his group in Japan conducted several studies with a specially-prepared whey protein isolate, treating patients with either hepatitis B or C. Improvements in liver function tests gave impetus for further studies using this glutathione precursor protein.

GSH and autoimmune hepatitis

When the immune system attacks its own body, the result is autoimmune disease. In the case of autoimmune hepatitis, the liver is the target, and liver failure can ensue. Studies of patients have noted both free radical damage and reduced GSH levels. Those with genetic errors in GSH metabolism are at greater risk of developing autoimmune hepatitis. Studies using glutathione-related treatment compounds have yet to be developed.

GSH and fatty liver

The development of a fatty liver, known as "steatohepatitis" is commonly seen in alcoholic hepatitis. However, cases of "non-alcoholic steatohepatitis (NASH)" are known, and may result from metabolic syndrome, diabetes, or obesity. This can lead to cirrhosis (hardening) of the liver and eventual liver failure.

Glutathione is clearly implicated in the pathogenesis of this disease. High levels of oxidative stress and concomitant low levels of glutathione are its hallmarks.

Investigators have looked into the use of antioxidants to treat fatty liver. The glutathione precursor NAC has shown promise, first with test tube studies, next in animal models, and now in human trials as well.

Whey proteins have also shown promise, initially in animal studies and later in humans. A group from Thailand was the first

Death rate:	20,000 per year and rising. May double in next ten years
Prevalence:	4 million Americans; four times more than AIDS
Percentage that will develop chronic hepatitis:	80%
Percentage that will develop cirrhosis:	20%
Percentage that will develop liver cancer:	5%
Success rate of Interferon treatment:	20%

TABLE 21: Hepatitis C: some important numbers

to demonstrate positive results in patients with NASH using a CRWPI (cysteine-rich whey protein isolate). Improvements in liver biochemical tests, blood glutathione and macrovascular steatosis (fat accumulation in the liver blood vessels) were all remarked on.

Case study

WHEN HE WAS YOUNG, Roger required multiple blood transfusions for hemophilia, a bleeding disorder. As a young adult his liver was tested for abnormal function and the results revealed that he had acquired hepatitis C, probably from contaminated blood. Worried about the side-effects of antiviral medications (as well as their limited success) he preferred to undergo unconventional treatment. His protocol included milk thistle (silymarin), turmeric (curcuma), alpha lipoic acid, methionine, N-acetylcysteine, and intravenous glutathione as well as a low-meat diet and avoidance of alcohol, acetaminophen and cigarettes. His liver function tests have since normalized.

Conclusion

The liver is the largest and one of the most complicated organs in your body. It is subject to a myriad of factors affecting health and illness (see Figure 21). GSH is a key constituent of proper liver function. Low GSH levels invite a host of toxicological and immunological diseases including viral hepatitis, alcoholic hepatitis, fatty liver disease and others. Higher levels of glutathione offer protection against these maladies.

THE LIVER & HEPATITIS

REFERENCES

ANKRAH NA, RIKIMARU T, EKUBAN FA, *Addae MM. Decreased cysteine & glutathione levels: possible determinants of liver toxicity in Ghanaian subjects.* Journal of Int. Medical Research 22:171-176, 1994

BARBARO G, DI LORENZO G, SOLDINI M, ET AL. *Hepatic glutathione deficiency in chronic hepatitis C: quantitative evaluation in patients who are hiv positive & hiv negative & correlations with plasmatic & lymphocytic concentrations & with the activity of the liver disease.* American Journal of Gastroenterology 91:2569-2573, 1996

BELOQUI O, PRIETO J, SUAREZ M, GIL B, QIAN CH, GARCIA N, CIVEIRA MP. *N-acetyl cysteine enhances the response to interferon-α in chronic hepatitis C: a pilot study.* Journal of Interferon Research 13:279-282, 1993

BRESCI G, PICCINOCCHI M, BANTI S. *The use of reduced glutathione in alcoholic hepatopathy.Minerva Medicine 82:753-755, 1991*

CHEN Y, DONG H, THOMPSON DC, SHERTZER HG, NERBERT DW, VASILIOU V. *Glutathione defense mechanism in liver injury: insights from animal models.* Food Chem Toxicol 60:38-44, 2013

Chitapanarux T, Tienboon P, Pojchamarnwiputh S, Leelarungrayub D. *Open-labeled pilot study of cysteine-rich whey protein isolate supplementation for non-alcoholic steatohepatitis patients.* J Gastroenterol Hepatol 24(6):1045-50, 2009

Choi J. *Oxidative stress, endogenous antioxidants, alcohol, & hepatitis C: pathogenic interactions & therapeutic considerations.* Free Radic Biol Med 52(7):1135-50, 2012

Chughlay MF, Kramer N, Spearman CW, Werfalli M, Cohen K. *N-acetylcysteine for non-paracetamol drug induced liver injury: a systematic review.* Br J Clin Pharmacol 81(6):1021-9, 2016

Chughlay MF, Kramer N, Werfalli M, Spearman W, Engel ME, Cohen K. *N-acetylcysteine for non-paracetamol drug induced liver injury: a systematic review protocol.* Syst Rev 4:84, 2015

Czuczejko J, Zachara BA, Staubach-Topczewska E, Halota W, Kedziora J. *Selenium, glutathione & glutathione peroxidases in blood of patients with chronic liver diseases.* Acta Blochim Pol 50(4):1147-54, 2003

Czaja AJ. *Nature & Implications of Oxidative & Nitrosative Stresses in Autoimmune Hepatitis. Dig Dis Sci 61(10):2784-2803, 2016*

De Andrade KQ, Moura FA, dos Santos JM, de Araujo OR, de Farias Santos JC, Goulart MO. *Oxidative Stress & Inflammation in Hepatic Diseases:* Therapeutic Possibilities of N-Acetylcysteine. Int J Mol Sci 16(12):30269-308, 2015

Dentico P, Volpe A, Buongiorno R, et al. *GSH in the treatment of chronic fatty liver diseases.* Recenti Prog Med. 1995 Jul-Aug;86(7-8):290-3.

El-Lakkany NM, Seif El-Din SH, Sabra AA, Hammam OA, Ebeid FA. *Co-administration of metformin & N-acetylcysteine with dietary control improves the biochemical & histological manifestations in rats with non-alcoholic fatty liver.* Res Pharm Sci 11(5):374-382, 2016

Engin A. *Non-Alcoholic Fatty Liver Disease.* Adv Exp Med Biol 960.443-467, 2017

Farinati F, Cardin R, De Maria N, et al. *Iron storage, lipid peroxidation & glutathione turnover in chronic anti-HCV positive hepatitis. Journal of Hepatology 22:449-456, 1995*

Ghosh N, Ghosh R, Mandal V, Mandal SC. *Recent advances in herbal medicine for treatment of liver diseases.* Pharm Biol 49(9):970-88, 2011

Hamad EM, Taha SH, Abou Dawood AG, Sitohy MZ, Abdel-Hamid M. *Protective effect of whey proteins against non-alcoholic fatty liver in rats.* Lipids Health Dis 10:57, 2011

Harrison PM, Wendon JA, Gimson AES, Alexander GJM, Williams R. *Improvement by acetylcysteine of hemodynamics & oxygen transport in fulminant hepatic failure.* New England Journal of Medicine 324:1852-1857, 1991

Heard K, Green J. *Acetylcysteine therapy for acetaminophen poisoning. Curr Pharm Biotechnol 13(10):1917-23, 2012*

Honda Y, et al. *Efficacy of glutathione for the treatment of non-alcoholic fatty liver disease:* an open-label, single arm, multicenter, pilot study. BMC Gastroenterol 17(1):96, 2017

Jewell SA, Di Monte D, Gentile A, Guglielmi A, Altomare E, Albano O. *Decreased hepatic glutathione in chronic alcoholic patients.* Journal of Hepatology 3:1-6, 1986

Kaffe ET, Rigopoulou EI, Koukoulis GK, Dalekos GN, Moulas AN. *Oxidative stress & antioxidant status in patients with autoimmune liver diseases.* Redox Rep 20(1):33-41, 2015

Kato T, Miyakawa H, Ishibashi M. *Frequency & significance of anti-glutathione S-transferase autoantibody (anti-GST A1-1) in autoimmune hepatitis.* J Autoimmun 22(3):211-6, 2004

Lieber CS. *Susceptibility to alcohol-related liver injury.* Alcohol 2(supple):315-326, 1994

Liu W, Baker SS, Baker RD, Zhu L. *Antioxidant Mechanisms in Nonalcoholic Fatty Liver Disease.* Curr Drug Targets 16(12):1301-14, 2015

Loguercio C, Federico A. *Oxidative stress in viral & alcoholic hepatitis.* Free Radic Biol Med 34(1):1-10, 2003

Loguercio C, Taranto D, Vitale LM, Beneduce F, Del Vecchio, Blanco C. *Effect of liver cirrhosis & age on the glutathione concentration in the plasma, erythrocytes, & gastric mucosa.* Free Radical Biology Medicine 20:483-488, 1996

Lozano-Sepulveda SA, Bryan-Marrugo OL, Cordova-Fletes C, Gutierrez-Ruiz MC, Rivas-Estilla AM. *Oxidative stress modulation in hepatitis C virus infected cells. World J Hepatol 7(29):2880-9, 2015*

Mokhtari V, Afsharian P, Shahhoseini M, Kalantar SM, Moini A. *A Review on Various Uses of N-Acetyl Cysteine. Cell J 19(1):11-17, 2017*

Mulder TP, Janssens AR, De Bruin WC, et al. *Plasma glutathione S-transferase alpha 1-1 levels in patients with chronic liver disorders.* Clin Chim Acta. 1997 Feb 3;258(1):69-77.

Nardi EA, Devito R, Ceccanti M. *High-dose glutathione in the therapy of alcoholic hepatopathy. Clinical Ter. 136:47-51, 1991*

Nguyen-Khac E, et al. *Glucocorticoids plus N-acetylcysteine in severe alcoholic hepatitis. N Eng J Med 365(19):1781-9, 2011*

Paracha UZ, Fatima K, Algahtani M, Chaudhary A, Abuzenadah A, Damanhouri

G, Qadri I. *Oxidative stress & hepatitis C virus.* Virol J 10:251, 2013

Pemberton PW, Aboutwerat A, Smith A, Burrows PC, McMahon RF, Warnes TW. *Oxidant stress in type I autoimmune hepatitis: the link between necroinflammation & fibrogenesis? Biochim Biophys Acta 1689(3):182-9, 2004*

Pradhan SC, Girish C. *Hepatoprotective herbal drug, silymarin from experimental pharmacology to clinical medicine.* Indian J Med Res 124(5):491-504, 2006

Pressman AH. *The GSH Phenomenon* St. Martin's Press, New York NY, 1997

Miscellaneous Proceedings *of the 16th International Congress of Nutrition.* Montreal, PR514, 1997

Rolo AP, Teodoro JS, Palmeira CM. *Role of oxidative stress in the pathogenesis of nonalcoholic steatohepatitis.* Free Radic Biol Med 52(1):59-69, 2012

Sagias FG, et al. *N-acetylcysteine improves the viability of human hepatocytes isolated from severely steatotic donor liver tissue.* N-acetylcysteine improves the viability of human hepatocytes isolated from severely steatotic donor liver tissue. Cell Transplant 19(11):1487-92, 2010

Salcedo M, et al. *Risk factors for developing de novo autoimmune hepatitis associated with anti-glutathione S-transferase T1 antibodies after liver transplantation.* Liver Transpl 15(5):539-9, 2009

Savolainen VT, Pjarinen J, Perola M, Penttila A, Karhunen PJ. *Glutathione S-transferase GST M1 "null" genotype & the risk of alcoholic liver disease.* Alcohol Clinical Experimental Research 20:1340-1345, 1996

Testino G, Leone S, Ansaldi F, Borro P. *Silymarin & S-adenosyl-L-methionine (SAMe): two promising pharmacological agents in case of chronic alcoholic hepathopathy. A review & a point of view.* Minerva Gastroenterol Dietol 59(4):341-56, 2013

Watanabe A, Okada K, Shimizu Y, Wakabayashi H, Higuchi K, Niiya K, Kuwabara Y, Yasuyama T, Ito H, Tsukishiro T, Kondoh Y, Emi N, Kohri H *Nutritional therapy of chronic hepatitis by whey protein (non-heated).* J Med. 2000;31(5-6):283-302

Watanabe A, Higuchi K, Yasumura Y, Shimizu Y, Kondo Y, Kohri H. *Nutritional modulation of glutathione level & cellular immunity in chronic hepatitis B & C.* Hepatology 24: pt2: 597A

Weiss L, Hildt E, Hofschneider PH. *Anti-hepatitis B virus activity of N-acetyl-L-cysteine (nac): New aspects of a well-established drug.* Antiviral Research 32:43-53, 1996

Wellington K, Jarvis B. *Silymarin: a review of its clinical properties in the management of hepatic disorders.* BioDrugs 15(7):465-89, 2001

Yuan L, Kaplowitz N. *Glutathione in liver diseases & hepatotoxicity.* Mol Aspects Med 30(1-2):29-41, 2009

10

Anemia

Introduction

Anemia, in general terms, is a condition where red blood cells are insufficient in number or activity to provide our cells and tissues with enough oxygen for normal function. The most common laboratory tests to confirm anemia are measurements of "hemoglobin" or "hematocrit", although more sophisticated tests exist, which may shed light on the cause of the anemia.

The incidence of anemia varies in different populations, depending on economic factors, sex, age, and pregnancy. Highest levels of anemia exist in pregnant women, menstruating women, children and the geriatric population. Although numbers vary depending on geographic location, it would be safe to say that between 10 and 20% of individuals suffer from anemia.

The treatment of anemia depends on what is causing it. Often an underlying nutrient deficiency may exist, the person may be losing blood (acutely or chronically), too few red blood cells may be manufactured by the body, or an underlying genetic defect is at play. The mainstay treatment for very severe anemia is blood cell transfusion, although this treatment is unacceptable in certain populations.

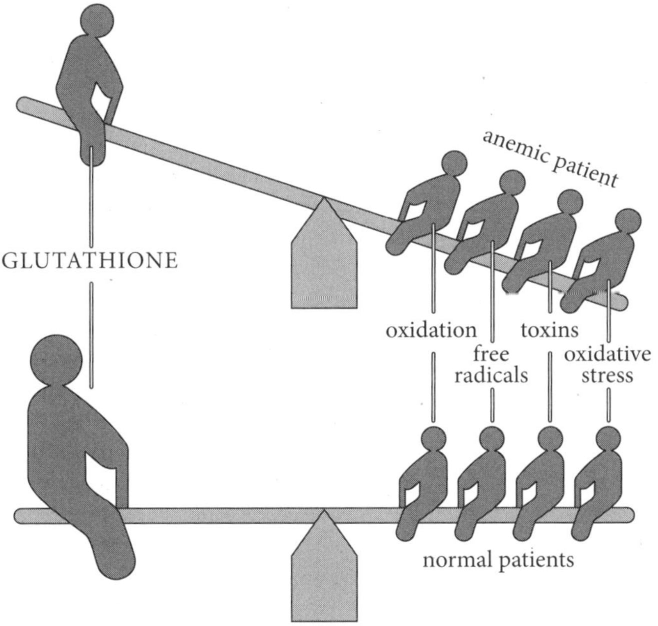

FIGURE 23: Tipping the balance away from anemia

There are several ways to classify anemia. Here, we will separate these into: 1) Destruction of red blood cells, 2) Decreased production of red blood cells, and 3) Blood loss (acute or chronic). Examples of these will be examined in turn, investigating the possible role of raising glutathione in improving the anemia.

Destruction of red blood cells (Hemolytic Anemia)

Sickle Cell Anemia, Falciform Anemia

Sickle cell disease is a condition in which red blood cells may be provoked into changing their appearance from a rounded disk shape to a sickle (falciform) shape. Normal disk-shaped blood cells easily slip through narrow blood vessels, but the crescent-shaped sickles have sharp edges which get trapped in narrow passageways and cause obstructions, decreased blood flow and damage from oxygen starvation of the affected tissues.

Sickling can be caused by a number of different events, most commonly: exercise, which can cause a shortage of oxygen; everyday stress; dehydration from either drinking less liquids or losing fluids to sweating, diarrhea or fever; infection; smoking and other toxic exposures.

A common feature to these events is the increased production of free radicals and oxidative stress, both of which tip the balance of oxidation and anti-oxidation. Red blood cells are very prone to oxidative damage and in the case of sickle cell disease, this damage is particularly severe.

The major substance produced by our body to prevent free-radical damage and oxidative stress, is the naturally occurring molecule glutathione. Glutathione is rapidly depleted in a sickle cell crisis and its protective effect greatly diminished.

Sickle cell patients have been well documented to have lower glutathione levels. Studies looking at raising glutathione levels in sickle cell patients have demonstrated much more favorable outcomes and prognosis.

Spherocytosis, Ovalocytosis

Like sickle cell disease, both spherocytosis and ovalocytosis are conditions of abnormally-shaped red blood cells. As the name implies, the red blood cells are either round (spheres) or oval in shape. These are not as stable as the normal cylinder-shape seen in healthy individuals, and are more prone to damage, destruction and removal from the bloodstream by the spleen (which serves as a filter). Many drugs and infections can trigger a breakdown of these abnormal red blood cells.

One of the mechanisms of destruction of these cells is through oxidative stress (abnormal oxidant/antioxidant balance). Not only have these patients been noted to have high levels of oxidation, this is also associated with low levels of antioxidants. More specifically, glutathione levels are reduced, increasing the vulnerability of these cells.

G6PD Deficiency, Favism

G6PD stands for "Glucose-6-Phosphate dehydrogenase", an enzyme important in red blood cell metabolism. When this enzyme is abnormally low, as is seen in certain hereditary diseases, the red cells become much more fragile when exposed to certain medications,

aplastic anemia	spherocytosis, ovalocytosis
fanconi anemia	G6PD deficiency, favism
lead exposure anemia	thalassemia
hydrocarbon exposure anemia	trauma, gi blood loss
marrow invasion	menstruation, parasitic infection
sickle cell disease	

Table 22: A sampling of anemias linked to glutathione deficiency

stress, infection, and in the case of Favism to "broad-beans" (Fava beans). Interestingly, G6PD deficiency is the most common human enzyme defect, being present in hundreds of millions of individuals.

The common mechanism in the pathway to destruction of these abnormal red blood cells is, again, oxidative stress. Dozens of studies have shown that these patients have abnormally high free radical damage and low glutathione protection. Strategies to raise glutathione levels, both in the laboratory and in humans, have shown improvement.

Thalassemia

Thalassemia is an inherited disorder of hemoglobin, the major oxygen-carrying protein in red blood cells. There are several types, the most common being "Alpha-thalassemia" and "Beta-thalessemia". It appears in higher frequency in peoples originating from the Mediterranean region.

Thalassemia patients have less hemoglobin and more fragile red blood cells. Besides anemia, they are more prone to iron overload, bone deformities and heart disease.

Glutathione is involved on several levels in the thalassemic patient. Of note, iron overload is a strong source of free-radical production and subsequent damage to tissues, cells and molecules like DNA. One unique feature of glutathione is its ability to chelate (bond directly to) excess iron and allow its elimination from the body. Efforts to raise glutathione levels in thalassemia patients have yielded promising results.

Toxin/Exposure	
benzene	many herbicides
chloramphenicol	mercury
carbamazepine	phenytoin
lead	phenylbutazone
many pesticides	radiation

Table 23: Short list of substances detoxified by glutathione that can potentiate aplastic anemia.

Decreased production of red blood cells

Aplastic Anemia

Blood cells are manufactured in the bone marrow, where the blood stem cells are found. When the marrow is damaged, all blood cells may be negatively affected, including red blood cells, white blood cells and platelets. This damage may come from a number of different sources, including exposure to chemicals, drugs, radiation, infection, and in certain hereditary diseases. In a great number of cases, the exact cause of aplastic anemia is never identified.

In the case of drugs and chemicals that can provoke aplastic anemia, the list of these substances that are detoxified by glutathione is well documented, including radiation exposure (see Table 23).

Another interesting observation made by geneticists is that many individuals who acquire aplastic anemia have abnormally functioning glutathione enzymes. This suggests that deficient glutathione function predisposes a person to the development of aplastic anemia.

Fanconi Anemia

Not to be confused with Fanconi Syndrome (a kidney disease), Fanconi Anemia is a genetic disease that resultS in a number of different problems, including anatomical abnormalities, a much higher risk of cancers (especially leukemia), and bone marrow failure leading to anemia.

It has been established that one of the mechanisms leading to problems in Fanconi Anemia is oxidative stress (the uncontrolled action of oxidation) which damages DNA, our blueprint for cellular growth and development. Recent studies in humans have successfully delayed clinical symptoms by utilizing glutathione precursors. This offers hope in retarding the onset of cancer and anemia in this disease.

Cancer

The details of the various roles of glutathione as they relate to cancer is beyond the scope of this chapter and can be found in Chapter 5. Cancer can lead to anemia through several mechanisms: direct invasion of the bone marrow reducing the manufacture of blood cells; depletion of nutrients needed for blood cell production; acute or chronic blood loss from the cancer, and; the potential adverse effects of chemotherapy and radiotherapy.

The medical literature is rich with clinical studies demonstrating the role of glutathione in addressing all these issues.

Blood loss

Acute Blood Loss

Sudden and severe blood loss is most common through accidental physical trauma (motor vehicle accidents, penetrating injuries, industrial accidents, etc.) or through gastrointestinal blood loss (stomach ulcers, esophageal hemorrhage, etc.).

Raising GSH levels doesn't address these issues directly, but does aid in recovery from them. It is well documented that a great percentage of patients in an ICU (intensive care unit) will be glutathione deficient. Low glutathione levels correlate with poorer outcomes. In contrast, raising GSH levels in surgical patients has been shown to speed up recovery and discharge from hospital.

Recently, the strategy of raising GSH concomitantly with erythropoietin (EPO) has shown favorable results in early studies. This medication is used to stimulate red blood cell synthesis. This has been demonstrated in both anemic patients and healthy athletes.

Chronic Blood Loss

A slow but steady loss of blood can be a result of many different medical conditions, including menstruation, parasitic infection, gastrointestinal lesions, and cancer. The topic of cancer has been briefly covered earlier. Glutathione depletion is a feature of numerous intestinal diseases, including Crohn's Disease, ulcerative colitis, esophagitis and more. Raising glutathione in these instances has shown promise in alleviating symptoms. See chapter 13.

One very interesting benefit of raised GSH is its reinforcement of the immune function. Improved GSH supplies help resist bacterial, viral, fungal and parasitical infections.

Many patients with anemia suffer from iron-deficiency anemia, for which the mainstay treatment is iron supplementation. This is not without adverse effects, mostly due to the strong oxidative properties of iron provoking free radical damage. Glutathione is key in neutralizing the oxidative damage following exposure to free radicals resulting from increased iron.

Conclusion

A large variety of conditions, both genetic and environmental, can lead to anemia. This can be from inadequate red blood cell production, red blood cell destruction, or direct blood loss. The treatment depends on the specific cause of the anemia. The mainstay of severe anemia treatment often entails blood transfusion.

A novel concept is the use of glutathione-enhancing substances. This can be achieved through non-pharmacological means. Glutathione depletion is well documented in many types of anemia. More importantly, the aspect of raising glutathione levels in anemia has shown promise in multiple clinical studies. Given the safety profile of natural glutathione enhancing substances, they can be viewed as an underutilized strategy in addressing this very common problem.

ANEMIA

REFERENCES

Abboud MM, Al-Awaid W. *Synchrony of G6PD activity and RBC fragility under oxidative stress exerted at normal and G6PD deficiency.* Clin Biochem 43(4-5):455-60, 2010

Aliciguzel Y, Asian M. *N-acetyl cysteine, L-cysteine, and beta-mercaptoethanol augment selenium-glutathione peroxidase activity in glucose-6-phosphate dehydrogenase-deficient human erythrocytes.* Clin Exp Med 4(1):50-5, 2004

Alsultan AI, Seif MA, Amin TT, Naboli M, Alsuliman AM, et al. *Relationship between oxidative stress, ferritin and insulin resistance in sickle cell disease.* Eur Rev Med Pharmacol Sci 14(6):527-38, 2010

Amer J, Atlas D, Fibach E. N-acetylcysteine amide (AD4) attenuates oxidative stress in beta-thalassemia blood cells. *Biochim Biophys Acta 1780(2):249-55, 2008*

Amer J, Dana M, Fibach E. *The antioxidant effect of erythropoietin on thalassemic blood cells.* Anemia 2010:978710, 2010

Amer J, Ghoti H, et al. *Red blood cells, platelets and polymorphonuclear neutrophils of patients with sickle cell disease exhibit oxidative stress that can be ameliorated by antioxidants.* Br. J Haematol 132(1):108-13, 2006

Babushok DV, Li Y, Roth JJ, et al. *Common polymorphic deletion of glutathione S-transferase theta predisposes to acquired aplastic anemia: Independent cohort and meta-analysis of 609 patients.* Am J Hematol 88(10):862-7, 2013

Ben Ameur S, Aloulou H, et al. *Hemolytic anemia and metabolic acidosis: think about glutathione synthetase deficiency.* Fetal Pediatr Pathol 34(1):18-20, 2015

Chan AC, Chow CK, Chiu D. *Interaction of antioxidants and their implication in genetic anemia.* Proc Soc Exp Biol Med 222(3):274-82, 1999

Darghouth D, Koehl B, Junot C, Romeo PH. *Metabolomic analysis of normal and sickle cell erythrocytes.* Transfus Clin Biol 17(3):148-50, 2010

Darghouth D, Koehl B, et al. *Pathophysiology of sickle cell disease is mirrored by the red blood cell metabolome.* Blood 117(6):e57-66, 2011

Emokpae MA, Uadia PO, Gadzama AA. *Correlation of oxidative stress and inflammatory markers with the severity of sickle cell nephropathy.* Ann Afr Med 9(3):141-6, 2010

Fibach E, Tan ES, Jamuar S, et al. *Amelioration of oxidative stress in red blood cells from patients with beta-thalassemia major and intermedia and E-beta-thalassemia following administration of a fermented papaya preparation.* Phytother Res 24(9):1334-8, 2010

Ghoti H, Amer J, Winder A, et al. *Oxidative Stress in red blood cells, platelets and polymorphonuclear leukocytes from patients with myelodysplastic syndrome.* Eur J Haematol 79(6):463-7, 2007

Gibson XA, Shartava A, McIntyre J et al. *The efficacy of reducing agents or antioxidants in blocking the formation of dense cells and irreversibly sickled cells in vitro.* Blood 91(11):4373-8, 1998

Gizi A, Papassotiriou I, et al. Assessment of oxidative stress in patients with sickle cell disease: *The glutathione system and the oxidant-antioxidant status.* Blood Cells Mol Dis 46(3):220-5, 2011

Gürer H, Ozgünes H, Neal R, et al. *Antioxidant effects of N-acetylcysteine and succimer in red blood cells from lead-exposed rats.* Toxicology 128(3):181-9, 1998

Hansen RM, Csuka ME, et al. *Gold induced aplastic anemia.* Complete response to corticosteroids, plasmapheresis, and N-acetylcysteine infusion. J Rheumatol 12(4):794-7, 1985

Hansen RM, Varma RR, Hanson GA. *Gold induced hepatitis and pure red cell aplasia.* Complete recovery after corticosteroid and N-acetylcysteine therapy. J Rheumatol 18(8):1251-3, 1991

Khalid S, Shaikh F, Moeen S. *Decreased activity of glutathione peroxidase with oral ferrous iron administration: A cause of oxidative stress.* Pak J Pharm Sci 31(2):405-409, 2018

Kalpravidh RW et al. *Glutathione redox system in β-thalassemia/Hb E patients.* ScientificWorldJournal 2013:543973, 2013

Monti D, Macchioni S, Guido M, et al. Resistance to apoptosis in Fanconi's anaemia. *An ex vivo study in peripheral blood mononuclear cells.* FEBS Lett 409(3):365-9, 1997

Muanprasat C, et al. *Protection against oxidative stress in beta thalassemia/hemoglobin E erythrocytes by inhibitors of glutathione efflux transporters.* PLoS One 8(1):e55685, 2013

Nur E, Brandjes DP, Teerlink T, Otten HM et al. *N-acetylcysteine reduces oxidative stress in sickle cell patients.* Ann Hematol 91(7):1097-105, 2012

Nur E, Verwijis M, de Waart DR, et al. *Increased efflux of oxidized glutathione (GSSG) causes glutathione depletion and potentially diminishes antioxidants defense in sickle erythrocytes.* Biochim Biophys Acta 1812(11):1412-7, 2011

Osman HG, Zahran FM, El-Sokkary AM,

Sabry AM. *Oxidative stress and antioxidant defense in Egyptian favism patients.* Eur Rev Med Pharmacol Sci 17(9):1211-7, 2013

Pace BS, Shartava A, Pack-Mabien A, Mulekar M et al. *Effects of N-acetylcysteine on dense cell formation in sickle cell disease.* Am J Hematol 73(1):26-32, 2003

Pagano G, Talamanca AA, et al. *Oxidative Stress in Fanconi anaemia: from cells and molecules towards prospects in clinical management.* Biol Chem 393(1-2):11-21, 2012

Ponte F, Sousa R, Fernandes AP, et al. *Improvement of genetic stability in lymphocytes from Fanconi anemia patients through the combined effect of α-lipoic acid and N-acetylcysteine.* Orphanet J Rare Dis 16,7:28, 2012

Rachmilewitz EA, Weizer-Stem O, et al. *Role of iron in inducing oxidative stress in thalassemia: Can it be prevented by inhibition of absorption and by antioxidants?* Ann NY Acad Sci 1054:118-23, 2005

Rehman S, Ahmed P, Saba N, et al. *Association of GSTM1 and GSTT1 deletion polymorphisms with Pakistani aplastic anemia patients and controls and meta-analysis. Ann Hematol 94(12):1965-71, 2015*

Sultanova UA, Karimov KhLA, Khuzhakhmedov ZdD. *[Lipid peroxidation and activity of antioxidative protection enzymes in patients with aplastic anemia]. Lik Sprava (3-4):27-31, 2009*

Thom GG, et al. *Characterization of S-glutathionyl hemoglobin in homozygous sickle cell disease.* J Pediatr Hematol Oncol 31(12):895-900, 2009

Tiwari AK, Mahdi AA, et al. *Oral iron supplementation leads to oxidative imbalance in anemic women: a prospective study.* Clin Nutr 30(2):188-93, 2011

Wright RO, Woolf AD, Shannon MW, Magnani B. *N-acetylcysteine reduces methemoglobin in an in-vitro model of glucose-6-phosphate dehydrogenase deficiency.* Acad Emerg Med 5(3):225-9, 1998

Youssry I, Hammoud R, et al. *Genetic polymorphisms of glutathione-S-transferase and microsomal epoxide hydrolase in Egyptian acquired aplastic anemia patients. J Pediatr Hematol Oncol 33(2):89-92, 2011*

Zimmerman CP, Natta C. *Glutathione peroxidase activity in whole blood of patients with sickle cell anaemia. Scand J Haematol* 26(3):177-181, 1981

11

AIDS

At the turn of the 21st century the spread of AIDS (Acquired Immune Deficiency Syndrome) was the most serious health crisis worldwide, reaching epidemic proportions. For years, in many American cities and other parts of the world, it was the leading cause of death for 25 to 45 year-olds. Due to widespread research into AIDS, the scientific community has learned more about viruses and the immune system in the last few years than in the previous ninety. Fortunately, this research has driven technological and medical advancements that have allowed many patients a reasonable chance to live much longer and better lives than was possible during the first spread of AIDS at the end of the twentieth century.

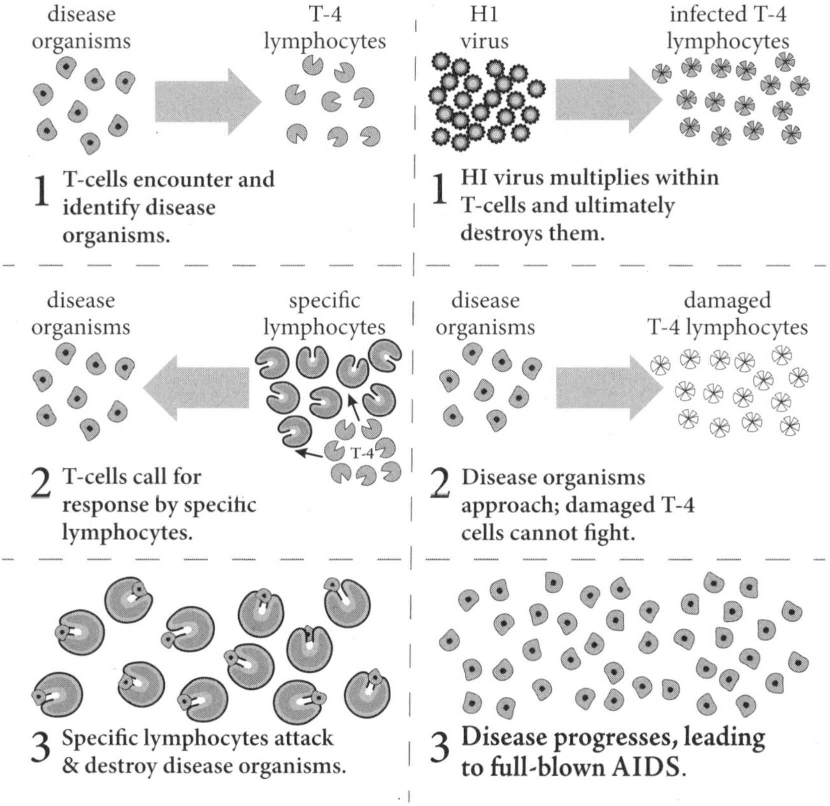

Figure 24: Normal immune response (left) and immune response of AIDS patients (right)

Human Immunodeficiency Virus (HIV)

AIDS is linked to the human immunodeficiency virus (HIV), which is particularly destructive to T-cell lymphocytes—a type of white blood cell necessary for effective immune response. There are three types: killer T-cells, helper T-cells and suppressor T-cells. Helper cells signal the presence of antigens so the body can effectively counter them. These are destroyed by HIV, preempting the build-up of killer cells that ordinarily threaten viruses. The result is immune-deficiency. The AIDS virus does not kill directly. It leaves the victim defenseless against even the most benign disease-causing organisms.

Long-term prospects for AIDS patients have greatly improved, and much can be done in the short-term. With good care the worst symptoms are avoided for years and the patient leads a productive life. As more is known about the disease and its spread, more effective treatments will emerge. There is widespread hope for a full-fledged cure within the next decade.

Many pharmacological and naturopathic medications are promoted as possible AIDS therapies, both for treatment and prevention. They have various levels of success and come at a cost—many pharmacological drugs are toxic, and while they help in their own ways to fight the disease, they exact a heavy physical and financial toll. There are no miracle cures. Some therapies help, some are hazardous. Nevertheless, a combination of treatments is more effective than any one alone, so most AIDS patients adopt one of several regimens known as 'drug cocktails.'

The worst aspects of the disease are secondary to HIV itself. Because the immune system has been compromised, it cannot adequately respond to most types of infection. It is these infections, not the HIV, that cause AIDS-related diseases.

The role of GSH in AIDS

Much attention is thus paid to the role of GSH in AIDS patients. Among other things, AIDS causes chronic inflammation and oxidative stress. This consumes GSH supplies and leads to dysfunction in CD4 helper immune cells. Once these T-cells lose their efficiency the patient becomes susceptible to opportunistic infections, including certain types of pneumonia, diarrhea and candida, as well as unusual cancers–the sorts of diseases to which healthy individuals are immune. This immunodeficiency becomes generalized and leads to malnutrition, wasting and death.

Researchers like Droge and Roederer have discovered that, among other biochemical changes, GSH concentrations are unusually low in AIDS patients. Some have noticed GSH levels in the blood fall to about 30% of normal. They suggest that this deficiency contributes to the typical feature of HIV infection–a progressive weakening of the immune system. Others give GSH a proactive role, claiming that the inflammatory cytokines that make HIV growth possible are inhibited when GSH concentrations are elevated. This effect was demonstrated by raising GSH levels with drugs like NAC (N-acetyl-cysteine). The same team in 1991 showed how the loss of glutathione in CD4 and CD8 T-cells corresponds to the progression of the disease.

In 1992, a team led by Gustavo Bounous investigated the properties of whey protein isolates at Montreal's McGill University. They developed a special method of extraction that preserved the GSH-enhancing, bioactive properties of the protein. Later the focus of many more clinical trials, this product eventually acquired a method-of-use patent for the treatment of HIV-seropositive patients.

Dr. Bounous and his colleagues saw that heightened GSH levels seemed to enhance the human immune system. Learning of the correlation between HIV progression and low GSH levels, they studied its effects on AIDS patients by giving their whey-protein isolate as a dietary supplement. The results

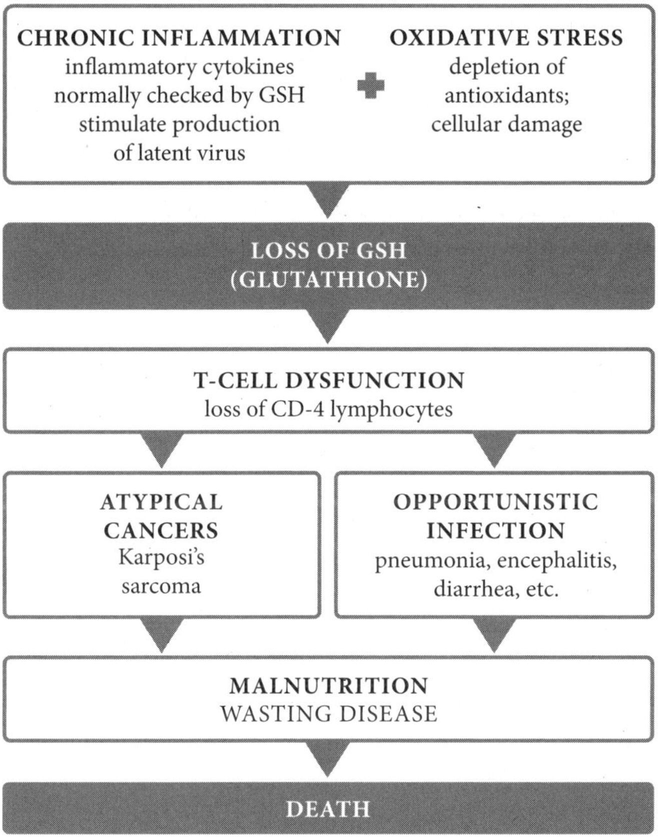

FIGURE 25: Role of glutathione loss in AIDS

were that it often diminished and sometimes reversed the wasting effects of AIDS. These patients also exhibited elevated CD4 T-cell counts and decreased viral load.

The availability of natural GSH precursors was welcome news to the AIDS research community. Bounous's discovery was presented at the Canadian Conference on HIV/AIDS Research in 1994 by Baruchel, Olivier and Mark Wainberg, the incumbent chairman of the International AIDS Research Association. Dr. Luc Montagnier (co discoverer of the AIDS virus) drew attention to the promising effects of this special protein isolate in his opening address at the Tenth International AIDS conference in Japan in 1994.

In a landmark 1997 paper, Herzenberg and Herzenberg categorically stated that GSH deficiency is associated with decreased survival in HIV disease. They improved survival rates by administering NAC (a GSH-promoting drug). Given the growing body of evidence demonstrating the benefits of raising GSH levels in AIDS patients, this represents a welcome addition to complementary therapy.

Case Study

The first member of this family of three to be diagnosed with AIDS was the father Bob, who developed pneumonia at age forty-four. His wife Joan developed swollen glands (lymphadenopathy), and tested positive shortly afterwards. Subsequently they discovered that their two-year old son Justin was also HIV-positive, though he was asymptomatic. Both Bob and Joan became progres-

sively unwell and Bob quit his job due to fatigue. Both were started on the antiviral drug AZT, but discontinued this therapy because of intolerable side-effects. Because she experienced vomiting and profound headaches on the drug, Joan decided not to allow her son to receive this therapy. Bob, Joan and Justin were started on a specially-prepared whey protein isolate. Both husband and wife noticed significant increase in their energy levels within weeks. Monitoring the family's blood tests over the next nine months, improvements in viral load, lymphocyte (white blood cell) count and specific CD4 lymphocyte values were noticed. Bob returned to work, Justin remained symptom-free and although Joan wanted another child, she was convinced not to pursue this idea.

Conclusion

AIDS attacks the immune system, is characterized by decreased GSH levels and generally lessens resistance to pathogens. In fact, GSH deficiency is associated with decreased survival in HIV disease. Studies have shown that supplementation aimed at maintaining GSH levels can diminish and sometimes reverse the wasting effect of AIDS. The patients in these experiments often also exhibited elevated CD-4 lymphocyte cell counts and decreased viral loads. As a result of these and many other AIDS trials, larger studies should establish glutathione supplementation as a mainstay of complementary therapy.

AIDS

REFERENCES

Adams JD, Jaresko GS, Louie SG et al. *Pneumocystis carinii pneumonia in HIV infected patients: effects of the diseases on glutathione & glutathione disulfide.* J Med 24(6):337-52, 1993

Baruchel S, Bounous G, Gold P. *Place for an antioxidant therapy in HIV infection.Oxidative Stress, Cell Activation & Viral Infection C Pasquier ed 1994*

Baruchel S, Viau G, Olivier R, Bounous G. *Nutriceutical modulation of glutathione with a humanized native milk serum protein isolate, Immunocal. Application in AIDS & cancer in: Oxidative Stress in Cancer, AIDS & Neurodegenerative Diseases.* Institute Pasteur Editors Montagnier L, Olivier R, Pasquier C Marcel Dekker, 1998

Baruchel S, Wainberg MA. *The role of oxidative stress in disease progression in individuals infected by HIV.* Journal of Leukocyte Biology 52:111-114, 1992

Bhaskar A, Munshi M, Khan Sz et al. *Measuring glutathione redox potential of HIV-1-infected macrophages.* J Biol Chem 290(2):1020-38, 2015

Borges-Santos MD, Moreto F, Pereira PC et al. *Plasma GSH of HIV patients responded positively & differently to dietary supplementation with cysteine or glutamine.* Nutrition 28(7-8):753-6, 2012

Bounous G, Baruchel S, Falutz J, Gold P. *Whey proteins as a food supplement in HIV-seropositive individuals.* Clinical Investigative Medicine 16(3):204-209, 1993

Buhl R, Jaffe HA, Holroyd KJ et al. *Systemic GSH deficiency in symptom-free HIV seropositive individuals.* Lancet ii:1294-1298, 1989

De Quay B, Malinverni R, Lauterburg BH. *Glutathione depletion in HIV-infected patients: role of cysteine deficiency & effect of oral N-acetylcysteine.* AIDS 6(6):815-9, 1992

Dröge W. *Cysteine & glutathione deficiency in AIDS patients: a rationale for the treatment with N-acetyl-cysteine.* Pharmacology 46(2):61-5, 1993

Droge W et al. *Functions of glutathione & glutathione disulfide in immunology & immunopathology.* FASEB J 8(14):1131-8, 1994

Dworkin BM, Rosenthal WS, Wormser GP et al. *Abnormalities of blood selenium & glutathione peroxidase activity in patients with acquired immunodeficiency syndrome & AIDS-related complex.* Biol Trace Elem Res 15:167-77, 1988

Fraternale A, Paoletti MF, Casablanca A et al. *GSH & analogs in antiviral therapy.* Mol Aspects Med 30(1-2):99-110, 2009

Fraternale A et al. *Antiviral & immunomodulatory properties of new pro-glutathione (GSH) molecules.* Curr Med Chem 13(15):1749-55, 2006

Harmsen MC, Swart PJ, De Bethune MP, PauwelsR, De Clercq E, The TH, Meijer DKF. *Antiviral effects of plasma & milk proteins: Lactoferrin shows potent activity against both human immunodeficiency virus & human cytomegalovirus replication in vitro.* The Journal of Infectious Diseases 172:380-388, 1995

Herzenberg LA, De Rosa SC, Dubs JG, Roederer M, Anderson MT, Ela SW, Deresinski SC, Herzenberg LA. *Glutathione deficiency is associated with impaired survival in HIV disease.* Proceedings of the National Academy of Science USA 94:1967-1972, 1997

Holroy KJ, Buhl R, Borok Z et al. *Correction of glutathione deficiency in the lower respiratory tract of HIV seropositive individuals by glutathione aerosol treatment.* Thorax 48(10):985-9, 1993

Kalebic T, Kinter A, Poli G, Anderson ME, Meister A, Fauci A. *Suppression of human immunodeficiency virus expression in chronically infected monocytic cells by GSH, GSH ester, & n-acetylcysteine.* Proceedings of the National Academy of Science USA 88:986-990, 1991

Kameoka M, Okada Y, Tobiume M, Kimura T, Ikuta K. *Intracellular GSH as a possible direct blocker of HIV Type 1 reverse transcription.* AIDS Research & Human Retroviruses 12(17):1635-1638, 1996

Look MP, Rockstroh JK, Rao GS et al. *Serum selenium, plasma glutathione (GSH) & erythrocyte GSH peroxidase (GSH-Px)-levels in asymptomatic versus symptomatic human immunodeficiency virus-1 (HIV-1)-infection.* Eur J Clin Nutr 51(4):266-72, 1997

Lopez Galera RM, Juarez-Gimenez JC et al. *Glutathione & cysteine in HIV-infected hemophiliacs.* Clin Chim Acta 254(1):63-72, 1996

Moreno YF, Sgarbieri VC, da Silva MN et al. *Features of whey protein concentrate supplementation in children with rapidly progressive HIV infection.* J Trop Pediatr 52(1):34-8, 2006

Morris D, Guerra C, Donohue C et al. *Unveiling the mechanisms for decreased glutathione in individuals with HIV infection.* Clin Dev Immunol 2012:734125, 2012

Morris D, Guerra C, Khurasany M et al. *Glutathione supplementation improves macrophage functions in HIV.* J Interferon Cytokine Res 33(5):270-9, 2013

Nguyen D, Hsu JW, Jahoor F, Sekhar RV. *Effect of increasing GSH with cysteine & glycine supplementation on mitochondrial fuel oxidation, insulin sensitivity & body composition in older HIV-infected patients.* J Clin Endocrinol Metab 99(1):169-77, 2014

Ogunro PS et al. *Plasma selenium concentration & glutathione peroxidase activity in HIV-1/AIDS infected patients: a correlation with the disease progression.* Niger Postgrad Med J 13(1):1-5, 2006

Palamara AT, Garaci E, Rotilio G et al. *Inhibition of murine AIDS by reduced GSH.* AIDS Res Hum Retroviruses 12(14):1373-81, 1996

Palamara AT, Perno CF, Aquaro S, Bue MC, Dini L, Garaci E. *Glutathione inhibits HIV replication by acting at late stages of the virus life cycle.* AIDS Research & Human Retroviruses 12(16):1537-1541, 1996

Raju PA, Herzenberg LA, Herzenber LA, Roederer M. *GSH precursor & antioxidant activities of N-acetylcysteine & oxothiazolidine carboxylate compared in in vitro studies of HIV replication.* AIDS Res Hum Retroviruses 10(8):961-7, 1994

Roberts RL, Aroda VR, Ank BJ. *N-acetylcysteine enhances antibody-dependent cellular cytotoxicity in neutrophils & monomuclear cells from health adults & human immunodeficiency virus-infected patients.* J Infect Dis 172(6):1492-502, 1995

Roederer M, Raju PA, Staal FJ et al. *N-acetylcysteine inhibits latent HIV expression in chronically infected cells.* AIDS Res Hum Retroviruses 7(6):563-7, 1991

Roederer M, Staal FJ, Anderson M et al. *Disregulation of leukocyte glutathione in AIDS.* Ann NY Acad Sci 677:113-25, 1993

Roederer M, Staal FJ, Ela SW, Herzenberg LA, Herzenberg LA. *N-acetylcysteine: potential for AIDS therapy.* Pharmacology 46(3):121-9, 1993

Roederer M, Staal FJT, Osada H, Herzenberg LA, Herzenberg LA. *CD4 & CD8 T cells with high intracellular glutathione levels are selectively lost as the HIV infection progresses.* International Immunology 3(9):993-937, 1991

Roederer M, Staal FJ, Raju PA, Ela SW, Herzenberg LA, Herzenberg LA. *Cytokine-stimulated human immunodeficiency virus replication is inhibited by N-acetyl-L-cysteine.* Proceedings of the National Academy of Science USA 87:4884-4888, 1990

Sbrana E, Paladini A, Bramanti E, Spinetti MC, Raspi G. *Quantitation of reduced glutathione & cysteine in human immunodeficiency virus-infected patients.* Electrophoresis 25(10-11):1522-9, 2004

Sekhar RV, Liu CW, Rice S. *Increasing glutathione concentrations with cysteine & glycine supplementation lowers inflammation in HIV patients.* AIDS 29(14):1899-900, 2015

Staal FJ. *GSH & HIV infection: reduced or increased oxidized?* Eur J Clin Invest 28(3):194-6, 1998

Staal FJ, Roederer M, Israelski DM et al. *Intracellular glutathione levels in T cell subsets decrease in HIV infected individuals.* AIDS Res Hum Retroviruses 8(2):305-11, 1992

Staal FJT, Ela SW, Roederer M, Anderson MT, Herzenberg LA, Herzenberg LA. *Glutathione deficiency & human immunodeficiency virus infection.* Lancet 339:909-912, 1992.

Treitinger A, Spada C, Masokawa IY et al. *Effect of N-acetyl-Lcysteine on lymphocyte apoptosis, lymphocyte viability, TNF-alpha & IL-8 in HIV-infected patients undergoing anti-retroviral treatment.* Braz J Infect Dis 8(5):363-71, 2004

Vallis KA. *Glutathione deficiency & radiosensitivity in AIDS patients.* Lancet 337:918-919, 1991

12

Lung Disease

One of the most distressing symptoms that anyone can experience is shortness of breath—dyspnea. Patients describe themselves as "not getting enough air." This triggers a series of physiological and behavioral reactions that increase heart rate, blood pressure and hormonal secretions, producing a feeling of general panic. Shortness of breath is a common symptom of many respiratory illnesses.

Just as the gut separates and absorbs food into the body, the lungs are a passage for the exchange of used air and fresh air. But there's a crucial difference between food and oxygen—we can't store oxygen. We must meet a moment-by-moment demand for this life-giving element, or die within minutes. The body responds instinctively and urgently to any interruption of this exchange.

Over 30 million Americans are affected by dozens of chronic lung diseases. Pulmonary (lung-related) medicine is vast and complicated. It deals with congenital problems like cystic fibrosis, acquired diseases like bronchitis, and self-inflicted problems like smoking. The importance of GSH in the respiratory system cannot be overstated. In this chapter we will discuss the following:

Antioxidants and the lungs

You'll see in these pages that most pulmonary diseases inflame the lung. Inflammation is either acute such as by exposure to toxins, or chronic , like cystic fibrosis. The processes of infection in asthma, bronchitis or pneumonia all lead to inflammation.

The body's inflammatory response itself generates free radicals, so traditional medications attempt to reduce this inflammation. In addition, antioxidants are used increasingly to complement conventional treatments. Researchers Morris and Bernard drew attention to this complementary treatment in an article called "Significance of glutathione in lung disease and implications for therapy," in which they underscored the weight of evidence supporting such research.

There is a fragile balance in the lungs between oxidants and antioxidants. Oxidative stress is high in the lungs and produces very large numbers of oxyradicals because it's the center of oxygen interchange—but for many

Asthma	Pulmonary fibrosis
Bronchitis, acute and chronic	Cancer
Chronic obstructive pulmonary disease (COPD)	Pneumonia
Emphysema	Toxic exposures
Adult respiratory distress syndrome (ARDS)	Tobacco abuse
Cystic fibrosis	

TABLE 24: Common and not-so-common ailments discussed in this chapter

other reasons too. White blood (immune) cells are highly active in the lining of the lungs. Their high metabolic rates release huge quantities of oxidative products. They also manufacture free radicals with which to attack biological and chemical invaders. Airborne pollutants are a further source of powerful free radicals. For all these reasons, antioxidants in the fluid lining of the lungs play a large part in our front-line defense against the environment.

When blood cells encounter bacteria they attack them with oxidizing peroxides and other caustic substances. The blood cells themselves, as well as the surrounding tissues, depend on glutathione to protect themselves from these oxidants. You will recall that tissue damage occurs either when oxidant levels grow too high or GSH levels are too low.

GSH is the most critical of all naturally-occurring antioxidants (see Chapter 1) and effectively supports exogenous antioxidants like vitamins C and E. Unlike glutathione, exogenous antioxidants are derived from the outside environment and are not native to the body, but both work together to soak up free radicals.

Generally, tissues and organs manufacture their own glutathione from dietary or drug-delivered precursors. However, the lining of the respiratory tree usually requires high levels of GSH and can absorb GSH directly. To take advantage of this unusual ability, a topical GSH aerosol has been used successfully to treat a number of diseases, including adult respiratory distress syndrome (ARDS), pulmonary fibrosis and HIV infection. In addition, the topical form of NAC (Mucomist)—a potent GSH precursor—has long been used to treat cystic fibrosis.

Oral and intravenous glutathione precursors receive a lot of attention from researchers, who have published many papers on the subject. Pulmonologists (lung doctors) are paying more and more attention to lung GSH content, and anticipating future applications. Ortolani and his team in Italy placed forty intensive care patients with respiratory difficulties on intravenous GSH, then compared their response to an equal number of untreated patients and found significant reductions in oxidative stress levels.

An experiment in preventive medicine was conducted by De Flora and his research team in Italy at the Institute of Hygiene and Preventive Medicine, University of Genoa. Patients were placed on a course of oral NAC tablets or placebo during the months of the

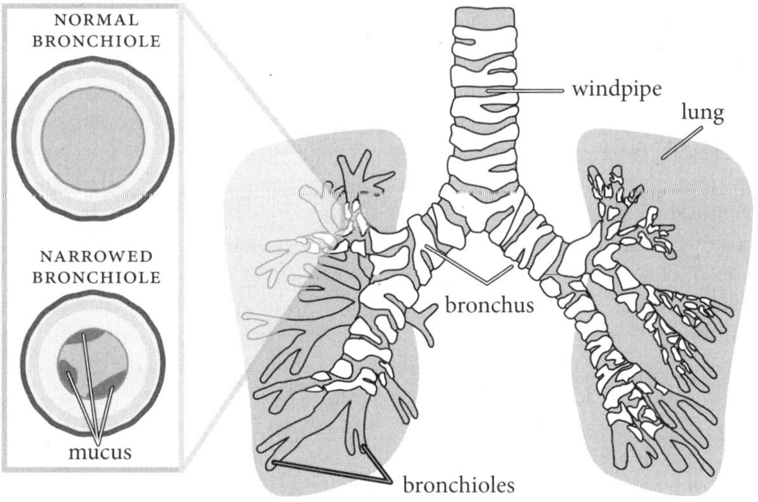

Figure 26: Asthma causes bronchioles to become narrow and restricts the passage of air into the lungs

influenza season. Although the number of people infected by the virus was unchanged, subjects receiving NAC experienced significantly fewer and less virulent symptoms.

Asthma

Bronchial asthma causes constriction of the bronchioles (airway passages). Figure 25 shows the windpipe and lungs, and cross-sections of normal and narrowed air passages. Asthma is always unpleasant and can be fatal. Asthma attacks vary in intensity, but all are characterized by tightness in the chest, shortness of breath, restlessness, coughing and wheezing. Although asthma is reversible and intermittent, it tends to recur and is generally considered a chronic condition. It is one of the most common causes of absenteeism and hospital admission in school-age children, who suffer from it more than anyone else. It currently affects about 1 in 13 people in America (over 8%) and is on the rise (probably due to air pollution).

Asthma is variable in frequency and severity and can be triggered by a very wide variety of stimuli, including allergens (things that provoke an allergic response). These include dust, pollen, dander (tiny particles of animal skin, fur and feather), certain foods and drugs, viral infections, emotional stress, anxiety and even plain old exercise. Muscles within the walls of the bronchioles flex and go into spasm, the walls thicken, air passages become clogged by mucus, and air is trapped in the deepest airways (the alveoli). The wheezing sound is caused by air passing with difficulty through these narrowed passages. In its severest form, breathing becomes impossible and the patient suffocates.

Asthma sufferers should make an effort to recognize and avoid situations that trigger their attacks, whether the cause is allergic, infectious, toxic, or emotional. They can also use preventative medications such as antihistamines and sodium cromoglycate, which minimize the effects of the allergic response.

Once an attack is underway, other drugs are required to reopen (dilate) the walls of the bronchioles. Bronchodilators such as salbutemol or albuterol are commonly used in inhalers. Steroids are also available, through inhalers or as pills. All of these minimize the swelling and inflammation of the bronchial walls. Once an attack begins, treatment must be immediate and aggressive. The longer it lasts, the more the symptoms advance and the longer they take to reverse. There's no time to waste.

It's long been thought that low levels of glutathione and glutathione peroxidase play a role in asthma, both at the outset and as it progresses. Studies of asthmatics have identified abnormalities in their red-blood GSH, white-blood cell GSH, serum GSH, platelet GSH and lung-fluid GSH. Low glutathione levels correspond directly to the severity of the asthma attack.

Dietary, environmental, and genetic factors can diminish the potency of antioxidant systems in the lung and increase the risk of asthma. This relationship between antioxidant levels and asthma is seen whenever free-radical activity is high, as in lead poisoning, excessive iron absorption and G6PD-deficiency[1], as well as in situations marked by low levels of vitamin C, vitamin E, and selenium (a component of glutathione peroxidase).

The pulmonologist Dr. Carol Trenga recently presented to the American Lung Association an antioxidant cocktail to aid asthmatics who were particularly sensitive to air pollutants. European physicians have long used GSH precursors in the treatment of asthma, particularly as a phlegm thinner (mucolytic) to break down thick secretions. In a double-blind study, inhaled bronchodilators were tested with and without NAC. The NAC (GSH-enhanced) group experienced greater improvement in lung function than the control group.

1 A genetic disorder that most often affects males. It happens when the body doesn't have enough of an enzyme called glucose-6-phosphate dehydrogenase (G6PD).

Case study

Jean-Pierre, a financial analyst, suffered from allergies and asthma his whole life. Summers were particularly bad and he often had to leave his native Montreal for weeks in August to escape the ragweed allergy season. In early summer, he was started on a program of NAC (N-acetylcysteine), L-cysteine, selenium, alpha-lipoic acid, multivitamins and stinging nettle (Urtica dioici). That season, he reported having to use his Ventolin inhaler (salbutemol, a bronchodilator for asthma) only two or three times a week, rather than two or three times a day, and his use of antihistamine drugs was at a minimum. He's even ventured to go camping with his girlfriend.

Bronchitis, Emphysema, and COPD

Bronchitis is an inflammation or obstruction of the bronchi, the larger airways of the lungs that eventually branch out to become the bronchioles (the site of asthma). Bronchitis resembles asthma in some ways, their common symptoms being shortness of breath, a phlegm-producing cough, chest discomfort and occasional wheezing. Bronchitis has two distinct forms—acute and chronic. They differ in important ways.

Acute bronchitis is almost always caused by a viral or bacterial infection. Coughing, chest pains, fever and chills are common complaints. In the healthy individual, it is usually a short-lived illness that clears up once the infection is overcome. If the infection is bacterial or mycoplasmal, antibiotics may be required. Occasionally inflammation remains, leading to a post-inflammatory cough that may persist for weeks. Inhaled steroids are often prescribed for this condition.

Like emphysema (described below), chronic bronchitis is an ongoing illness requiring frequent medical attention. Although it may be exacerbated by infectious disease, chronic bronchitis is usually caused by long-term exposure to lung irritants—toxins, allergens or repeated bouts of acute bronchitis. By far the most common cause of chronic bronchitis is cigarette smoke.

Lungs exposed to tobacco smoke are subject to several pathological processes. One of the most damaging is the dysfunction or loss of cilia lining the airways. Cilia are microscopic hair-like structures that trap and remove dust, mucus and other debris. A single puff of a cigarette can paralyze these hairs, increasing the chances of subsequent lung injury and infection.

As chronic bronchitis progresses, the lung's ability to exchange oxygen and carbon dioxide diminishes. The attempt to compensate for the loss of pulmonary function increases energy demands, causing the chest muscles to work harder and the heart to pump faster. This in turn can lead to secondary diseases such as pulmonary hypertension, heart failure and emphysema.

Emphysema progresses slowly over time and is usually the result of prior lung disease. Typical symptoms are a chronic cough and shortness of breath. Although it may occasionally be caused by hereditary factors, environmental exposures, chronic asthma or chronic bronchitis, emphysema most often results from years of heavy smoking. It is the most common cause of death from respiratory disease in North America.

Emphysema shares many symptoms with chronic bronchitis. In fact, the two diseases usually overlap to some degree. They are often classed together under the heading COPD (chronic obstructive pulmonary disease). However, they differ anatomically. Emphysema results in irreversible damage to alveoli—tiny sac-like structures where the actual exchange of oxygen and carbon dioxide occurs. Alveoli are counted in the millions, like bubbles in a bath. Emphysema causes them to burst one by one, and then coalesce into fewer, larger sacs. As a result, their total surface area dwindles, reducing the volume of air that can be exchanged with each breath.

Most lung diseases are characterized by

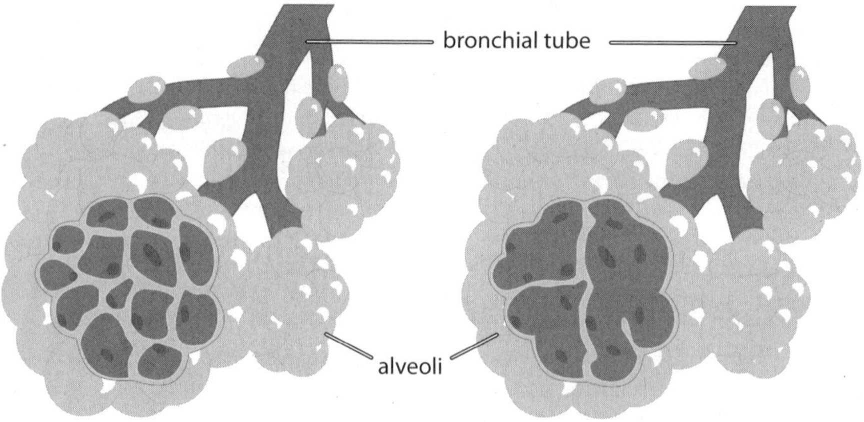

FIGURE 27: Normal alveoli (left) and alveoli with emphysema (right)

weak antioxidant activity and impaired glutathione-related enzyme systems. Starting from that well-studied fact, a group of French researchers used GSH screening as a way to predict possible pulmonary disease. They tested subjects for the absence of a gene (GSTM1) responsible for a specific GSH enzyme (about 47% of the French population lacks this gene). They found that heavy smokers with moderate chronic bronchitis were missing this gene 66% of the time and that smokers with severe chronic bronchitis were deficient in 71% of cases. They concluded that factors diminishing GSH function—in this case a hereditary factor—put individuals at greater risk of respiratory problems.

Other studies determined that COPD patients were highly sensitive to low GSH levels after even gentle exercise, demonstrating the precarious balance of glutathione in their bodies, and the great importance of maintaining adequate stores.

Hansen and his team at Odense University in Denmark conducted a double-blind study of the general well-being of patients with mild chronic bronchitis. They gave them oral NAC during the winter months, and placebo to a similar group. Of the two, the GSH-enhanced group did much better on a GHQ (general health questionnaire). Other research teams have studied the use of oral NAC as a preventative measure. Although it didn't significantly reduce the number of chronic bronchitis attacks, it greatly reduced their symptoms and their number of days off work.

In a large, open study of over two thousand patients, Volkl and Schneider from Hanover Medical School in Germany showed that the use of NAC led to clear improvements in symptoms and pulmonary function. The four-week study included patients with acute and chronic bronchitis, bronchial asthma and emphysema. All groups experienced similar relief from their disease.

Smoking and GSH

There is no doubt that cigarette smoking is a major risk factor for chronic bronchitis, emphysema, COPD, cancer and cardiovascular disease. One way in which cigarette smoke damages the body is by severely intensifying oxidative stress in the lungs.

A single puff of cigarette smoke contains billions of free radicals and can literally "burn up" antioxidants. That isn't the worst of it. Additional oxidative stress results from the lung inflammation that's also triggered by smoking. The total oxidative damage caused by smoke corresponds directly to the impairment of individual patients—as measured by lung injury, respiratory compromise, morbidity and mortality.

Pharmacologists are investigating the use of inhaled GSH to prevent the onset or progression of emphysema in smokers. As a GSH precursor, NAC is receiving equal attention. Double blind studies in smokers using NAC demonstrate their lungs' enhanced ability to clear away thick secretions in their airways.

Balansky at the Institute of Hygiene and Preventive Medicine in Italy exposed rats to high levels of cigarette smoke. This decreased their body weight, causing intense pathological damage of the terminal airways, inflammation of the bronchial and bronchiolar linings, alveolar damage, emphysema, white blood cell abnormalities and pre-cancerous lesions. Rats given daily NAC at the same time suffered significantly less damage, demonstrating the protective role of GSH against lung damage and the onset of cancer.

Smokers are also more susceptible to infectious bronchitis and pneumonia. Chronic bronchitis in smokers increases bacterial colonization. Treatment with NAC has decreased both the frequency of infectious episodes and the virulence of the bacteria.

Adult Respiratory Distress Syndrome (ARDS)

ARDS is acute, life-threatening respiratory failure following injury to the lung. It leads to profound shortness of breath (dyspnea), fluid accumulation in the lungs (pulmonary edema) and oxygen starvation (hypoxemia). This all-too-common medical emergency is triggered by several acute processes that directly or indirectly damage the lung. They include bacterial or viral pneumonias, inhalation of stomach contents or other toxins, direct trauma to the chest, sepsis (overwhelming infection of multiple organs), profound circulatory shock, drowning and many other medical conditions. With appropriate therapy the survival rate is about 50%. Long-term complications include the eventual development of pulmonary fibrosis.

ARDS is a very complicated inflammatory process of which swelling (edema) is only one symptom. In the past, physicians treated this disorder aggressively with corticosteroids, because of their well-known anti-inflammatory properties. Sadly, randomized trials have shown that steroids are relatively ineffective in this disease. A hunt is on for useful treatments.

For several reasons, ARDS patients experience high levels of oxidative stress and subsequent depletion of antioxidants and glutathione. One cause may be the release of free radicals by endotoxins at the injury site. These are found in the residue of certain bacteria when they die. However, oxidative stress probably comes most from inflammation. Some white blood cells (neutrophils) are highly active at sites of inflammation, producing very large amounts of reactive oxygen species as weapons. These include free oxygen radicals, hydrogen peroxide, 'hot' oxygen, and others.

In light of the severe oxidant-antioxidant imbalance and glutathione depletion that comes with ARDS, many researchers have turned to NAC. Bernard and his team at Vanderbilt University tested the usefulness of intravenous NAC for the lungs. Both in the lab and in clinical trials they found increased oxygen delivery, improved lung compliance (elasticity) and an improvement in the condition of pulmonary edema patients. Trials with another GSH precursor—OTZ (Procysteine)—produced similar results while reducing the duration of lung injury.

In a larger double-blind study, Suter's group at the University of Geneva used intravenous NAC on intensive care patients. Compared to a control group, the NAC patients showed significant improvement in oxygenation and required less time on mechanical ventilators (life support).

Pulmonary fibrosis

Pulmonary fibrosis is also called fibrosing alveolitis or interstitial fibrosis, among other things. It is a non-specific condition in which the lungs react to damage by producing scar tissue (fibrosis). This stiffens the lung, so that it can't properly clear its secretions. Fibrosis also interferes with gas exchange.

Its causes include numerous bacterial, viral or fungal infections as well as inhaled toxins, dusts (organic and inorganic) and chemicals. Occasionally, stomach contents are inhaled, damaging the lungs. Other diseases may also be involved, such as certain autoimmune disorders[2] including sarcoidosis (inflammation of multiple systems) and collagen-vascular diseases (rheumatoid arthritis, lupus, polyarteritis nodosa, scleroderma and dermatomytosis). This disease is often an unwanted consequence of radiation therapy or chemotherapy. Conventional treatments have limited success.

Oxidative stress plays an important role in the causes and conditions of many types of pulmonary fibrosis. Behr and his group of pulmonologists at the University of Munich studied this in laboratory cultures (in vitro) as well as in pulmonary fibrosis patients (in vivo). Since pulmonary fibrosis is an inflammatory disorder, any treatment needs to suppress the immune inflammatory response. With the help of NAC, patients' pulmonary function tests improved and the number of oxidative breakdown products fell. By using aerosolized NAC, Borok from the NIH (National Institute of Health) reversed the oxidant-antioxidant imbalance in pulmonary fibrosis patients. Both NAC and aerosol GSH have proven successful at this. Clearly, both oral and inhaled NAC can successfully raise pulmonary glutathione levels.

Fibroblasts form most connective tissue in animals, but when they grow excessively in both number and activity, they produce the fibrous scar tissue that results in pulmonary fibrosis. Tissue cultures made from these cells revealed that when GSH was present the excessive growth slowed down, suggesting that it may delay the progress of pulmonary fibrosis.

Case study

With a background in law from her native France, Nona became actively involved with business and philanthropic pursuits in Canada. She was a 41 year-old mother of three when she was diagnosed with Hodgkin's disease. She required both chemotherapy and radiotherapy, and although these treatments cured the Hodgkin's disease, they left her lungs scarred with pulmonary fibrosis. As her breathing deteriorated she dropped everything that interested her and ended up at home, dependent on an oxygen tank and many medications. Despite conventional treatment, her pulmonary function tests (PFT's) continued to fall. Then, as an experiment, she started taking a cysteine-rich whey protein isolate. Six weeks later she returned to her lung doctor claiming she could breathe again. The physician repeated the pulmonary function tests, which showed her lungs back at about 90% of normal values. To eliminate the possibility of a possible placebo effect and to eliminate other possible explanations, he withdrew the protein supplement. She subsequently deteriorated again. Three weeks after restarting daily use of the product, her PFT's went back up to 95% of normal values and she promised herself never to stop again.

---

[2] mistaken immune response to healthy processes

Cystic fibrosis

Cystic fibrosis affects many organ systems, the lungs in particular. It's also called mucoviscidosis because it secretes a sticky mucus which neither lubricates the nose, throat, airways and intestines, nor flows freely. Cystic fibrosis is one of the most common inherited diseases in North America and affects some 30,000 people. Survivors live to an age of about 28 years, depending on the extent of pulmonary involvement.

Cystic fibrosis is most often classified as a disorder of the exocrine glands, and primarily affects the pancreas in fibrocystic pancreatic disease, the sweat glands, and pulmonary mucus production in mucoviscidosis. The problem stems from an inherited defect in the gene responsible for secreting certain fluids from these glands.

The disease often appears early in life. Cystic fibrosis babies have very frequent digestive difficulties since their pancreas doesn't make enough digestive juice. This leads to malabsorption (poor ability to use nutrients) and malnutrition. Their skin loses large amounts of salt and they may sweat profusely. The lungs secrete a very thick (viscous) mucus that can obstruct airways, causing coughing, wheezing, and recurrent lung infections. Comprehensive and intensive therapy with health workers specialized in nursing, nutrition, physical therapy and respiratory therapy is essential.

Dr. Larry Lands, director of the cystic fibrosis clinic at McGill University in Montreal, aptly points out that inflammation is central to cystic fibrosis, that inflammation always precedes lung infection, and that lung infection almost inevitably follows severe inflammation. Continued inflammation depletes even more antioxidants and glutathione, resulting in a vicious circle.

The loss of GSH in cystic fibrosis is noticeable in the fluid lining of the lungs (epithelial lining fluid), and also in blood serum, red blood cells and elsewhere. All indications are that ongoing oxidative stress depletes the entire body.

Cystic fibrosis patients are at further risk of antioxidant depletion because they also suffer from impaired pancreatic function, leading to bad digestion and poor absorption of essential nutrients. Many researchers are investigating the use of supplemental antioxidants in this disease. Lands' team is investigating a whey-based, cysteine-rich GSH precursor.

NAC has long been packaged in an aerosol form to break down mucus accumulation in cystic fibrosis patients. It can be used in the same way for asthma, bronchitis, COPD, emphysema, pneumonia and other situations where thick secretions impair pulmonary function.

Case study

Eight year-old Zach, a cystic fibrosis patient, loved baseball. He was smaller than the rest of the kids but it was shortness of breath and recurrent respiratory problems, that kept him off the team, not his height. He took care of his nutritional needs and was good about taking his additional vitamin and antioxidant supplementation. His parents learned how to provide him with home aerosol treatments by mask. He has been using both oral and nebulized (by mask) Mucomyst (N-acetylcysteine). Although he's mainly a "bench-warmer," Zach is back on the team.

Conclusion

An impressive amount of research has clarified the critical importance of antioxidants and glutathione in all these pulmonary diseases. Unlike most other tissues, the lungs can use GSH as-is—through direct contact—rather than having to first absorb the ingredients and then make it. There are many ways to deliver glutathione to the lungs, including oral, intravenous and inhaled therapies. In the next few years even more products will begin to raise glutathione levels in acute, chronic and critical care patients.

LUNG DISEASE

REFERENCES

Balansky RM, De Flora S. *Chemoprevention by n-acetylcysteine of urethane-induced clastogenicity & lung tumors in mice.* Int. J. Cancer 77: 302-305, 1998

Balansky RB, D'Agostinin F, Zannacchi P, De Flora S. *Protection of n-acetylcysteine of the histopathological & cytogenetical damage produced by exposure of rats to cigarette smoke.* Cancer Lett. 64: 123-131, 1992

Baranova H, Perriot J, Albuisson E, et al. *Peculiarities of the GSTM1 0/0 genotype in French heavy smokers with various types of chronic bronchitis.* Human Genetics 99: 822-826, 1997

Behr J, Degenkolb B, Maier K, et al. *Increased oxidation of extracellular GSH by bronchoalveolar inflammatory cells in diffuse fibrosing alveolitis.* Eur. Respir. J. 8: 1286-1292, 1995

Behr J, Maier K, Degenkolb B, et al. *Antioxidative & clinical effects of high-dose n-acetylcysteine in fibrosing alveolitis. Adjunctive therapy to maintenance immunosuppression. American J. Respir.* Crit. Care Med. 156: 1897-1901, 1997

Bernard GR. *Potential of n-acetylcysteine as treatment for the adult respiratory distress syndrome.* Eur. Respir. J. Suppl. 11: 496S-498S, 1990

Bernard GR. *N-acetylcysteine in experimental & clinical acute lung injury.* American J. Med. 91:(3c): 54S-59S, 1991

Bernard GR, Wheeler AP, Arons MM, et al. *A trial of antioxidants n-acetylcysteine & procysteine in ARDS. The antioxidant in ARDS Study Group.* Chest 112: 164-172, 1997

Bibi H, Schlesinger M, Tabachnik E, et al. *Erythrocyte glutathione peroxidase activity in asthmatic children.* Ann. Allergy 61: 339-340, 1988

Biljak VR et al. *Glutathione cycle in stable chronic obstructive pulmonary disease.* Cell Biochem Funct 28(6):448-53, 2010

Biswas SK, Rahman I. *Environmental toxicity, redox signaling & lung inflammation: the role of glutathione.* Mol Aspects Med 30(1-2):60-76, 2009

Blasi F, Page C, Rossolini GM et al. *The effect of N-acetylcysteine on biofilms: Implications for the treatment of respiratory tract infections.* Respir Med 117:190-7, 2016

Borok Z, Buhl R, Grimes GJ, et al. *Effect of GSH aerosol on oxidant-antioxidant imbalance in idiopathic pulmonary fibrosis.* Lancet 338: 215-216, 1991

Brigham KL. *Oxidant stress & adult respiratory distress syndrome.* Eur. Respir. J. Suppl. 11: 482s-484s, 1990

Brown RK, Kelly FJ. *Evidence for increased oxidative damage in patients with cystic fibrosis.* Pediatr. Res. 36: 487-493, 1994

Buhl R, Meyer A, Vogelmeier C. *Oxidant-protease interaction in the lung. Prospects for antioxidant therapy.* Chest 110 (6 Suppl): 267S-2727S, 1996

Buhl R, Vogelmeier C. *Therapy of lung diseases with anti-oxidants.* Pneumologie 48: 50-56, 1994

Buhl R, Vogelmeier C, Critinden, et al. *Augmentation of glutathione in the fluid lining the epithelium of the lower respiratory tract by directly administering glutathione aerosol.* Proc. Natl. Acad. Sci. USA 87: 4063-4067, 1990

Bunnel E, Pacht ER. *Oxidized glutathione is increased in the alveolar fluid of patients with the adult respiratory distress syndrome.* American Rev. Respir. Dis. 148: 1174-1178, 1993

Calabrese C, Tosco A, Abete P et al. *Randomized, single blind, controllet trial of inhaled glutathione vs placebo in patients with cystic fibrosis.* J Cyst Fibros 14(2):203-10, 2015

Cantin A, Crystal RG. *Oxidants, antioxidants & the pathogenesis of emphysema.* Eur. J. Dis. Suppl. 139:7-17, 1985

Cantin A, Hubbard RC, Crystal RG. *Glutathione deficiency in the epithelial lining fluid of the lower respiratory tract in idiopathic pulmonary fibrosis.* American Rev. Respir. Dis. 139: 370-372, 1989

Cantin A, Larivee P, Begin RO. *Extracellular glutathione suppresses human lung fibroblast proliferation.* American J. Respir. Cell. Mol. Biol. 3: 79-85, 1990

Cato A, Goldstein I, Millman. *A double-blind parallel study of acetylcysteine-isoproterenol & saline-isoproterenol in patients with chronic obstructive lung disease.* J. Int. Med. Res. 5: 175-183, 1977

Cao T, Xu N, Wang Z, Liu H. *Effects of Glutathione S-Transferase Gene Polymorphisms & Antioxidant Capacity per Unit Albumin on the Pathogenesis of Chronic Obstructive Pulmonary Disease.* 2017:6232397, 2017

Castillo RL, Carrasco RA, Alvarez PI et al. *Relationship between severity of adult community-acquired pneumonia & impairment of the antioxidant defense system.* Biol Res. 46(2):207-13, 2013

Cazzola M, Calzetta L, Page C. et al. *Influence of N-acetylcysteine on chronic bronchitis or COPD exacerbations: a meta-analysis.* Eur Respir Rev 24(137):451-61, 2015

Ciofu O, Lykkesfeldt J. *Antioxidant supplementation for lung disease in cystic fibrosis.* Cochrane Database Syst Rev (8):CD007020, 2014

Conaway CC, Jiao D, Kelloff GJ, et al. *Chemopreventive potential of fumaric acid, n-acetylcysteine, N-(4-hydroxyphenyl) retinamide & beta-carotene for tobacco-nitrosamine-induced lung tumors in A/J mice.* Cancer Lett. 124: 85-93, 1998

Cotgreave IA, Moldeus P. *Lung protection by thiol-containing antioxidants.* Bull. Eur. Physiopathol. Respir. 23: 272-277, 1987

Dai X, Bowatte G, Lowe AJ et al. *Do Glutathione S-Transferase Genes Modify the Link between Indoor Air Pollution & Asthma, Allergies & Lung Function?* A Systematic Review. Curr Allergy Asthma Rep 18(3):20, 2018

D'Agostini F, Bagnasco M, Giunciuglio D, et al. *Inhibition by oral n-acetylcysteine of doxorubicin-induced clastogenicity & alopecia, & prevention of primary tumors & lung metastasis in mice.* Int. J. Oncol. 13: 217-224, 1998

Davreux CJ, Soric I, Nathens AB, et al. *N-acetyl cysteine attenuates acute lung injury in the rat.* Shock 8: 432-438, 1997

De Flora S, Grassi C, Carati L. *Attenuation of influenza-like symptomatology & improvement of cell-mediated immunity with long-term n-acetylcysteine treatment.* Eur. Respir. J. 19: 1535-1541, 1997

Demling R, Ikegami K, Lalonde C. *Increased lipid peroxidation & decreased antioxidant activity correspond with death after smoke exposure in the rat.* J. Burn Care Rehabil. 16(2 Pt 1): 104-110, 1995

Demling R, Lalonde C, Picard L, Blanchard J. *Changes in lung & systemic oxidant & antioxidant activity after smoke inhalation.* Shock 1: 101-107, 1994

Dickerhof N, Pearson JF, Hoskin TS et al. *Oxidative stress in early cystic fibrosis lung disease is exacerbated by airway glutathione deficiency.* Free Radic Biol Med 113-236-243, 2017

Dickerhof N, Turner R, Khalilova I et al. *Oxidized glutathione & uric acid as biomarkers of early cystic fibrosis lung disease.* J Cyst Fibros 16(2):214-221, 2017

Eiserich JP, van der Vliet, et al. *Dietary antioxidants & cigarette smoke-induced biomolecular damage: a complex interaction.* American J. Clin. Nutr. 62(6 Suppl): 1490S-1500S, 1995

Fitzpatrick AM, Jones DP, Brown LA. *Glutathione redox control of asthma: from molecular mechanisms to therapeutic opportunities.* Antioxid Redox Signal 17(2):375-408, 2012

Fowdar K, Chen H, He Z et al. *The effect of N-acetylcysteine on exacerbations of chronic obstructive pulmonary disease:* A meta-analysis & systematic review. Heart Lung 46(2):120-128, 2017

Goldstein RH, Fine A. *Potential therapeutic initiatives for fibrogenic lung diseases.* Chest 108: 848-855, 1995

Gould NS, Min E, Gauthier S et al. *Lung glutathione adaptive responses to cigarette smoke exposure.* Respir Res 12:133, 2011

Greene LS. *Asthma & oxidant stress: nutritional, environmental & genetic risk factors.* J. American Coll. Nutr. 14: 317-324, 1995

Gressier B, Lebegue S, Gosset P, et al. *Protective role of glutathione on alpha ! proteinase inhibitor inactivation by the myeloperoxidase system. Hypothetic study for the therapeutic strategy in the management of smoker's emphysema.* Fundam. Clin. Pharmacol. 8: 518-524, 1994

Grunwell JR, Gillespie SE, Ward JM et al. *Comparison of Glutathione, Cysteine, & Their Redox Potentials in the Plasma of Critically Ill & Healthy Children.* Front Pediatr 3 :46, 2015

Hansen NC, Skriver A, Brorsen-Riis L, et al. *Orally administered n-acetylcysteine may improve general well-being in patients with mild chronic bronchitis.* Respir. Med. 88: 531-515, 1994

Hasselmark L, Malmgren R, Unge G, Zetterstrom O. *Lowered platelet glutathione peroxidase activity in patients with intrinsic asthma.* Allergy 45: 523-527, 1990

Hull J, Vervaart P, Grimwood K, Phelan P. *Pulmonary oxidative stress response in young children with cystic fibrosis.* Thorax 52: 557-560, 1997

Hunninghake GW, Kalica AR. *Approaches to the treatment of pulmonary fibrosis.American J. Respir. Crit. Care Med. 151(3 Pt 1): 915-918, 1995*

Ikegami K, Lalonde C, Young YK, et al. *Comparison of plasma reduced glutathione & oxidized glutathione with lung & liver tissue oxidant & antioxidant activity during acute inflammation.Shock 1: 307-312, 1994*

Kadrabova J, Mad'aric A, Kovacikova Z, et al. *Selenium status is decreased in patients with intrinsic asthma.Biol. Tr. Elem. Res. 52: 241-248, 1996*

Kelly FJ, Cotgrove M, Mudway IS. *Respiratory lining tract fluid antioxidants: the first line of defense against serious gaseous pollutants.Cent. Eur. J. Public Health 4 Suppl: 11-14, 1996*

Kettle AJ, Turner R, Gangell CL et al. *Oxidation contributes to low glutathione in the airways of children with cystic fibrosis.Eur Respir J 44(1):122-9, 2014*

Khatri SB, Peabody J, Burwell L et al. *Systemic antioxidants & lung function in asthmatics during high ozone season: a closer look at albumin, glutathione, & associations with lung function.* Clin Transl 7(4):314-8, 2014

LANDS LC, ISKANDAR M, BEAUDOIN N ET AL. *Dietary supplementation with pressurized whey in patients with cystic fibrosis.J Med Food 13(1):77-82, 2010*

LANDS LC, GREY VL, GRENIER. *Total plasma antioxidant capacity in cystic fibrosis. Pediatr. Pulmonol. 29: 81-87, 2000*

LAURENT T, MARKERT M, FEIHL F, ET AL. *Oxidant-antioxidant balance in granulocytes during ARDS. Effect of n-acetylcysteine.Chest 109: 163-166, 1996*

LI F, LI S, CHANG H ET AL. *Quantitative assessment of the association between the GSTM1-null genotype & the risk of childhood asthma.* Genet Test Mol Biomarkers 17(9):656-61, 2013

LI XF, OUYANG B, WU JF ET AL. *[N-acetylcysteine (NAC) inhibited pulmonary fibrosis in acute respiratory distress syndrome (ARDS)].* Zhongguo Wei Zhong Bing Ji Jiu Yi Xue 23(10):559-601, 2011

LOTHIAN B, GREY V, KIMOFF RJ, LANDS LC. *Treatment of obstructive airway disease with a cysteine donor protein supplement:* A case report. Chest: 117:914-916, 2000

MACNEE W. *Chronic obstructive pulmonary disease from science to the clinic: the role of glutathione in oxidant-antioxidant balance.* Monaldi. Arch. Chest Dis. 52: 479-485, 1997

MACNEE W, BRIDGEMAN MM, MARSDEN M, ET AL. *The effects of n-acetylcysteine & glutathione on smoke-induced changes in lung phagocytes & epithelial cells.* American J. Med. 91(3C): 60S-66S, 1991

MARSON FA, BERTUZZO CS, RIBEIRO AF, RIBEIRO JD ET AL. *Polymorphisms in the glutathione pathway modulate cystic fibrosis severity: a cross-sectional study.* BMC Med Genet 15-27, 2014

MATERA MG, CALZETTA L, CAZZOLA M. *Oxidation pathway & exacerbations in COPD: the role of NAC.* Expert Rev Respir Med 10(1):89-97, 2016

MEYER A, BUHL R, KAMPF S, MAGNUSSEN H. *Intravenous n-acetylcysteine & lung glutathione of patients with pulmonary fibrosis & normals.* American J. Respir. Crit. Care Med. 152: 1055-1060, 1995

MEYER A, BUHL R, MAGNUSSEN H. *The effect of oral n-acetylcysteine on lung glutathione levels in idiopathic pulmonary fibrosis.* Eur. Respir. J. 7: 431-436, 1994

MISSO NL, POWERS KA, GILLON RL, ET AL. *Reduced platelet glutathione peroxidase activity & serum selenium concentration in atopic asthmatic patients.* Clin Exp Allergy. 1996 Jul;26(7):838-47.

MORADI M ET AL. *The role of glutathione-S-transferase polymorphisms on clinical outcome of ALI/ARDS patient treated with N-acetylcysteine.* Respir Med 103(3):434-41, 2009

MORENO-SOLIS G, DELA TORRE-AGUILAR MJ, TORRES-BORREGO J ET AL. *Oxidative stress & inflamatory plasma biomarkers in respiratory syncytial virus bronchiolitis.* Clin Respir J 11(6):839-846, 2017

MORRIS PE, BERNARD GR. *Significance of glutathione in lung disease & implications for therapy.* American J. Med. Sci. 307: 119-127, 1994

NASH EF, STEPHENSON A, RATIEN F, TULLIS E. *Nebulized & oral thiol derivatives for pulmonary disease in cystic fibrosis.* Cochrane Database Syst Rev (1):CD007168, 2009

NOVAK Z, NEMETH I, GYURKOVITS K, ET AL. *Examination of the role of oxygen free radicals in bronchial asthma in childhood.* Clin. Chim. Acta. 201: 247-251, 1991

OLIVIERI D, MARISCO SA, DEL DONNO M. *Improvement of mucociliary transport in smokers by mucolytics.* Eur. J. Respir. Dis. Suppl. 139: 142-145, 1985

ORTOLANI O, GRATINO F, LEONE D, ET AL. *Usefulness of the prevention of oxygen radical damage in the critical patient using the parental administration of reduced glutathione in high doses.* Boll. Soc. Ital. Biol. Sper. 68: 239-244, 1992

PACHT ER, TIMERMAN AP, LYKENS MG, MEROLA AJ. *Deficiency of alveolar fluid glutathione in patients with sepsis & the adult respiratory distress syndrome.* Chest 100: 1397-1403, 1991

PARR GD, HUITSON A. *Oral Fabrol (oral n-acetylcysteine) in chronic bronchitis.* Br. J. Dis. Chest 81: 341-348, 1987

PATTERSON CE, RHOADES RA. *Protective role of sulfhydryl reagents in oxidant lung injury.Exp. Lung Res. 14 Suppl: 1005-1019, 1988*

PEARSON DJ, SUAREZ-MENDEZ VJ, DAY JP, MILLER PF. *Selenium status in relation to reduced glutathione peroxidase activity in aspirin-sensitive asthma.Clin Exp. Allergy 21: 203-208, 1991*

PIACENTINI S, POLIMANTI R, SIMONELLI I ET AL. *Glutathione S-transferase polymorphisms, asthma susceptibility & confounding variables: a meta-analysis.* Mol Biol Rep 40(4):3299-313, 2013

PORTAL BC, RICHARD MJ, FAURE HS, ET AL. *Altered antioxidant status & increased lipid peroxidation in children with cystic fibrosis.American J. Clin. Nutr. 61: 843-847, 1995*

POWELL CV, NASH AA, POWERS HJ, PRIMHAK RA. *Antioxidant status in asthma.Pediatr. Pulmonol. 18: 34-38, 1994*

RAHMAN I, MACNEE W. *Role of oxidants/ antioxidants in smoking-induced lung diseases.Free Radic. Biol. Med. 21: 6669-681, 1996*

RASMUSSEN JB, GLENNOW C. *Reduction in days of illness after long-term treatment with n-acetylcys-*

teine controlled-release tablets in patients with chronic bronchitis. Eur. Respirol. J. 4:351-355, 1988

Reynaert NL. *Glutathione biochemistry in asthma.* Biochim Biophys Acta 1810(11):1045-51, 2011

Riise GC, Larsson S, Larsson P, et al. *The intrabronchial microbial flora in chronic bronchitis patients: a target for n-acetylcysteine therapy?Eur. Respir. J. 7: 94-101, 1994*

Rogers A, Bunyavanich S.Unravelling gene-by-environment effects in asthma & allergy: *the glutathione pathway as an early success story.Clin Exp Allergy 41(11):1502-4, 2011*

Rogers DF, Jeffery PK.Inhibition by oral n-acetylcysteine of cigarette smoke-induced "bronchitis" in the rat.Exp. Lung Res. 10: 267-283, 1986

Roum JH, Buhl R, McElvaney, et al.Systemic deficiency of glutathione in cystic fibrosis.J. Appl. Physiol. 75: 2419-2424, 1993

Sadowska AM. *N-Acetylcysteine mucolysis in the management of chronic obstructive pulmonary disease.* Ther Adv Respir Dis 6(3):127-35, 2012

Sanguinetti CM. *N-acetylcysteine in COPD: why, how, & when?* Muldiscip Respir Med 11:8, 2016

Santus P, Corsico A, Solidoro P et al. *Oxidative stress & respiratory system: pharmacological & clinical reappraisal of N-acetylcysteine.* COPD 11(6):705-17, 2014

Sala R, Moriggi E, Corvasce G, Morelli D. *Protection by n-acetylcysteine against pulmonary endothelial cell damage induced by oxidant injury.* Eur. Respir. J. 6: 440-446, 1993

Simon LM, Suttorp N. *Lung cell oxidant injury: decrease in oxidant mediated cytotoxicity by n-acetylcysteine.* Eur. J. Dis. Suppl. 139: 132-135, 1985

Suter PM, Domenighetti G, Schaller, et al. *N-acetylcysteine enhances recovery from acute lung injury in man. A randomized, double-blind, placebo-controlled clinical study.Chest 105: 190-194, 1994*

Tanswell AK, Freeman BA. *Antioxidant therapy in critical care medicine.New Horiz. 3: 330-341, 1995*

Tattersall AB, Bridgman KM, Huitson A. *Irish general practice study of acetylcysteine (Fabrol) in chronic bronchitis. J. Int. Med. Res. 12: 96-101. 1984*

Teramoto S, Fukuchi Y, Uejima Y, et al. *Superoxide anion formation & glutathione metabolism of blood in patients with idiopathic pulmonary fibrosis.Biochem. Mol. Med. 55: 66-70, 1995*

Tse HN, Raiteri L, Wong KY et al. *Benefits of high-dose N-acetylcysteine to exacerbation-prone patients with COPD.* Chest 146(3):611-623, 2014

Tse HN, Raiteri L, wong KY et al. *High-dose N-acetylcysteine in stable COPD: the 1-year, double-blind, randomized, placebo-controlled HIACE study.* Chest 144(1):106-118, 2013

Van Zandwijk N. *N-acetylcysteine (nac) & glutathione: antioxidant & chemopreventative properties, with special reference to lung cancer.* J. Cell. Biochem. Suppl. 22: 24-32, 1995

Van Zandwijk N. *N-acetylcysteine for lung cancer protection.* Chest 107: 1437-1441, 1995

Vina J, Servera E, Aseni M, et al. *Exercise causes blood glutathione oxidation in chronic obstructive pulmonary disease: prevention by O2 therapy.* J. Appl. Physiol. 81: 2198-2202. 1996

Vlahos R, Bozinosvki S. *Glutathione peroxidase-1 as a novel therapeutic target for COPD.* Redox Rep 18(4):142-9, 2013

Volkl KP, Schneider B. *Therapy of respiratory tract diseases with n-acetylcysteine. An open therapeutic observation study of 2,512 patients.* Fortschr. Med. 110: 346-350, 1992

Wagner PD, Mathieu-Costello O, Bebout BE, et al. *Protection against pulmonary O2 toxicity by n-acetylcysteine.* Eur. Respir. J. 2: 116-126, 1989

White CW, Repine JE. *Pulmonary antioxidant defense mechanisms. Exp. Lung Res. 8: 81-96, 1985*

Winklhofer-Roob BM. *Oxygen free radicals & antioxidants in cystic fibrosis: the concept of an oxidant-antioxidant imbalance.* Acta. Paediatr. Suppl. 83: 49-57, 1994

Witschi H, Espiritu I, Yu M, Willits NH. *The effects of phenethyl isothianate, n-acetylcysteine & green tea on tobacco smoke-induced lung tumors in strain A/J mice Carcinogenesis 19: 1789-1794, 1998*

Zinellu A, Fois AG, Sotgia S et al. *Plasma protein thiols: an early marker of oxidative stress in asthma & chronic obstructive pulmonary disease.* Eur J Clin Invest 46(2):181-8, 2016

13

Digestive Diseases

This chapter describes the latest research on glutathione in the digestive tract.

A string of connected organs, the digestive tract (see Figure 28) stretches from the mouth to the bowels. Through it we eat, digest and eliminate waste. It is prone to many digestive disorders, caused by such factors as genetics, stress, toxins, infectious disease and pharmaceutical drugs.

In the mouth and salivary organs, glutathione helps protect from periodontal disease, stomatitis and gingivitis. In the esophagus it counters inflammation. In the stomach, it fights against gastritis, peptic ulcer and cancer, and in the liver against hepatitis and organ failure. GSH also defends the pancreas against inflammation and the large intestine (bowel) from colitis, inflammatory bowel disease, ulcerative colitis, Crohn's disease and cancer.

Gastritis

Gastritis is an inflammation of the stomach lining (gastric mucosa). Acute gastritis produces a short-lived inflammation with symptoms of pain, heartburn, occasional nausea, vomiting and loss of appetite. Chronic gastritis is more prolonged. It has fewer symptoms but more readily progresses to serious illnesses such as anemia, stomach ulcer and stomach cancer. As the population ages, gastritis is becoming so common that some scientists consider it a part of the aging process.

One of many possible causes of gastritis is generalized stress. It may be a psychological reaction to daily life or be the physically induced trauma of major illness, head

Organ	Common Disorders
mouth and salivary organs	periodontal disease • stomatitis, gingivitis • parotitis
esophagus	esophagitis • cancer • hiatus hernia • Barrett's esophagus
stomach	gastritis • peptic ulcer • cancer
liver	hepatitis • liver failure
gall bladder	gallstones (cholelithiasis)
pancreas	pancreatitis • cancer
small intestines	gastroenteritis, celiac disease • gluten intolerance • intestinal ischemia
large intestines (bowel)	colitis • inflammatory bowel disease • ulcerative colitis Crohn's disease • cancer, polyps • malabsorption syndromes

TABLE 25: *The digestive tract: organs and their disorderst*

Stress and anxiety	Alcohol
Trauma, burns	Vitamin C
Aspirin	Extreme foods
Anti-inflammatories	Tobacco
Corticosteroids	Blood type O
Caffeine	Helicobacter pylori

TABLE 26: Some risk factors for developing ulcers

injury or burns. A long list of toxins has also been implicated, the most common ones being coffee, alcohol, tobacco, over-spiced foods and certain infectious diseases. Some often-used pharmaceutical drugs may also induce gastritis, notably: aspirin, corticosteroids, and anti-inflammatory medications. Mixing these drugs may be especially damaging. Always consult your physician before combining them.

Stomach ulcers

Stomach ulcers (peptic ulcers) are spots where the stomach lining has been eroded, leaving an open wound. This can vary in depth and may develop into a hole through the stomach wall (perforated ulcer). Most ulcers occur in the stomach or duodenum and they are rarely found elsewhere along the digestive tract. About one in ten North Americans will suffer at some point in their life from an ulcer, leading to symptoms like those seen in gastritis—abdominal pain, heartburn, and even melena (black or maroon-colored stools caused by oxidized blood leaking into the digestive tract). A bleeding ulcer may also lead to anemia—a low hemoglobin (red blood) count.

Ulcers were once thought to be caused by excessive acid levels of digestive juices, but many ulcer patients have normal acid levels. We now know that ulcers also develop when the stomach lining fails to protect itself from these strong acids. There are various possible causes for this failure.

Several factors contribute to these defenses. Mucus production, biochemical cellular barriers and adequate replacement of damaged mucosal cells all play a role in the maintenance of a healthy stomach lining. Immunological factors are only just now being understood. For example, they seem

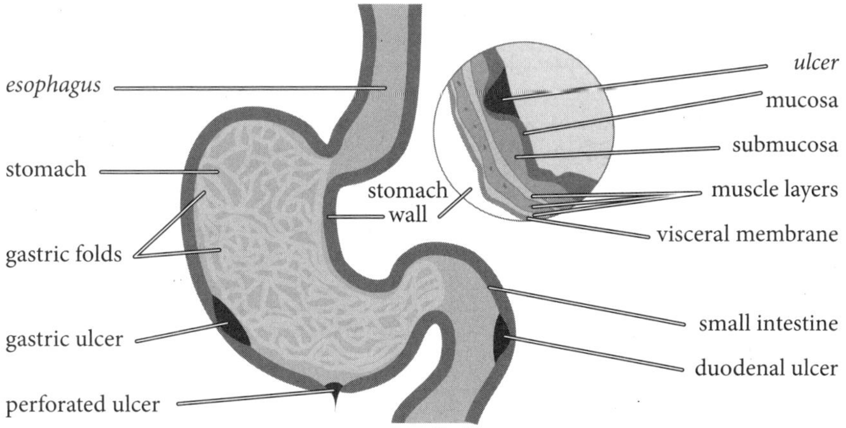

FIGURE 28: Ulcers of the stomach and duodenum

to explain why blood Type 'A' individuals are likely to develop stomach ulcers whereas those with blood type 'O' are more prone to duodenal ulcers.

Many factors can disrupt the protective lining. Over-secretion or overproduction of stomach acids is one. The same drugs that cause gastritis may also lead to ulcers, either by increasing acid production or by modifying the protective factors. These drugs include corticosteroids, aspirin, and dozens of anti-inflammatory drugs known by a variety of brand names.

Similarly to gastritis, other risk factors include cigarette smoking, alcohol abuse, high caffeine intake. Dietary factors include overindulgence in fatty foods and highly spiced foods, such as whole chili peppers. High dosages of vitamin C (ascorbic acid) have also been implicated. Stress and anxiety have traditionally been identified as causes, but now seem less significant.

Medical science has recently discovered an infectious agent involved with ulcer formation—the bacteria Helicobacter pylori, found in 70-90% of ulcer cases. A short course of antibiotics may cure the problem, but a significant portion of the population has H. pylori in the digestive tract without ever developing ulcers. Other immunological or physiological factors must come into play before this infection becomes pathological.

Case study

Kurt was a 53 year-old vice-president of sales for a large manufacturing company. Among the seventy-hour weeks, two-martini lunches, coffees well into the night, a pack-and-a-half-a-day cigarette habit, and the stress of a poor sales quarter, he developed severe stomach pains. He was lucky. Medical investigation determined that he only had gastritis (stomach inflammation) but that if his present lifestyle continued, he would likely develop an ulcer. Unwilling to quit smoking or working so much, he agreed to a reduction in alcohol and coffee and to visit a nutritionist. After three weeks on silymarin, melatonin, glutamine, chamomile, selenium, multiple vitamins including B-complex, C and E, he felt "infinitely better," even though sales were still down. He laughs about this now and is thinking of quitting smoking and starting regular exercise. Kurt now believes that if he feels better in his body, his performance at work will improve.

Stomach cancer

Stomach cancer (gastric carcinoma) often begins at the site of a stomach ulcer. It is generally believed that ulcers do not necessarily cause stomach cancer, but that stomach cancer is often preceded by a particular type of ulcer. In America, it is the seventh most common cause of cancer death. However, the incidence of stomach cancer varies enormously around the world. In Japan, Chile and Iceland it's one of the most common causes of mortality. Scientists have suggested that this may be due to differences in diet or environment. The theory is supported by the fact that certain occupational hazards, such as exposure to coal dust or heavy metals like mercury and lead, also increase the chances of contracting this disease.

Other risk factors include certain types of

Medical Conditions	Toxins	Foods
stomach ulcer	alcohol	barbecued
chronic gastritis	tobacco	smoked
stomach polyps	aflatoxins	pickled
	heavy metals	highly salted

TABLE 27: *Some potential causes of stomach cancer*

prepared food and molds. Some moldy foods include a carcinogen called aflatoxin. This byproduct of fungi can be found growing in nuts, seeds, corn and other dried foods.

H. pylori bacteria have also been implicated in stomach cancer. Chronic gastritis (stomach inflammation) and polyps

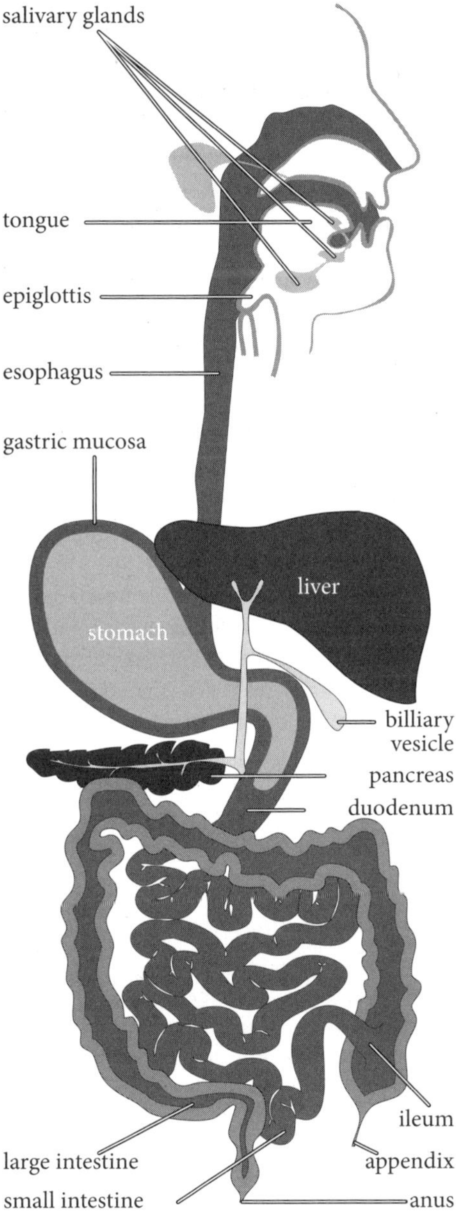

FIGURE 29: The Digestive Tract

(abnormal protruding growths) may also become cancerous. These conditions, as well as stomach ulcer, toxins like alcohol, tobacco, aflatoxins and foods that are barbecued, smoked, pickled and highly salted, may all contribute to the development of cancer.

GSH and the stomach

Glutathione's ability to protect the stomach is being widely researched. Its therapeutic role is promising and it has been shown to protect the stomach in several different ways. It is a primary shield against oxidative stress, it detoxifies potentially harmful substances—even carcinogens—and regulates immune mechanisms, ensuring a more effective response to these threats.

Acute gastritis

It has recently been shown that GSH levels rise when the lining of the stomach faces a toxic challenge. Several groups of researchers demonstrated this, using alcohol to provoke an anti-toxic response. Low to moderate levels of alcohol led to an adaptive elevation in GSH levels, but high levels of alcohol overwhelmed and eventually damaged this system.

An even more direct clinical application of glutathione's protective role in the stomach was brought to light by Balint in Hungary. His team studied an all-too-common problem—gastric side-effects of anti-inflammatory drugs such as indomethacin and piroxicam (trade names: Indocid, Feldene etc.). Subjects given small amounts of glutathione or cysteine at the same time as the drug itself had significantly fewer side-effects. This is a great example of a natural therapy and traditional medicine complementing each other.

It's known that patients with chronic inflammation of the stomach lining (gastritis) and those carrying the bacteria Helicobacter pylori suffer increased free-radical damage and GSH consumption. Both conditions may lead to ulcer disease and probably also increase the risk of stomach cancer.

Ulcer disease may also be caused in part

by high levels of lipid peroxidation, as well as disruption of the antioxidant defense mechanisms in the stomach lining (gastric mucosa). There is certainly a close relationship between GSH-dependent enzymes and the development of gastric ulcers. Glutathione and its related enzymes are found only in very low concentrations within the ulcer. Correspondingly, they rise again when the ulcerated tissue heals. Laboratory animals given drugs to lower their GSH levels suffered from significantly higher oxidative damage to the stomach lining.

Traditionally, Helicobacter pylori-related ulcers are treated with antibiotics (Amoxicillin, Biaxin, Flagyl, etc.) and proton-pump inhibitors (Losec, Pantoloc, etc.). This is more effective when applied along with antioxidants. A newer medication (Rebamipide, developed in Japan) works partly as a free radical scavenger and slows down GSH loss. Studies using Rebamipide along with conventional drugs show improved healing.

A Swiss group from the University of Zurich studied tobacco smokers with ulcers. Combining conventional treatment with the potent GSH precursor NAC (n-acetylcysteine), produced good results. This makes sense because smokers in general suffer from much higher levels of oxidative stress than non-smokers, and benefit more obviously from high antioxidant levels. Furthermore, Davydenko's team in the Ukraine believe that antioxidant therapy should continue even after conventional treatment has stopped.

When we look at cancer cells in the stomach, as well as the normal cells immediately surrounding them, we find several recurring characteristics. Cells are heavily damaged by oxidative stress, their antioxidant defenses are diminished and the power-plants of each cell (the mitochondria) are defective—possibly due to free radical damage. Notably, GSH-related enzyme systems are impaired. There is little doubt that low glutathione levels go hand-in-hand with increased risk of cancer. The following research results speak for themselves.

Katoh at the National Institute of Environmental Health Sciences in North Carolina showed a particular relationship between GSH levels and the development of gastric cancer. For genetic reasons, some people have inactive or inefficient sub-types of GSH enzymes. They are at greater risk of contracting both stomach and bowel cancer.

A group from Italy studied glutathione levels in patients with stomach cancer and came to the unequivocal conclusion that the 'decrease of this tripeptide' (glutathione) was 'dramatical.' Their work suggests that any therapeutic approach should include such glutathione precursors as cysteine.

A Japanese team reached similar conclusions while investigating gastric ulcers. They found that levels of gastric mucosal GSH 'are closely related to the etiology and course of gastric ulcer.' Various researchers and theorists have suggested that the antioxidant capacity of the cancerous tissues has been impaired and that, even more significantly, the body's entire antioxidant defense mechanism may be breaking down.

Pancreatitis

The pancreas is an important organ with several functions, the two most crucial being: a) to secrete digestive enzymes that help prepare food for intestinal absorption, and b) to produce hormones such as insulin and glucagon that are critical to the metabolism of sugars and carbohydrates.

Pancreatitis is an inflammation of the pancreas leading to pain (often severe), as well as digestive and metabolic abnormalities. It can be potentially life-threatening, and, if it becomes chronic, may lead to other illnesses, like diabetes.

Acute pancreatitis is an abrupt onset of pancreatitis most commonly caused by blockage of the passage to the intestines. This usually happens when gall-stones form and get lodged there, and sometimes at the site of a tumor. The pancreatic juices contain powerful digestive enzymes which may back up when blocked, and start to digest the pancreas itself.

Other causes of acute pancreatitis include certain viral and bacterial infections, specific drugs, high fat levels in the blood including cholesterol or triglycerides (hyperlipidemia), abdominal trauma, and critically low blood pressure (severe hypotension).

Chronic pancreatitis develops over months or years, usually after repeated bouts of acute pancreatitis. The most common trigger by far for this type of pancreatitis is alcoholism. Chronic pancreatitis may impair normal functions, such as insulin secretion, leading, among other potential problems, to secondary diabetes.

Many studies suggest that oxyradicals and free radicals are involved in the development of all types of pancreatitis. The importance of GSH in the antioxidant defense of the pancreas cannot be overstated. Braganza's team at the Royal Infirmary in Manchester, UK, found GSH depletion in all early stages of acute pancreatitis. They surmise that low GSH levels may predict the vulnerability of other organs to pancreatitis. Schoenberg at Germany's University of Ulm suggests that GSH supplementation may be a way to avoid extra-pancreatic complications.

Researchers at the Royal Infirmary developed the 'Manchester oxidant stress hypothesis' to describe the development of pancreatitis. They suggest that falling GSH levels enable the eventual breakdown of cells, and oxidant stress (caused mainly by toxins) opens the door to chronic pancreatitis. This team developed an antioxidant cocktail of methionine, vitamin C and selenium in placebo-controlled, retrospective cross-sectional trials.

At Germany's University of Dusseldorf, Luthen's team used oxothiazolidine carboxylate (OTC)—a potent GSH-enhancing drug—to reduce the severity of pancreatitis. They found critical GSH loss in biliary pancreatitis (blockage due to a gall stone), and believe that when anti-oxidative defenses are weak, GSH depletion triggers early activation of auto-digestive enzymes. Walling considers GSH depletion a key factor when external toxins cause chronic pancreatitis.

The most common cause of chronic pancreatitis is alcoholic pancreatitis. Sufferers are particularly deficient in levels of vitamins E and A, selenium and glutathione peroxidase. Researchers have suggested that these patients needed higher daily requirements to ward off such oxidative stress.

Another variety of this disease is hereditary pancreatitis—an inherited disease that was examined at the Cleveland Clinic Foundation. A correlation was found between the disease and diminished antioxidant defenses, most notably GSH, selenium and vitamin E. The close relationship of these three antioxidants is described in Chapters 1 and 4. The researchers at Cleveland proposed that supplementation therapy with natural products would decrease the frequency of attacks.

The main complication leading to death from pancreatitis is multiple organ failure. Here, the integrity of cell membranes breaks down, leading to leakages both into and out of these cells. Wang and his team at Sweden's Lund University successfully used NAC (N-acetylcysteine, a potent GSH-raising drug) to prevent damage to most tissues. Gukovsky at the University of California also found that NAC led to significant improvement in acute pancreatitis patients.

Inflammatory bowel diseases

Inflammatory bowel disease includes ulcerative colitis and Crohn's Disease. Both are described here.

Ulcerative colitis

Colitis is a general term for inflammation of the bowel. Ulcerative colitis (UC) is a chronic inflammatory disease of the large bowel (colon) leading to ulcers in the mucous membranes lining it and causing pain, bloody diarrhea, gas, bloating and many other symptoms. Fever, weight loss,

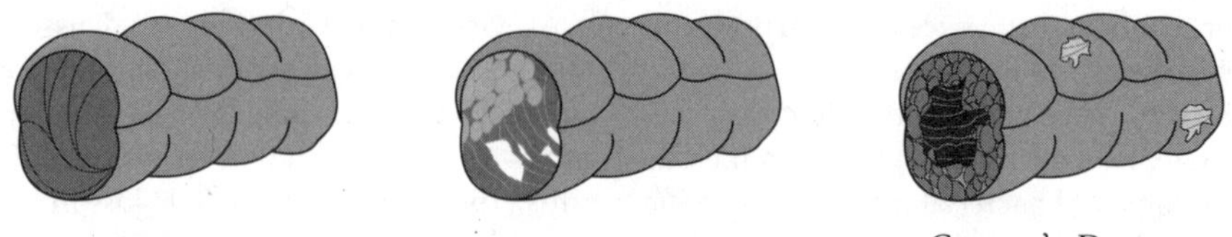

NORMAL
undamaged, unobstructed passage

ULCERATIVE COLITIS
inflamed 'cobblestones', ulcerated lining

CROHN'S DISEASE
ulcerated, obstructed passage, perforated walls

FIGURE 30: Ulcerative colitis and Crohn's Disease

joint pains and even visual problems may accompany the digestive issues.

Ulcerative colitis tends to develop early on in life, usually between the ages of 15 and 30. It ranges in severity from a single brief attack to a progressive illness complicated by severe blood loss (hemorrhaging), a perforated bowel or the spread of infection into the bloodstream (sepsis). Ulcerative colitis patients bear a higher risk of subsequent colon cancer. However ulcerative colitis is rarely fatal and most of those affected lead fairly normal lives.

The cause of this disease is still unclear but it has a small tendency to run in families. Various possibilities have been proposed, including infectious agents, immunological abnormalities, dietary factors, toxins, allergies and stress. However, these hypotheses remain unproven.

The large and small intestines lie in the lower abdomen like a loosely-folded fire hose that leads a long and winding path from the stomach to the anus (see Figure 28). Ulcerative colitis produces ulcers that eat away at the intestinal wall. Crohn's Disease is an inflammation that leads to swelling and tenderness in the intestinal wall. Figure 27 shows the different ways ulcerative colitis and Crohn's Disease affect the intestines.

Case study

28 year-old Debbie, a massage therapist, had ulcerative colitis but had so far managed to avoid surgery. She maintained a sensible diet, continuing the medications her doctor had prescribed and avoiding foods that disagreed with her. However, the previous few years had been fraught with repeated bouts of cramps, diarrhea and occasionally bloody stools. Eventually, she was unable to get through a workday without numerous visits to the washroom. A dietary consultant added to her diet a high-dose antioxidant mixture containing selenium, L-glutamine, and—when her stool was firmer—psyllium husks. Her blood loss has abated, and she now visits the washroom at lunchtimes only.

CROHN'S DISEASE

Crohn's disease (CD) is similar in many ways to ulcerative colitis (see above). However, this is potentially more severe. In ulcerative colitis, small ulcers are scattered in the lining of the large bowel. In contrast, Crohn's disease is less selective. It can affect any part of the digestive system from mouth to anus. It is most common in the ileum (the end of the small intestine where it joins the large intestine; see Figure 28). The disease occurs in heavy patches, while areas between diseased patches are only mildly affected. It is most common in the gut, where the intestine wall may grow extremely thick following repeated inflammation. Deep ulcers may pass right through the lining, perforating the gut tissues.

With repeated or prolonged inflammation of the intestine, the entire thickness of the intestinal wall is affected. As the walls thicken, the intestinal passage becomes narrow and obstructed. Symptoms can include spasms of abdominal pain, diarrhea, appetite loss, anemia and weight loss. The elderly are more prone to inflammation of the rectum. Young and old alike may suffer from chronic abscesses, deep fissures (cracks) and fistulas (abnormal passageways) in the anus. Because the entire digestive system is susceptible, complications are more profound than those following ulcerative colitis. They include bowel obstruction, infection, malabsorption, and elevated cancer risk—as much as 20 times greater than healthy individuals.

Like ulcerative colitis, the exact cause of Crohn's disease is unknown, but there tends to be a stronger familial tendency. Some researchers think this may also be an autoimmune disease. Studies suggest that sufferers may benefit by avoiding certain food additives, allergens and cigarettes.

GSH IN INFLAMMATORY BOWEL DISEASE

It is clear from observing patients with inflammatory bowel disease that inflamed cells in the lining of the intestines are a hotbed of free radicals. However, there is still debate as to whether the free radicals cause the damage characterizing these diseases, or result from it. Samples of tissue inflamed by ulcerative colitis and Crohn's disease show consistent evidence of severe oxidative stress. The degree of oxidative damage can even be correlated to the degree of inflammation. Of all the antioxidants that can prevent or retard this damage, GSH is the main one.

Researchers from around the world, including Bhaskar from India and Australia's Buffington, have scrutinized tissues affected by inflammatory bowel disease and Crohn's disease. All have remarked on a significant depletion of glutathione and alteration of its enzymes. In the past, most researchers believed that GSH depletion was more likely to be a consequence of ongoing inflammation and oxidative stress than a contributing cause of the problem. But today, opinions may be changing. More recent findings by B. Sido of the German University of Heidelberg reported not only diminished GSH levels but also diminished activity of the enzymes involved in GSH production. This implies that declining glutathione production may actually contribute to the development of the disease. Genetic testing of glutathione enzyme abnormalities has validated this suggestion.

Antioxidant therapy has thus emerged as a treatment for inflammatory bowel disease. One of the more traditional groups of medications applied to these diseases are the aminosalicylates (sulfasalazine, Asacol, Dipentum, etc.). These are potent antioxidants, but are also pharmaceutical drugs. More natural, less toxic products would be preferable.

Cruz, Galvez and their team from Spain's University of Granada, were able to protect inflamed bowels with a flavonoid called rutoside. (Flavonoids are a variety of crystalline compounds found in plants.) This worked with both acute and chronic disease. They explained their success by pointing to rutoside's tendency to maintain or increase GSH content in the gut.

Crohn's disease (CD) is more likely to lead to malnutrition than ulcerative colitis. The reasons are complex but are summarized by the fact that Crohn's is more deeply involved in the bowel. The nutritional status of those suffering from this disease has been investigated at great length and reveals general GSH depletion throughout the body. These findings have also been reported in children with CD, possibly due to ongoing oxidative stress.

Numerous scientists have suggested oral GSH supplementation as a treatment for UC and CD. We presented evidence in Chapters 1 and 4 that oral glutathione is not effective in raising total body GSH. However, digestive tissues seem able to make use of it. The tissues most positively affected by oral GSH are those in direct contact with it. The intestinal lining (mucosa) is one. Alton Meister—often called the father of glutathione research—suggests that both oral GSH and GSH excreted in the bile can protect the intestinal mucosa. There, it has been shown that depletion of gut glutathione leads to severe damage of this sensitive lining.

For a long time European researchers have

taken the lead in using glutathione-elevating substances to address medical issues. In the World Journal of Gastroenterology, Guijarro and his team published a double-blind study that successfully showed improvement in ulcerative colitis patients receiving NAC. Romagnoli similarly showed significant results in Crohn's patients using NAC.

Celiac disease, gluten intolerance

Celiac disease (CD) is a digestive illness triggered in some people by foods containing the protein 'gluten' and a component of gluten called 'gliadin.' Celiac disease was previously called 'sprue' or 'coeliac sprue'. The medical term is 'gluten-sensitive enteropathy.' Less severe forms of the disease are often referred to as 'gluten intolerance' or 'gluten sensitivity.'

Gluten protein is found in wheat, barley and rye. The mainstay of treatment is avoidance of these products. However, these are extremely popular grains that appear in many types of foods as well as baked goods. For this reason, individuals with celiac disease must watch out for gluten-containing foods, and carefully read product labels.

In sensitive individuals, gluten triggers an immune response in the small intestine. Over time this leads to inflammation and tissue damage, poor absorption of nutrients and symptoms that range from cramps, bloating and diarrhea to more serious complications, including weight loss, anemia, osteoporosis and lymphoma. Considered a type of autoimmune disease, celiac disease can lead to a host of other complaints including fatigue, headaches, rashes, joint pain and more.

Clinical trials of celiac disease using antioxidant vitamins have been promising, but have not as yet answered an important question: whether the antioxidants work by simply correcting a problem of malabsorption, or by addressing a deeper, underlying problem of oxidative stress.

Celiac disease and glutathione

Since celiac disease is an immune-related disease, it's no surprise to find both GSH and oxidative stress implicated. Various studies have demonstrated that gluten/gliadin disturbs the pro-oxidant/antioxidant balance of affected individuals by overproducing free radicals and depleting antioxidants—notably GSH. This is particularly apparent in children. Correction of celiac disease at a young age is necessary to avoid cases of 'failure to thrive.'

Conclusions

GSH and stomach disease

Evidence suggests that glutathione defends the stomach lining against various threats, including toxins, oxidative stress and carcinogens. This has prompted scientists to seek ways of raising GSH levels in humans for both preventive and curative purposes. Elevated GSH levels may protect against gastritis, ulcer and cancer and can certainly complement conventional treatments for these diseases.

Pancreatitis

It's known that pancreatitis leads to high levels of oxidative stress and glutathione depletion, and antioxidant therapy is being used to treat pancreatitis and prevent its recurrence. Although antioxidant therapy is a safe complementary treatment for chronic pancreatitis, its wider adoption as a standard healthcare tool will take time. The lynchpin of such an approach is the search for tools to enhance (modulate) intracellular glutathione levels. As these tools evolve, further research will focus on how to use them most effectively.

Inflammatory bowel disease

Imbalance in the formation of free radicals and a poor supply of antioxidant micronutrients may cause or encourage tissue injury in inflammatory bowel disease. Levels of glutathione and its related compounds are significantly lower in these diseases. Different antioxidants including GSH, GSH monoesters, NAC (N-acetylcysteine), vitamin C (ascorbate), vitamin E (tocopherol), SOD (superoxide dismutase) and others have been used with varying success. Whether GSH loss is a cause or consequence of these inflammatory disorders, they are alleviated by therapies that raise or sustain GSH levels. Recent research suggests that raising glutathione levels may be a novel approach to the treatment of both ulcerative colitis and Crohn's disease.

Celiac disease, gluten intolerance

This immune-related disease has shown high levels of oxidation and low levels of glutathione as part of its pathophysiology. Active investigation into replenishing both antioxidants and glutathione are forthcoming.

DIGESTIVE DISEASES

REFERENCES

Stomach disease

Altomare E, Grattagliano I, Didonna D, et al. *Gastric & intestinal ethanol toxicity in the rat. Effect on glutathione level & role of alcohol & acetaldehyde metabolisms.* Ital. J. Gastroenterol. Hepatol. 30:82-90, 1998

Arivazhaga S, Kavitha K, Nagini S. *Erythrocyte lipid peroxidation & antioxidants in gastric cancer patients.* Cell. Biochem. Funct. 15:15-18, 1997

Balint GA. *A novel approach to reduce the unwanted gastric side-effects of orally administered non-steroidal anti-inflammatory drugs in rats.* Exp. Toxicol. Pathol. 49:61-63, 1997

Bell W. Obst B, Sewing KF, Wagner S. *Helicobacter pylori reduces intracellular glutathione in gastric epithelial cells.* Dig Dis Sci 45(9):1769-73, 2000

Davydenko OM, Kolomoiets MIU, Davydenko IS. *Free-radical oxidation, the glutathione system & the status of the gastric mucosa in peptic ulcer in adolescents & young people under dynamic restorative treatment.* Lik Sprava 7-8:60-64, 1994

De Bruyne E, Ducatelle R, Foss D et al. *Oral glutathione supplementation drastically reduces Helicobacter-induced gastric pathologies.* Sci Rep 6:20169, 2016

Eapen CE, Madesh M. Balasubramanian KA, et al. *Mucosal mitochondrial function & antioxidant defenses in patients with gastric carcinoma.* Sc&. J. Gastroenterol. 33:957-981, 1998

Farinati F, Della Libera G, Cardin R, et al. *Gastric antioxidant, nitrites, & mucosal lipoperoxidation in chronic gastritis & Helicobacter pylori infection.* J. Clin. Gastroenterol. 22:275-281, 1996

Flahou B et al. *Gastric epithelial cell death caused by Helicobacter suis & Helicobacter pylori y-glutamyl transpeptidase is mainly glutathione degradation-dependent.* Cell Microbiol 13(12):1933-55, 2011

Giorgi G, Micheli L, Segre G, Pecchi A *Glutathione (GSH) in human stomach mucosa.Riv. Eur. Sci. Med. Farmacol. 11:163-167, 1989*

Guilarro LG, Matte J, Gisbert JP, et al. *N-acetyl-cysteine combined with mesalamine in the treatment of ulcerative colitis: a r&omized, placebo-controlled pilot study.* World J Gastroenterol 14(18):2851-2857, 2008.

Hahm KB, Lee KJ, Kim YS, et al. *Augmented eradication rates of Helicobacter pylori by new combination therapy with lansoprazole, amoxicillin, & rebamipide.* Dig. Dis. Sci. 43:235-240, 1998

Hirokawa K, Kawasaki H. *Changes in glutathione in gastric mucosa of gastric ulcer patients.* Res Commun Mol Pathol Pharmacol 88(2):163-76, 1995

Hirokawa K, Kawasaki H. *Changes in glutathione in gastric mucosa of gastric ulcer patients.* Res. Commun. Mol. Pathol. Pharmacol. 88: 163-176, 1995

Katoh T, Nagata N, Kuroda Y, et al. *Glutathione S-transferase M1 (GSTM1) & T1 (GSTT1) genetic polymorphism & susceptibility to gastric & colorectal adenocarcinoma.* Carcinogenesis 17:1855-1859, 1996

Kikkawa S, Kadohara M, Kawasaki H. *Superoxide dismutase & glutathione in the gastric mucosa of patients with chronic liver disease.* Res Commun Chem Pathol Pharmacol 78(3):289-309, 1992

Kurokawa T, Joh T, Ikai M, et al. *Rebamipide protects against oxygen radical-mediated gastric mucosal injury in rats.* Dig. Dis. Sci. 43 (9 Suppl): 113S-117S, 1998

Kuyumcu A et Al. *Improved oxidative status*

in major abdominal surgery patients after N-acetyl cysteine supplementation. Nutr J 14:4, 2015

Matthews GM, Butler RN. *Cellular mucosal defense during Helicobacter pylori infection: a review of the role of glutathione & the oxidative pentose pathway.* Helicobacter 10(4):298-306, 2005

Meng X, Liu Y, Liu B. *Glutathione S-transferase M1 null genotype meta-analysis on gastric cancer risk.* Diagn Pathol 9:122, 2014

Moghadasian MH, Godin DV. *Ethanol-induced gastrointestinal damage. Influence of endogenous antioxidant components & gender.* Digestive Disease Sci. 41:791-797, 1996

Oijen AH, Verhulst ML, Roelofs HM et al. *Eradication of Helicobacter pylori restores glutathione S-transferase activity & glutathione levels in antral mucosa.* Jpn J Cancer Res 92(12):1329-34, 2001

Pasechnikov VD, Mosin VI, Vigranskii AO. *Lipid peroxidation & the antioxidant enzyme system of the gastric mucosa in peptic ulcer.* Ter. Arkh 60: 30-33, 1988

Romagnoli C, Marcucci T, et al. *Role of N-acetylcysteine & GSH redox system on total & active MMP-2 in intestinal myofibroblasts of Crohn's disease patients.* Int J Colorectal Dis 28(7):915-924, 2013.

Savoye G, Miralles-Barrachina O et al. *Low levels of gastric mucosal glutathione during upper gastric bleeding associated with the use of nonsteroidal anti-inflammatory drugs.* Eur J Gastroenterol Hepatol 13(11):1309-13, 2001

Soliman NA, Zineldeen DH, Katary MA, Ali DA. *NAC a possible protector against indomethacin-induced peptic ulcer: crosstalk between antioxidant, anti-inflammatory, & antiapoptotic mechanisms.* Can J Physiol Pharmacol 95(4):396-403, 2017

Sakuri K, Osaka T, Yamasaki K. *Protection by rebamipide against acetic acid-induced colitis in rats: relationship with its antioxidative activity.* Dig. Dis. Sci. 43 (9 Suppl): 125S-133S, 1998

Tripathi S et al. *Association between gastric mucosal glutathione-S-transferase activity, glutathione-S-transferase gene polymorphisms & Helicobacter pylori infection in gastric cancer.* Indian J Gastroenterol 30(6):257-63, 2011

Verhulst ML, Van Oijen AH, Roelofs HM et al. *Antral glutathione concentration & glutathione S-transferase activity in patients with & without Helicopter pylori.* Dig Dis Sci 45(3):629-32, 2000

Wang Q, Chen Y, Zhang Y et al. *Quantitative assessment of the influence of glutathione S-transferase T1 null variant on gastric cancer risk.* Tumour Biol 35(1):849-58, 2014

Yoshikawa T, Minamiyama Y, Ichkawa H, et al. *Role of lipid peroxidation & antioxidants in gastric mucosal injury induced by the hypoxanthine-xanthine oxidase system in rats.* Free Radic. Biol. Med. 23: 243-250. 1997

Zala G, Flury R, Wust, et al. *Omeprazole/amoxicillin: improved eradication of Helicobacter pylori in smokers because of n-acetylcysteine.* Schweiz. Med. Wochenschr. 124: 1391-1397, 1994

Pancreatitis

Alsfasser G, Gock M, Herzog L et al. *Glutathione depletion with L-buthionine-(S,R)-sulfoximine demonstrates deleterious effects in acute pancreatitis of the rat.* Dig Dis Sci 47(8):1793-9, 2002

Atayoglu K et al. *Effect of N-acetylcysteine on neutrophil functions during experimental acute pancreatitis.* Ulus Travma Acil Cerrahi Derg 23(2):100-106, 2017

Braganza JM, Scott P, Bilton D, et al. *Evidence of early oxidative stress in acute pancreatitis. Clues for correction.* Int. J. Pancreatol. 17:69-81, 1995

Demols A, Van Laethem JL, Quertinmont E et al. *N-acetylcysteine decreases severity of acute pancreatitis in mice.* Pancreas 20(2):161-9, 2000

Du BQ, Yang YM, Chen YH, Liu XB, Mai G. *N-acetylcysteine improves pancreatic microcirculation & alleviates the severity of acute necrotizing pancreatitis.* Gut Liver 7(3):357-62, 2013

Grady T, Saluja A, Kaiser A, Steer M. *Edema & intrapancreatic trypsinogen activation precede glutathione depletion during caerulein pancreatitis.* Am J Physiol 271(1 Pt 1), 1996

Huang ZW, Tang JZ, Chen Y et al. *[Protective effect of reduced glutathione on multiple organ function in patient with acute pancreatitis]* Zhongguo Wei Zhong Bing Ji Jiu Yi Xue 17(11):673-4, 2005

Gukovsky I, Gukovskaya AS, Blinman TA, et al. *Early NF-kappa B activation is associated with hormone-induced pancreatitis.* American J. Physiol. 275(6 pt 1): G1402-1414, 1998

Luthen R, Grendell JH, Haussinger D, Niederau C. *Beneficial effects of L-2-oxothiazolidine-4-carboxylate on cerulein pancreatitis in mice.* Gastroenterology 112:1681-1691, 1997

Luthen R, Grendell JH, Niederau C, Haussinger D. *Trypsinogen activation & glutathione content are linked to pancreatic injury in models of biliary acute pancreatitis.* Int. J. Pancreatol. 24: 193-202, 1998

Luthen R, Niederau C, Grendell JH. *Intrapancreatic zymogen activation & levels of ATP & glutathione during caerulein pancreatitis in rats.* Am. J. Physiol. 268(4 pt 1): G592-604, 1995

Mathew P, Wyllie R, Van Lente F, et al. *Antioxidants in hereditary pancreatitis.* American

J. Gastroenterology 91: 1558-1562, 1996

McCloy R. *Chronic pancreatitis at Manchester UK. Focus on antioxidant therapy.* Digestion 59 (Suppl 4): 36-48, 1998

Milnerowicz H et al. *The antioxidant profiles, lysosomal & membrane enzymes activity in patients with acute pancreatitis.* Mediators Inflamm 2014:376518, 2014

Moreno ML, Escobar J, Finamor I, Martinez-Ruiz A, Sastre J. *Disulfide stress & its targets in acute pancreatitis.* Inflamm Allergy Drug Targets 13(5):312-22, 2014

Moreno ML, Escobar J, Izquierdo-Alvarez A et al. *Disulfide stress: a novel type of oxidative stress in acute pancreatitis.* Free Radic Biol Med 70:265-77, 2014

Mumcu S, Alhan E et al. *Effects of N-acetylcysteine on acute necrotizing pancreatitis in rats.* Eur Surg Res 37(3):173-8, 2005

Onur E, Paksoy M, Baca B, Akoglu H. *Hyperbaric oxygen & N-acetylcysteine treatment in L-arginine-induced acute pancreatitis in rats.* J Invest Surg 25(1):20-8, 2012

Rahman SH, Ibrahim K, Larvin M et al. *Association of antioxidant enzyme gene polymorphisms & glutathione status with severe acute pancreatitis.* Gastroenterology 126(5):1322-22, 2004

Rahman SH, Srinivasan AR, Nicolaou A. *Transsulfuration pathway defects & increased glutathione degradation in severe acute pancreatitis.* Dig Dis Sci 54(3):675-82, 2009

Ramudo L, Manso MA. *N-acetylcysteine in acute pancreatitis.* World J Gastrointest Pharmacol 1(1):21-6, 2010

Schoenberg MH, Buchler M et al. *Lipid peroxidation & glutathione metabolism in chronic pancreatitis.* Pancreas 10(1):36-43, 1995

Schoenberg MH, Birk D, Berger HG. *Oxidative stress in acute & chronic pancreatitis. American J. Clin. Nutr. 62(Supl 6): 1306S-1314S, 1995*

Schoenberg MH, Buchler M, Younes M, et al. *Effect of antioxidant treatment in rats with acute hemorrhagic pancreatitis.Dig. Dis. Sci. 39: 1034-1040, 1994*

Sevillano S, De la Mano AM, De Dios I et al. *Major pathological mechanisms of acute pancreatitis are prevented by N-acetylcysteine.* Digestion 68(1):34-40, 2003

Sevillano S, de la Mano AM, Manso Ma et al. *N-acetylcysteine prevents intra-acinar oxygen free radical production in pancreatic duct obstruction-induced acute pancreatitis.* Biochim Biophys Acta 1639(3):177-84, 2003

Turkyilmaz S, Usta A, Cekic AB et al. *N-acetylcysteine amid reduces pancreatic damage in a rat model of acute necrotizing pancreatitis.* J Surg Res 203(2):383-9, 2016

Verlaan M, Roelofs HM, van-Schaik A et al. *Assessment of oxidative stress in chronic pancreatitis patients.* World J Gastroenterol 12(35):5705-10, 2006

Walling MA. *Xenobiotic metabolism, oxidant stress & chronic pancreatitis. Focus on glutathione.* Digestion 59(Suppl 4): 13-24, 1998

Wang XD, Deng XM, Haraldson P, et al. *Antioxidant & calcium channel blockers counteract endothelial barrier injury induced by acute pancreatitis in rats.* Sc&. J. Gastroenterol. 30:1129-1136, 1995

Wereszcynska-Siemiatkowska U et al. *The importance of interleukin 18, glutathione peroxidase, & selenium concentration changes in acute pancreatitis.* Dig Dis Sci 49(4):642-50, 2004

Inflammatory bowel disease

Achitei D, Ciobica A, Balan G et al. *Different Profile of pheripheral antioxidant enzymes & lipid peroxidation in active & non-active inflammatory bowel disease patients.* Dig Dis Sci 58(5):1244-9, 2013

Ahnfelt-Ranne I, Nielsen OH, Christensen A, et al. *Clinical evidence supporting the radical scavenger mechanism of 5-aminosalicylic acid.* Gastroenterology 98:1162-1169, 1990

Alzoghaibi MA. *Concepts of oxidative stress & antioxidant defense in Crohn's disease.* World J Gastroenterol 19(39):6540-7, 2013

Bhaskar L, Ramakrishna BS, Balasubramanian KA. *Colonic mucosal antioxidant enzymes & lipid peroxide levels in normal subjects & patients with ulcerative colitis.* J. Gastroent. Hepatol. 10:140-143, 1995

Buffington GD, Doe WF. *Depleted mucosal antioxidant defenses in inflammatory bowel disease.* Free Radic. Biol. Med. 19: 911-918, 1995

Bulger EM, Helton WS. *Nutrient antioxidants in gastrointestinal diseases.* Gastrenterol. Clin. North America 27: 403-419, 1998

Chu FF, Esworthy RS, Doroshow JH. *Role of Se-dependent glutathione peroxidases in gastrointestinal inflammation & cancer.* Free Radic Biol Med 36(12):1481-95, 2004

Cruz T, Galvez J, Ocete MA, et al. *Oral administration of rutoside can ameliorate inflammatory bowel disease in rats.* Life Sci. 62:687-695, 1998

Geerling BJ, Badart-Smook A, Stockbrugger RW, Brummer RJ. *Comprehensive nutritional status in patients with long-st&ing Crohn's disease currently in remission.American J. Clin. Nutr. 67: 919-926, 1998*

Grisham MB. *Oxidants & free radicals in inflamm. bowel disease.* Lancet 344(8926): 859-861, 1994

GROSS V, ARNDT H, &US, ET AL. *Free radicals in inflammatory bowel diseases pathophysiology & therapeutic implications.* Hepato-gastroenterology 41: 320-327, 1994

HAGEN TM, WIERZBIKA GT, BOWMAN BB, ET AL. *Fate of dietary glutathione: disposition in the gastrointestinal tract.* American J. Physiol. 259:G530-G535, 1990

HARRIS ML, SCHILLER HJ, REILLY PM, ET AL. *Free radicals & other reactive oxygen metabolites in inflammatory bowel disease: cause, consequence, or epiphenomenon?* Pharmac. Ther. 53:375-408, 1992

HOFFENBER EJ, DEUTSCH J, SMITH S, SOKOL RJ. *Circulating antioxidant concentrations in children with inflammatory bowel disease. American J. Clin.* Nutr. 65:1482-1488, 1997

HOLMES EW, YONG SL, EIZENHAMER D, KESHAVARIAN A. *Glutathione content of colonic mucosa: evidence for oxidative damage in active ulcerative colitis.* Dig. Dis. Sci. 43:1088-1095, 1998

IANTOMASI T, MARRACCINI P, FAVILLI F, ET AL. *Glutathione metabolism in Crohn's disease. Biochem. Med. Metab. Biol. 53: 87-91, 1994*

IBORRA M, MORET I, RAUSELL F ET AL. *Role of oxidative stress & antioxidant enzymes in Crohn's disease.* Biochem Soc Trans 39(4):1102-6, 2011

JEFFERIES H, BOT J, COSTER J ET AL. *The role of glutathione in intestinal dysfunction.* J Invest Surg 16(6):315-23, 2003

KRZYSTEK-KORPACKA M ET AL. *Impaired erythrocyte antioxidant defense in active inflammatory bowel disease: impact of anemia & treatment.* Imflamm Bowel Dis 16(9):1467-75, 2010

LIH-BRODY L, POWELL SR, COLLIER KP, ET AL. *Increased oxidative stress & decreased antioxidant defenses in mucosa of inflammatory bowel disease.* Digestive Diseases & Sciences, 41:2078-2086, 1996

MARTENSSON J, JAIN A, MEISTER A. *Glutathione is required for intestinal function.* Proc. Natl. Acad. Sci. USA 87: 1715-1719, 1990

PATLEVIC P ET AL. *Reactive oxygen species & antioxidant defense in human gastrointestinal diseases.* Integr Med Res 5(4):250-258, 2016

PÉREZ S ET AL. *Redox signaling in the gastrointestinal tract.* Free Radic Biol Med 104:75-103, 2017

PINTO MA, LOPES MS, BASTOS ST ET AL. *Does active Crohn's disease have decreased intestinal antioxidant capacity?* J Crohn's colitis. 7(9):e358-66, 2013

QIAN J, SONG Z, LV Y ET AL. *Glutathione S-Transferase T1 Null Genotype is Associated with Susceptibility to Inflammatory Bowel Disease.* Cell Physiol Biochem 41(6):2545-2552, 2017

ROMAGNOLI C, MARCUCCI T, PICARIELLO L ET AL. *Role of N-acetylcysteine & GSH redox system on total & active MMP-2 in intestinal myofibroblasts of Crohn's disease patients.* Int J Colorectal Dis 28(7):915-24, 2013

SIDO B, HACK V, HOCHLEHNERT A, ET AL. *Impairment of intestinal glutathione synthesis in patients with inflammatory bowel disease.* Gut 42: 485-492, 1998

STOCCO G, PELIN M, FRANCA R ET AL. *Pharmacogenetics of azathioprine in inflammatory bowel disease:* a role for glutathione-S-transferase? World J Gastroenterol 20(13):3534-41, 2014

SOKOL RJ, HOFFENBERG EJ. *Antioxidants in pediatric gastrointestinal disease.* Pediatr. Clin. North America 43: 471-488, 1996

SZCZEKLIK K ET AL. *Alterations in glutathione peroxidase & superoxide dismutase activities in plasma & saliva in relation to disease activity in patients with Crohn's disease.* J Physiol Pharmacol 67(5):709-715, 2016

CELIAC DISEASE

BODA M, NEMETH I. *Decrease in the antixodant capacity of red blood cells in children with celiac disease.* Acta Paediatr Hung 32(3):241-55, 1992

KATAR M, OZUGURLU AF, OZYURT H, BENLI I. *Evaluation of glutathione peroxidase & superoxide dismutase enzyme polymorphisms in celiac disease patients.* Genet Mol Res 13(1):1030-7, 2014

MORETTI S, MRAKIC-SPOSTA S, RONCORONI L ET AL. *Oxidative stress as a biomarker for monitoring treated celiac disease.* Clin Transl Gastroenterol 9(6):157, 2018

SEVINC E, SEVINC N, AKAR HH ET AL. *Plasma glutamine & cystine are decreased & negatively correlated with endomysial antibody in children with celiac disease.* Asia Pac J Clin Nutr 25(3):452-6, 2016

STOJILIKOVIC V ET AL. *Glutathione redox cycle in small intestinal mucosa & peripheral blood of pediatric celiac disease patients.* An Acad Bras Cienc 84(1):175-84, 2012

STOJILIKOVIC V ET AL. *Antioxidant status & lipid peroxidation in small intestinal mucosa of children with celiac disease.* Clin Biochem 42(13-14), 2009

STOJILIKOVIC V ET AL. *Antioxidant enzymes, glutathione & lipid peroxidation in peripheral blood of children affected by coeliac disease.* Ann Clin Biochem 44(Pt 6):537-43, 2007

VARKONYI A, BODA M, ENDREFFY E ET AL. *Coeliac disease: always something to discover.* Sc& J Gastroenterol Suppl 228-122-g, 1998

WAHAB PJ, PETERS WH, ROELOFS HM, JANSEN JB. *Glutathione S-transferases in small intestinal mucosa of patients with coeliac disease.* Jpn J Cancer Res 92(3):279-84, 2001

14

Kidney Failure & Dialysis

The kidney (renal) system is responsible for filtering the blood and disposing of waste products, toxins and excess fluid in the form of urine. It also maintains water balance and regulates various chemical levels and blood pressure. If the kidneys cannot do their job, waste products and toxins accumulate in the blood. This affects other organ systems, often producing neurological and circulatory problems. Any sort of acute (sudden) or chronic (gradual/prolonged) illness can interfere with kidney function and lead to long-term disease. Kidney disease may also shorten life expectancy.

Chronic kidney disease (CKD) is surprisingly common in North America. Thirty million American adults (a full 15% of the population, or one in seven) are estimated to have CKD. Mexican and Canadian statistics are similar. Individuals with kidney (renal) failure are at much higher risk of premature death from heart disease and all other causes.

Acute kidney failure can be triggered by all sorts of conditions. For example, a massive hemorrhage (blood loss), a heart attack or an overwhelming infection (sepsis) can suddenly and severely restrict blood flow, quickly injuring sensitive kidney tissues.

The most common medical conditions leading to chronic renal failure are hardening of the arteries (atherosclerosis), high blood pressure and diabetes. These long-term diseases damage the circulation involved with the kidneys. Serious damage is also caused by organic and inorganic toxins, such as poisonous mushrooms, solvents, wood alcohol, antifreeze and heavy metals, either inhaled or ingested. There are many other causes of kidney failure, including chronic toxic exposure, inherited kidney diseases, vascular diseases and autoimmune diseases.

Kidney disease and renal failure are often triggered by other disorders, so the initial or potential cause must be identified. Diabetics should carefully control their sugar levels. Hypertensive patients must keep blood pressure down, and we all need to eliminate ongoing exposure to toxins. Some drugs help manage chemical imbalances, circulatory problems and accumulation of waste products. Proper nutrition and dietary management are particularly important, and

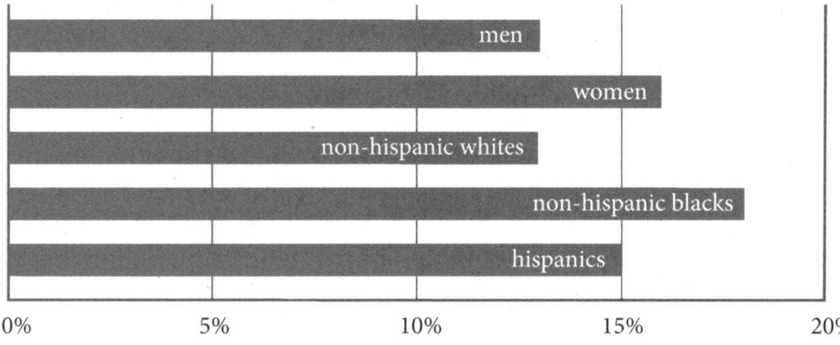

FIGURE 31: Prevalence of CKD among US adults aged 18 years or over, by sex and race/ethnicity

reduced protein intake is often advised in cases of renal failure.

If these measures aren't enough, a kidney transplant may be required. A less traumatic alternative is dialysis, but it's highly intrusive and uses artificial devices to perform the kidney's functions. Two types of dialysis are commonly used—hemodialysis and peritoneal dialysis. Like chemical and radiation therapy for cancer patients, these procedures are life-saving but punishing. They exact a heavy toll on the body's antioxidant defenses.

Hemodialysis

In hemodialysis, blood is shunted out of the body to a mechanical filtering device. There it is cleansed, chemically balanced and returned to the person's circulatory system. The procedure is repeated several times a week and each session takes several hours, during which the patient is physically attached to the machine.

Peritoneal dialysis

Peritoneal dialysis cleans blood without removing it from the body by using the peritoneal membrane (inner lining of the abdomen) as a filter. This membrane has many of the characteristics of the kidney's filtering system. Once a plastic tube has been implanted in the abdominal wall, patients usually carry out the procedure for themselves. A special dialysis solution (dialysate) is passed through the tube and into the abdomen. Waste material from the blood filters through the small vessels of the peritoneal membrane and is trapped by the fluid. After a few hours, the dialysate is drained and discarded. This procedure may be repeated several times a day.

GSH and renal failure

One cause of toxicity in the kidneys and failure is exposure to heavy metals such as mercury, cadmium and lead (see Chapter 2). The body detoxifies these substances principally with GSH-related enzymes that bind glutathione to these metals by a process known as "chelation," after which they are easily and safely removed. Kidney cells are protected by high levels of GSH. While treating for severe mercury toxicity, tests in laboratory trials and with kidney patients show that adding NAC (a GSH-enhancing drug) to the dialysate helps chelate inorganic mercury and remove it from the solution.

Acute renal failure occurs most commonly when the kidneys suffer from poor blood flow (ischemia). Laboratory studies at the University of Texas and elsewhere have shown that damage suffered during ischemic renal failure is lessened by the infusion of NAC. This appears to result from either an improved supply of antioxidants to the tissue or the detoxification of noxious metabolites like nitric oxide—or both.

Many pharmaceutical drugs are implicated in kidney failure. Common medications such as ibuprofen, acetaminophen and even vitamin D place high demands on the kidneys and can damage them. Many anti-cancer agents used in chemotherapy do the same. The immunosuppressant cyclosporin[1] can also damage the kidneys. Research indicates that elevated antioxidant defenses help protect the body from cyclosporin toxicity.

A rarer cause of kidney failure is polycystic kidney disease—the growth of cysts that eventually impair kidney function. Experiments were carried out to artificially lower GSH levels with the drug BSO. This caused the disease to worsen, and suggests that the presence of GSH plays a protective role.

The most common cause of poor blood

[1] used after organ transplantation and in certain kidney diseases such as the nephrotic syndrome

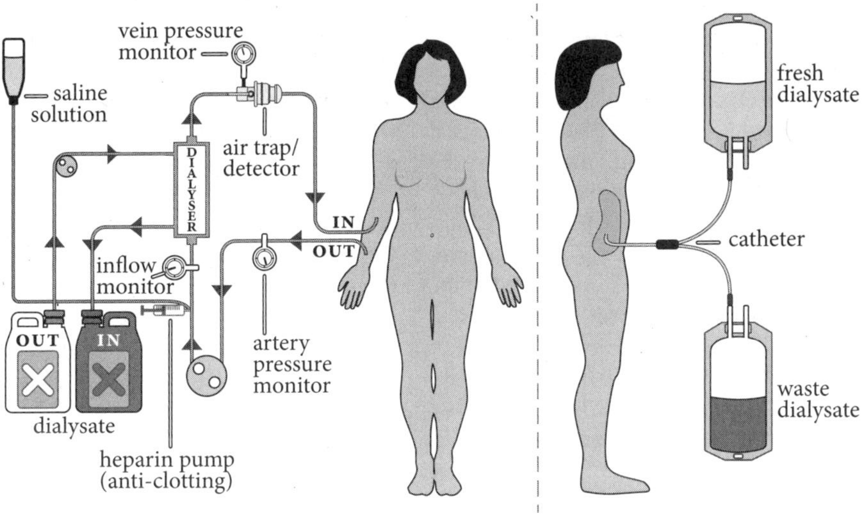

FIGURE 32: Hemodialysis (left) and peritoneal dialysis (right)

flow is atherosclerosis—a plaque build-up that blocks blood vessels. While GSH detoxifies pharmaceutical drugs and heavy metals, and fights such threats as polycystic kidney disease, it also fights plaque by inhibiting lipid peroxidation (see Chapter 7).

Oxidative stress can easily be measured from blood samples. The correlation of impaired glutathione levels and kidney function is strong enough to consider GSH measurements as a way to follow the progress of a patient's disease.

Attempts to raise glutathione levels in renal failure are in their early stages but have already yielded promising results, and there is optimism about further studies. Both Pache de Faria et al (2014) and Danilovic (2011) et al have published results showing improvement in kidney function using the glutathione precursor NAC.

GSH and dialysis

Renal failure patients suffer from a profound imbalance of oxidants and antioxidants that grows worse as the kidney fails. In spite of their life-saving action, both peritoneal dialysis and especially hemodialysis can worsen kidney malfunction by increasing oxidative stress levels. Because dialysis is not optional for these patients, its side-effects must be addressed.

Some researchers think that dialysis damages the anti-oxidant system and leads to a dramatic fall in levels of the GSH enzymes that protect us from lipid peroxidation. This results in long-term complications such as accelerated atherosclerosis. In fact, cardiovascular disease is the major cause of morbidity and mortality in patients with end-stage renal failure. Abundant evidence shows that antioxidant support might benefit these patients. A strong link between kidney function and glutathione availability has led some scientists to suggest that glutathione peroxidase levels may be used to measure kidney function.

To test this hypothesis, elderly patients undergoing continuous peritoneal dialysis were analyzed in two ways: first by their ability to absorb and process certain nutrients (especially serum albumin and iron); secondly by measuring glutathione peroxidase (antioxidant) levels. Test results revealed a strong association between the two. Clearly, the ability of kidney patients to fight oxidation is progressively and profoundly compromised. Unchallenged oxidative stress leads to untold damage.

To get a clearer picture of this process in peritoneal dialysis patients, researchers examined the cells of their peritoneal membrane. They found that when the patients were exposed to the life-saving dialysate fluid, GSH levels fell significantly. To counteract this decline, OTZ (a pharmaceutical precursor of GSH) was added to the dialysate fluid. This helped restore GSH to protective levels in these tissues.

The link between GSH status and oxidative stress in dialysis patients is not only widely accepted, it is also considered highly significant. In patients with renal failure, oxidative stress damages the circulating red blood cells (erythrocytes) causing low hemoglobin levels (anemia). Such damage is normally kept to a minimum by glutathione—the principal antioxidant in this struggle. GSH acts on the surface of the wall of the red blood cell to preserve its integrity. Since hemodialysis causes significant oxidative changes and damages red blood cells, it is important that patients undergoing this procedure maintain high GSH levels. Drugs like NAC and OTZ effectively raise glutathione levels and improve a patient's ability to fight oxidative stress, but there are also safer, dietary ways to raise GSH levels. These are described in Chapter 4.

Many dialysis patients are treated for their anemia (shortage of red blood cells) with erythropoietin. This drug is meant to stimulate the production of red blood cells, but provides an additional benefit. It turns out that younger cells have higher levels of GSH and are thus more resistant to lipid peroxidation and cell-wall breakdown. Studies have shown that antioxidants given to patients on erythropoietin may enhance the effectiveness of the drug, making it possible to lower dosage. This was demonstrated by giving patients intravenous GSH during dialysis sessions.

An important double-blind study of hemodialysis patients was conducted by Costagliola's team in Italy. Patients were given intravenous GSH while others received placebo. To test for anemia, doctors measured red blood cell, hemoglobin and hematocrit levels—all known to fall in dialysis patients. Those receiving GSH maintained higher levels than those on placebo. Their levels of oxidative stress also fell. Similar but separate Italian studies led by Usberti also resulted in lessened anemia. These findings show that elevating GSH levels helps manage the anemia to which dialysis patients are particularly prone.

This has led dialysis researchers to suggest that oral antioxidants must be considered for these patients. This is an effective way to potentially raise glutathione. In addition, it's well understood how nutritionally compromised many of these individuals are. Sohrabi and his team (2016) published a report using oral whey protein in hemodialysis patients, with positive outcomes. Tomayko and his team (2015) used both soy and whey to achieve similar results. Others have used oral NAC with favorable outcomes.

Since poor antioxidant and detoxification defenses are implicated in kidney disease and the complications of dialysis, there's reason to believe that GSH supplementation may help individuals like George, a 62 year old former country and western singer.

Case study

George had struggled with diabetes for over thirty years. Following only moderate success controlling his sugar levels, he developed progressive kidney failure and subsequent anemia. In a few short years he went from being an active, gregarious entertainer to a listless, sofa-ridden recluse. His energy level and concentration deteriorated, and his local hospital clinic in Hawaii was obliged to monitor his condition closely. His biliary urea nitrogen (BUN) and creatinine levels crept higher and higher—signs of diminishing kidney function—and his red blood cell (hemoglobin) value continued to fall. His physician placed him on a waiting list to undergo preparation for dialysis.

After learning about GSH, George started taking 20 grams per day of a whey protein isolate high in GSH precursors. Within three weeks his BUN and creatinine levels began to fall—a sure sign of improved kidney function. After a further three weeks his hemoglobin climbed by one full gram per deciliter (g/dL) of blood and he was again singing at his friends' parties. His wife was uncomfortable about his exposure to alcohol and cigarettes but three months later his renal function tests and hemoglobin levels had improved so much his physician put plans for dialysis on hold.

Protein intake and renal failure

Diseased kidneys have trouble clearing away breakdown products, many of which are left over from the digestion of dietary protein. Large amounts of protein lead to high levels of urea-nitrogen in the blood—a condition called uremia, with further health problems. Therefore, protein intake is restricted and monitored. Renal failure patients are encouraged to eat plenty of carbohydrates, but as an important nutrient, protein cannot be avoided. Since kidney failure patients often can consume it only in limited quantities, it should be of the highest quality.

A measure of food protein quality is biological value (BV). It rates the usefulness and quantity of biochemicals made available to the body by a particular food protein. BV especially reflects the ratio of essential to non-essential amino acids. We need a continuous supply of essential amino acids in our diet. We need non-essential amino acids too, but don't necessarily have to eat them—our body can manufacture them from the essential ones. For dialysis patients, proteins rich in essential amino acids are preferable because of their higher biological value. Some patients undergoing dialysis become protein deficient (hypoalbuminemic). For them, the quality of dietary protein is even more important.

The natural protein with the highest biological value is whey protein—ideal for kidney patients. Also, the amino acids found in some whey proteins are GSH precursors (building blocks). Their presence or absence depends principally on how the whey protein is prepared and stored. See Chapter 4 for more about whey protein.

Conclusion

GSH is important in the prevention and treatment of renal failure, in the anemia that often accompanies kidney failure and dialysis, and in the cardiovascular complications of kidney disease. GSH-modifying agents offer promising treatments for both short and long-term complications of kidney failure. GSH acts both as a detoxifier and as an antioxidant, preventing lipid peroxidation. Because some whey proteins contain additional nutritional benefits and act as glutathione precursors, they are a useful complement to traditional therapy.

KIDNEY FAILURE & DIALYSIS

REFERENCES

Andreoli SP. *Reactive oxygen molecules, oxidant injury and renal disease.* Pediatr. Nephrol. 5: 733-742, 1991

Bonnefont-Rousselot D, Jaudon MC, Issad B, et al. *Antioxidant status of elderly chronic renal patients treated by continuous ambulatory peritoneal dialysis. Nephrol.* Dial. Transplant. 12: 1399-1405, 1997

Bossola M, Muscaritoli M, Tazza L, Giungi S, et al. *Malnutrition in hemodialysis patients: what therapy?* AM J Kidney Dis 46(3):371-86, 2005

Breborowicz A, Rodela H, Martis L, Oreopoulos DG. *Intracellular glutathione in human peritoneal mesothelial cell exposed in vitro to dialysis fluid.* Int. J. Artif. Organs 19: 268-275, 1996

Canestrari F, Galli F, Giorgini A, et al. *Erythrocyte redox state in uremic anemia: effects of hemodialysis and relevance of glutathione metabolism.* Acta. Haematol. 91: 187-193, 1994

Cavdar C, Cansari T, Semin I, et al. *Lipid peroxidation and antioxidant activity in chronic hemodialysis patients treated with recombinant human erythropoietin.* Scand. J. Urol. Nephrol. 31: 371-375, 1997

Ceballos-Pict I, Witko-Sarsat V, Merad-Boudia M, et al. *Glutathione antioxidant system as a marker of oxidative stress in chronic renal failure.* Free Radic. Biol. Med. 21:845-853, 1996

CDC (Centers for Disease Control and Prevention. *Chronic kidney disease surveillance system website.* www.cdc.gov/ckd. Accessed 2017.

Chen CK, Liaw JM, Juang JG, Lin TH. *Antioxidant enzymes and trace elements in hemodialyzed patients.* Biol. Trace Elem. Res. 58: 140-157, 1997

Costagliola C, Romano L, Scibelli G, et al. *Anemia and chronic renal failure: a therapeutic approach by reduced glutathione parenteral administration.* Nephron 61: 404-408, 1992

Costagliola C, Romano L, Sorice P, Di Benedetto A. *Anemia and chronic renal failure: the possible role of the oxidative state of glutathione.* Nephron 52: 11-14, 1989

Cristol JP, Bose JY, Badiou S, et al. *Erythropoietin and oxidative stress in haemodialysis: beneficial effects of vitamin E supplementation.* Nephrol. Dial. Transplant. 12: 2312-2317, 1997

Danilovic A, Lucon AM, Srougi M, et al. *Protective effect of N-acetylcysteine on early outcomes of deceased renal transplantation.* Transplant Proc 43(5):1443-9, 2011

Demirci S. et al. *The importance of oxidative stress in patients with chronic renal failure whose hypertension is treated with peritoneal dialysis.* Cell Biochem Funct 29(3):249-54, 2011

Diamond GL, Zalups RK. *Understanding renal toxicity of heavy metals.* Toxicol. Pathol. 26: 92-103, 1998

DiMari J, Megyesi J, Udvarhelyi N, et al. *N-acetyl cysteine ameliorates ischemic renal failure.American J. Physiol. 272(3 Pt 2): F292-F298, 1997*

Drai J, Bannier E, Chazot C, Hurot JM, et al. *Oxidants and antioxidants in long-term haemodialysis patients.* Farmaco 56(5-7):463-5, 2001

Durak I, Karabacak HI, Buyukkocak S, et al. *Impaired antioxidant defense system in the kidney tissues from rabbits treated with cyclosporin.* Protective effects of vitamins E and C. Nephron 78: 207-211, 1998

Epperlein MM, Nourooz-Zadeh J, Jayasena SD, et al. *Nature and biological significance of free radicals generated during bicarbonate hemodialysis.* J. American Soc. Nephrol. 9: 457-463, 1998

Ferguson CL, Cantilena LR Jr. *Mercury clearance from human plasma during in vitro dialysis: screening systems for chelating agents.* J. Toxicol. Clin. Toxicol. 30: 423-441, 1992

Hsu SP, Chiang CK, Yang SY, Chien CT. *N-acetylcysteine for the management of anemia and oxidative stress in hemodialysis patients.* Nephron Clin Pract 116(3):c207-16, 2010

Jin B, Wu BW, Zhang JJ, Luo XP, Shi HM. *Preventive effect of reduced glutathione on contrast-induced nephropathy in elderly patients undergoing coronary angiography or intervention: a randomized, controlled trial.* Braz J Med Biol Res 48(9):839-42, 2015

Johnson-Davis KL, Fernelius C, Eliason NB, Wilson A, Beddhu S, Roberts WL. *Blood enzymes and oxidative stress in chronic kidney disease: a cross sectional study.* Ann Clin Lab Sci 41(4):331-9, 2011

Lucchi L, Bergamini S, Iannone A, Perrone S, Stipo L, Olmeda F, Tomasi A, Albertazzi A. *Erythrocyte susceptibility to oxidative stress in chronic renal failure patients under different substitutive treatments.* Artif Organs 29(1):67-72, 2005

Lund ME, Banner W Jr, Clarkson TW, Berlin M. *Treatment of acute methylmercury ingestion by hemodialysis with n-acetylcysteine (Mucomyst) infusion and 2,3-dimercaptopropane sulfonate.* J. Toxicol. Clin. Toxicol. 22: 31-49, 1984

Locatelli F, Canaud B, Eckardt KU, Stenvinkel P, Wanner C, Zoccali C. *Oxidative stress in end-stage renal disease: an emerging threat to patient outcome.* Nephrol Dial Transplant 18(7):1272-80, 2003

Martin-Mateo MC, Del Canto-Jafiez E, Barrero-Martinez MJ. *Oxidative stress and enzyme activity in ambulatory renal patients undergoing continuous peritoneal dialysis.* Renal Failure 20: 117-124, 1998

Martin-Mateo MC, Sanchez-Portugal M, Iglesias S, et al. *Oxidative stress in chronic renal failure.Renal Failure 21: 155-167, 1999*

Meisinger C et al. *Chronic kidney disease and risk of incident myocardial infarction and all-cause and cardiovascular disease mortality in middle-aged men and women from the gereal population.Eur Heart J, 27(10):1245-1250, 2006.*

Mimic-Oka J, Simic T, Elkmescic V, Dragicevic P. *Erythrocyte glutathione peroxidase and superoxide dismutase activities in different stages of chronic renal failure.* Clin Nephrol. 44: 44-48, 1995

Moberly JB, Logan J, Borum PR, et al. *Elevation of whole-blood glutathione in peritoneal dialysis patients by L-2-oxothiazolidine-4-carboxylate, a cysteine prodrug (Procysteine).* J. American Soc. Nephrol. 9: 1093-1099, 1998

Modaresi A, Nafar M, Sahraei Z. *Oxidative*

stress in chronic kidney disease. Iran J Kidney Dis 9(3):165-79, 2015

Montazerifar F, Hashemi M, Karajibani M, Sanadgol H, Dikshit M. *Evaluation of lipid peroxidation and erythrocyte glutathione peroxidase and superoxide dismutase in hemodialysis patients.* Saudi J Kidney Dis Transpl 23(2):274-9, 2012

Nascimiento MM, Suliman ME, Silva M, et al. *Effect of oral-N-acetylcysteine treatment on plasma inflammatory and oxidative stress markers in peritoneal dialysis patients: a placebo-controlled study.* Perit Dial Int 30(3):336-42, 2010

NIH (National Institutes of Health). *2016 USRDS annual data report: Epidemiology of kidney disease in the United States.* Nat Instit Diabetes Digest Kidney Dis; 2016.

Ong-awyooth L, Ong-ajyooth S, Tiensong K, et al. *Reduced free radical scavengers and chronic renal failure.* J. Med. Assoc. Thai. 80: 101-108, 1997

Pache de Faria Guimaraes L, Seguro AC, et al. *N-acetyl-cysteine is associated to renal function improvement in patients with nephropathic cystinosis.* Pediatr Nephrol 29(6):1097-102, 2014

Pasaoglu H, Muhtaroglu S, Gunes M, Utas C. *The role of the oxidative state of glutathione and glutathione-related enzymes in anemia of hemodialysis patients.* Clin. Biochem. 29: 567-572, 1996

Peti A, Csiky B, Guth E, et al. *Effect of Oxidative Stress in Hemodialysed Patients.* EJIFCC 22(2):45-51, 2011

Ratliff BB, Abdulmahdi W, Pawar R, Wolin MS. *Oxidant Mechanisms in Renal Injury and Disease.* Antioxid Redox Signal 25(3):119-46, 2016

Roozbeh J, et al. *Comparative effects of sylmarin and vitamin E supplementation on oxidative stress markers, and hemoglobin levels among patients on hemodialysis.* Ren Fail 33(2):118-23, 2011

Ross EA, Koo LC, Moberly JB. *Low whole blood and erythrocyte levels of glutathione in hemodialysis and peritoneal dialysis patients.* American J. Kidney Disease 30: 489-494, 1997

Roxborough HE, Mercer C, McMaster D, et al. *Plasma glutathione peroxidase activity is reduced in haemodialysis patients.* Nephron 81: 278-283, 1999

Saitoh T, Satoh H, Nobuhara M, et al. *Intravenous glutathione prevents renal oxidative stress after coronary angiography more effectively than oral N-acetylcysteine.* Heart Vessels 26(5):465-72, 2011

Salom MG, Ramirez P, Carbonell LF, et al. *Protective effect of N-acetyl-L-cysteine on the renal failure induced by inferior cava occlusion.* Transplantation 65: 1315-1321, 1998

Schiavon R, Biasioli S, De Fanti E, et al. *The plasma GSH peroxidase enzyme in hemodialyzed subjects.* ASAIO J 40:968-971, 1994

Schiavon R, Guidi GC, Biasioli S, et al. *Plasma glutathione peroxidase activity as an index of renal function.* Eur. J. Clin. Chem. Clin. Biochem. 32: 759-765, 1994

Sohrabi Z, Eftekhari MH, et al. *Intradialytic Oral Protein Supplementation and Nutritional and Inflammantion Outcomes in Hemodialysis: A Randomized Controlled Trial.* Am J Kidney Dis 68(1):122-30, 2016

Soldini D, Zwahlen H, Gabutti L, Marzo A, Marone C. *Pharmacokinetics of N-acetylcysteine following repeated intravenous infusion in haemodialysed patients.* Eur J Clin Pharmacol 60(12):859-64, 2005

Stepniewska J, *Dolegowska B, et al.* Erythrocyte antioxidant defense system in patients with chronic renal failure according to the hemodialysis conditions. Arch Med Res 37(3):353-9, 2006

Stepniewska J, Golembiewska E, Dolegowska B, Domanski M, Ciechanowski K. *Oxidative stress and antioxidative enzyme activities in chronic kidney disease and different types of renal replacement therapy.* Curr Protein Pept Sci 16(3):243-8, 2015

Suvakov S, Damjanovic T, et al. *Glutathione S-transferase A1, M1, P1 and T1 null or low-activity genotypes are associated with enhanced oxidative damage among haemodialysis patients.* Nephrol Dial Transplant 28(1):202-12, 2013

Suliman ME, et al. *Influence of nutritional status on plasma and erythrocyte sulphur amino acids, sulph-hydryls, and inorganic sulphate in end-stage renal disease.* Nephrol Dial Transplant 17(6):1050-6, 2002

Sung CC, Hsu YC, Chen CC, Lin YF, Wu CC. *Oxidative stress and nucleic acid oxidation in patients with chronic kidney disease.* Oxid Med Cell Longev, 2013

Tamma G, Valenti G. *Evaluating the Oxidative Stress in Renal Diseases: What Is the Role for S-Glutathionylation?* Antioxid Redox Signal 25(3):147-64, 2016

Tesauro M, Nistico S, Noce A, et al. *The posible role of glutathione-S-transferase activity in diabetic nephropathy.* Int J Immunopathol Pharmacol 28(1):129-33, 2015

Tomayko EJ, Kistler BM, Fitschen PJ, Wilund KR. *Intradialytic protein supplementation reduces inflammation and improves physical function in maintenance hemodialysis patients.* J Ren Nutr 25(3):276-83, 2015

Torres VE, Bengal RJ, Litwiller RD, Wilson DM. *Aggravation of polycystic kidney disease in Han:SPRD rats by buthionine sulfoxamine.* J. American Soc. Nephrol. 8: 1283-1291, 1997

Tucker PS, Dalbo VJ, Han T, Kingsley

MI. *Clinical and research markers of oxidative stress in chronic kidney disease.* Biomarkers 18(2):103-15, 2013

Usberti M, Lima G, Arisi M, et al. *Effect of exogenous reduced glutathione on the survival of red blood cells in hemodialyzed patients.* J. Nephrol. 10: 261-265, 1997

Wang C, Wang W, Ma S, Lu J, Shi H, Ding F. *Reduced Glutathione for Prevention of Renal Outcomes in Patients Undergoing Selective Coronary Angiography or Intervention.* J Interv Cardiol 28(3):249-56, 2015

Whitin JC, Tham DM, Bhamre S, et al. *Plasma glutathione peroxidase and its relationship to renal proximal tubule function.* Mol. Genet. Metab. 65: 238-245, 1998

Yeh EL, Chen CH, Huang SC, Huang YC. *A higher glutathione demand may be necessary for assisting hemodialysis patients to cope with increased oxidative stress.* Nephrology (Carlton). 2019 Mar 19. doi: 10.1111/nep.13588

Yoshimura S, Suemizu H, Nomoto Y, et al. *Plasma glutathione peroxidase deficiency caused by renal dysfunction.* Nephron 73: 207-211, 1996

Zachara BA, Adamwicz A, Trafikowska U, et al. *Selenium and glutathione levels, and glutathhione peroxidase activities in blood components of uremic patients on hemodialysis supplemented with selenium and treated with erythropoietin.* J Trace Elem Med Biol 15(4):201-8, 2001

Zachara BA. *Selenium and selenium-dependent antioxidants in chronic kidney disease.* Adv Clin Chem 68:131-51, 2015

Zachee P, Ferrant A, Daelmans R, et al. *Reduced glutathione for the treatment of anemia during hemodialysis: a preliminary communication.* Nephron 71: 343-349, 1995

15

Ears, Nose & Throat

Specialists in ear, nose and throat (ENT) have only recently become aware of the role of glutathione in the diseases they treat. Given the critical roles of GSH as the body's most important naturally occurring antioxidant, its ability to detoxify substances encountered in the environment and its immune-sustaining abilities, glutathione research is now finally picking up in these fields as well.

Glutathione in the upper respiratory tract

All the food we eat, fluids we drink and air we breathe pass through the nose, mouth and throat, which make up the upper respiratory tract. The importance of GSH in the lower respiratory tract (lungs) is well known. Since the upper tract is our front-line contact with the external environment, it is fitting that glutathione would protect us here against infections and toxins.

The respiratory tract is lined with a complicated fluid mixture of biochemicals and immune cells, called the respiratory tract lining fluid (RTLF). Glutathione is the main antioxidant in this fluid and provides our initial defense against inhaled toxins. Institutions like the Inhalation and Toxicology Research Institute in Albuquerque, New Mexico started researching the role of antioxidant enzyme activities in RTLF in the early 1990's. More recent work at the University of California (Davis) has elaborated further on the role of antioxidants in this fluid.

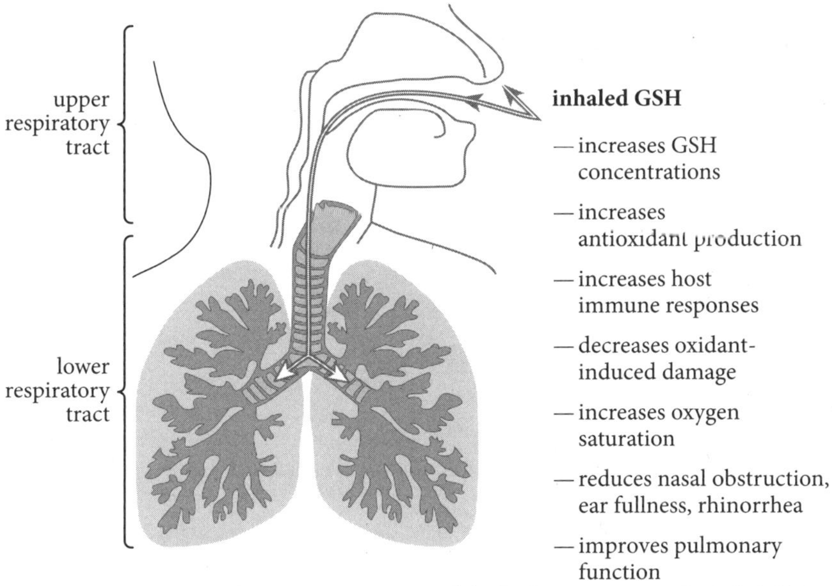

FIGURE 33: The respiratory tract and the healing trajectory of inhaled GSH

This research project is only one of several focusing on the importance of glutathione in respiratory tract lining fluids, where it protects from xenobiotics (foreign substances) and infection. In severe or prolonged illness, these GSH levels may become depleted, enabling the disease to progress and cause further complications. Furthermore, Krishna and his team at the University of Kentucky showed that this glutathione defense system weakens with age, and more rapidly in men than women.

Testa and Mesolella from the University of Naples' Institute of Otolaryngology used a GSH nasal aerosol spray in their studies. Statistical results from their experiments show that this treatment significantly improved nasal obstruction, rhinorrhea (runny nose) and ear fullness. Although most of the tissues that comprise the human body can only use the glutathione manufactured in the body's own cells (from GSH precursors), the lining of the nose is an exception. It is one of the few human tissues that readily absorb glutathione.

Sinusitis

Infection or inflammation of the sinus cavities in the bones of the face is one of the most common reasons people go to the doctor. As many as 50 million Americans are affected each year, most commonly by bacterial or viral infection, allergies and impaired mucus flow. Most treatments are designed to either destroy the infection or improve drainage of mucus from the sinuses. The sinus cavities are near the front of the head, behind the forehead, nose region and cheeks, as shown in Figure 33.

Physicians have long used the drug NAC (N-acetylcysteine) for the treatment of disorders involving thickened lung secretions (cystic fibrosis, chronic bronchitis). It is now also used for upper airway problems, such as sinusitis. NAC breaks down mucus and raises glutathione levels at the same time. NAC also affects "biofilms"—a complicated layering of bacteria and biochemicals that lie over mucosal tissues in the body (See Figure 36 (Chapter 16). The mucolytic action of NAC breaks up these biofilms, making it easier for immune defenses and antibiotics to work more effectively. American, French, Italian, Korean and Scandinavian research teams have all studied the efficacy of NAC and other antioxidants in the treatment of sinusitis.

The Amsterdam group led by Westerveld showed that glutathione levels fall during

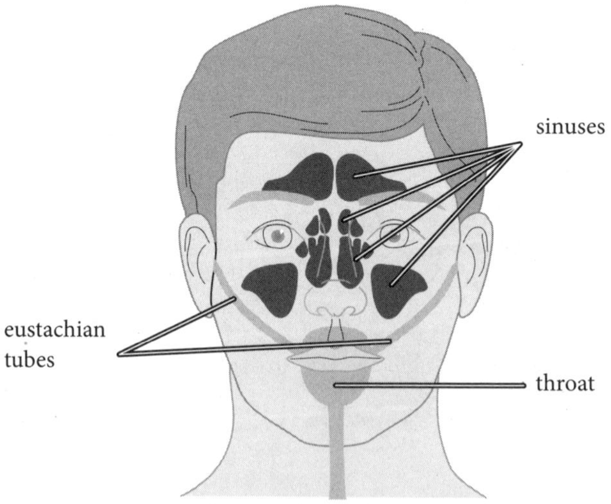

FIGURE 34: Sinus cavities: the eustachian tubes connect the middle ear and the throat

Rhinitis	Menière's Disease
Allergic Rhinitis	Laryngeal conditions
Chronic Rhinosinusitis	Noise-induced Hearing Loss
Nasal Polyps	Toxin-induced Hearing Loss
Otitis Media	Presbycusis (age-related hearing loss)
Tonsillitis	Sinusitis

TABLE 28: ENT conditions associated with glutathione abnormalities

chronic sinusitis, and concluded that this fall is part of a generally decreased antioxidant defense, which then makes the disorder worse.

As mentioned previously, glutathione can be directly absorbed by certain mucosal tissues, including those in the nose and throat. This approach is increasingly applied to sinusitis. In other scenarios, oral NAC is being actively investigated for the treatment of sinus problems.

Ear infection, Otitis

Infection of the middle ear (otitis media) is extremely common, especially among children. It is caused mostly by a combination of fluid buildup and infection in the middle ear. The triggering event is often a viral infection, but the site is commonly superinfected (one infection on top of another) by bacteria, and even fungi. For many years the standard treatment was with antibiotics, but doctors are increasingly reluctant to over-prescribe these drugs nowadays—especially for ear infections. Decongestants can help drain fluid from the middle ear, through the eustachian canal and into the throat.

More and more evidence shows that free radicals play a large part in the development of inflammation leading to middle-ear infections. Examination of GSH levels in these tissues shows that they fluctuate according to how infected or inflamed the site is. Scientists have examined the effects of both ways of raising glutathione levels—topical and ingested, and have found both to be effective against oxidative stress.

Patients with middle-ear infections sometimes have tubes inserted through the eardrum to drain accumulated fluid and prevent subsequent infection. This intrusion by a foreign object does the job, but at a cost. The body responds by treating the insertion as an inflammatory process. The procedure also promotes a high oxygen state in the middle ear. These two factors lead to free radical and oxyradical formation, causing changes in the cells lining the middle ear and leading to scarring and fibrosis. Ovesen and his team of ENT researchers at Aarhus University in Denmark passed liquid NAC through these small tubes. The drug reduced inflammation and prevented the long-term scarring that normally follows.

Italian researchers used another approach to raise glutathione levels in the ear. Testa and his group gave glutathione nasal sprays to patients with chronic otitis media. Compared to placebo, the improvement was significant.

Oral NAC has also received much attention in treating middle ear infections. Studies have shown that using this glutathione precursor can improve outcome, increase the effectiveness of antibiotics and reduce the need to re-insert drainage tubes.

Deafness & Hearing Loss

Almost 30 million North Americans experience sufficient hearing loss to interfere with their ability to converse. This is almost one in ten. One in a hundred is deaf and cannot hear at all. Almost one in three people over 65 experience some form of hearing loss, and this figure increases with age.

The many causes of impaired hearing all fit broadly into two categories: conductive hearing loss caused by a mechanical problem in the middle ear and external canal, and sensorineural hearing loss, a problem of the inner ear or auditory nerve. In the latter case the problem may be sensory—in the cochlea, the actual organ of hearing—or neural, affecting the auditory nerve. Causes of hearing loss include physical trauma, exposure to repeated loud noise, infection, tumors and malignancies, obstruction of the ear canal, genetic defects, toxins and drugs, various neurological diseases and the aging process in general.

Noise exposure

Noise-induced hearing loss accounts for about one third of all hearing loss cases, and is particularly unfortunate because it is mostly avoidable. It may affect 15% of Americans between the ages of 20 and 70 years. All that's required to prevent noise-induced hearing loss is appropriate caution. Teenagers often are fed and enjoy damaging levels of noise. Preventive aids such as earplugs can help. So can turning down the volume.

People working in noisy environments and those with noisy hobbies risk their hearing. Most of us have experienced buzzing, ringing or hissing in the ears after leaving a concert or construction site. Hearing loss is sometimes temporary, lasting minutes or days before it returns to normal. This is a 'temporary threshold shift,' caused by injury to the sensitive hair cells in the cochlea—the spiral shaped organ in the middle ear. Severe, repeated or prolonged exposure to excessive noise can destroy these neurological hair cells, leading to permanent hearing damage.

Interestingly, the cochlea can be trained to withstand greater noise levels and suffer less damage. This is known as 'sound conditioning' or 'toughening.' Priming the ear to low level noise before exposing it to higher levels seems to protect against hearing loss. Researchers at the Albert Einstein College of Medicine in New York examined the biochemical changes found in sound conditioning. They saw that certain enzymes that raise GSH levels or keep glutathione in a reduced (non-oxidized) state were stimulated by low-noise exposure. This suggests that whatever protects or increases the glutathione system in the cochlea also protects against noise-induced hearing loss.

Other studies of glutathione and noise exposure lend support to this model. A team at the Kresge Hearing Research Institute at the University of Michigan chemically depleted glutathione levels using the drug BSO, with the result that noise-induced hearing loss was more profound. The same team went on to raise GSH levels with OTC (a GSH precursor), with the result that hearing loss was minimized.

Dr. Denis McBride, from the Office of Naval Research in Arlington, Virginia, found that delivering antioxidants directly to the cochlea through a small tube (within six hours of exposure) could prevent permanent damage following noise exposure. Other researchers suggest that workers with prolonged noise exposure would gain long-term benefits from elevated glutathione levels.

Many studies using diverse animals such as mice, rats, rabbits, guinea pigs and chinchilla (a classic "test" animal for hearing experiments) have shown that the use of NAC and other glutathione precursors served to protect against noise-induced hearing loss.

Given the importance of this pathology to those in the industrial, military and music industries, the question is whether these animal studies will be as successful in humans. Since around 2010 a number of groups have looked into this, using NAC. Chinese, American, Iranian, Swedish, and Belgian scientists funded from both industrial and military sources have successfully demonstrated the usefulness of glutathione precursors in this preventable problem.

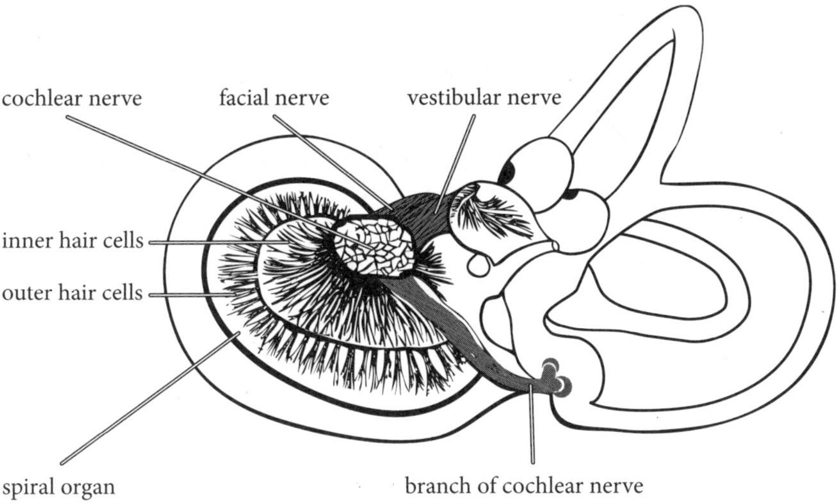

FIGURE 35: Cochlea hairs: the most common site of hearing damage

As has been noted in a number of other pathologies, people who have inborn errors of glutathione metabolism are also prone to noise-induced hearing loss. This may someday be a screening tool to help workers be properly informed before entering noisy work environments.

Hearing loss induced by drugs or toxins

Exposure to a variety of pharmaceutical chemicals may lead to sensorineural hearing loss.[1] They include high doses of aspirin, several antibiotics, a number of diuretics (medication for high blood pressure), quinine, and several chemotherapy agents.

One of these chemotherapy drugs is cisplatin, a common cancer treatment that can also damage auditory neurons.[2] Researchers have shown that this damage is caused by free radicals in the tissue. Studies that lowered GSH levels showed increased damage, while those raising GSH reduced the damage. It seems that raised glutathione levels protect patients from both the hearing damage and the kidney damage that can result from this treatment.

Similar studies have been conducted in relation to aminoglycoside antibiotics (including gentamycin, kanamycin, amikacin and others) and loop diuretics (lasix, furosemide, ethacrynic acid and others). Research teams from the USA (University of Michigan, Southern Illinois University), Japan (Hiroshima General Hospital), and Germany (Universitats HNO) all found that substances that raise glutathione activity have a protective effect against the hearing loss associated with these drugs. Maruzi from the Houston Medical Center even suggests that deafness following acute meningitis may be caused by free radicals in the inflamed tissue, and that antioxidants preventing lipid peroxidation in the auditory nerve would protect the patient.

The glutathione precursor NAC is commonly used in hospitals to prevent complications from radiological dyes used in some X-ray techniques. It is also a standard treatment for acetaminophen toxicity. NAC has more recently garnered attention for its ability to reduce the toxicity of pharmaceutical drugs. This includes intravenous

[1] caused by a lesion or disease of the inner ear or the auditory nerve.
[2] hearing nerve cells

antibiotics in dialysis patients (aminoglycosides, amikacin, etc.), as well as multidrug treatment of tuberculosis and for uraemic peritonitis patients. The scope of glutathione-precursors in complementary medical treatment continues to expand.

Conclusion

Glutathione plays several roles in the upper respiratory tract. Its suppression of free radicals, detoxification of environmental xenobiotics and reinforcement of the immune system makes it an excellent tool against airway irritation caused by pollution, sinusitis, otitis and other infections and inflammations of our ears, nose and throat. Having long utilized NAC in pulmonary disease, the medical profession is now pursuing its use in ear, nose and throat diseases. An interesting clinical application of elevated GSH is the treatment and prevention of noise-induced hearing loss as well as that caused by certain ototoxic drugs.

EARS, NOSE & THROAT

REFERENCES

Angeli SI, Bared A, Ouyang X et al. *Audioprofiles & antioxidant enzyme genotypes in presbycusis.* Laryngoscope 122(11):2539-42, 2012

Asher BF, Guilford FT. *Oxidative Stress & Low Glutathione in Common Ear, Nose, & Throat Conditions: A Systematic Review.* Altern Ther Health Med 22(5):44-50, 2016

Babic I et al. *Therapeutic efficacy of azithromycin & acetylcysteine in chronic otitis media with effusion.* Fur Arch Otorhinolaryngol 274(3):1351-1356, 2017

Bared A, Ouyang X, Angeli S et al. *Antioxidant enzymes, presbycusis, & ethnic variability.* Otolaryngol Head Neck Surg 143(2):263-8, 2010

Bebear JP, Darrouzet V. *Efficacy of n-acetylcysteine by oral route in chronic sinusitis.* Rev. Laryngol. Otol. Rhinol. 109: 185-186, 1988

Bielefeld EC, Hynes S et al. *A comparison of the protective effects of systemic administration of a pro-glutathione drug & a Src-PTK inhibitor against noise-induced hearing loss.* Noise Health 7(29):24-30, 2005

Boner AL, Vallette EA, Andrioli A, et al. *A combination of cefuroxime & n-acetylcysteine for the treatment of maxillary sinusitis in children with respiratory allergy.* Int. J. Clin. Pharmacol. Ther. Toxicol. 22: 511-514, 1984

Burduk PK, Betlejewski S, Drewa G. *Antioxidants enzymes activity & concentration of lipid peroxidation products in chronic tonsillitis before & after surgery.* Otolaryngol Pol 59(5):693-7, 2005

Calabrese V, Cornelius C, Maiolino L et al. *Oxidative stress, redox homeostasis & cellular stress response in Ménière's disease: role of vitagenes.* Neurochem Res 35(12):2208-17, 2010

Campbell KC, Larsen DL, Meech RP et al. *Glutathione ester but not glutathione protects against cisplatin-induced ototoxicity in a rat model.* J Am Acad Audiol 14(3):124-33, 2003

Celik M, Tuncer A, Soyer OU et al. *Oxidative stress in the airways of children with asthma & allergic rhinitis.* Pediatr Allergy Immunol 23(6):556-61, 2012

Cemek M, Caksen H, Cemek F et al. *Investigation of antioxidant status in children with acute otitis media & tonsillitis.* Int J Pediatr Otorhinolaryngol 68(11):1381-5, 2004

Chapple IL. *Reactive oxygen species & antioxidants in inflammatory diseases. J. Clin. Periodontol. 24: 287-296, 1997*

Cross CE, Van der Vilet A, O'Neil CA, et al. *Oxidants, antioxidants, & respiratory tract lining fluids.* Environ. Health Perspect. 102(Suppl 10): 185-191, 1994

Cvetkovic T et al. *Investigation of oxidative stress in patients with chronic tonsillitis.* Auris Nasus Larynx 36(3):340-4, 2009

Dagli M, Eryilmaz A, Besler T et al. *Role of free radicals & antioxidants in nasal polyps.* Laryngoscope 114(7):1200-3, 2004

Dahl AR, Hadley WM. *Nasal cavity enzymes involved in xenobiotic metabolism: effects on the toxicity of inhalants.* Crit. Rev. Toxicol. 21: 345-372, 1991

Domenech M, Garcia E. *N-Acetyl-l-Cysteine & Cysteamine as New Strategies against Mixed Biofilms of Nonencapsulated Streptococcus pneumoniae & Nontypeable Haemophilus Influenzae.* Antimicrob Agents Chemother 61(2), 2017

Doosti A, Lotfi Y, Moossavi A et al. *Compar-*

ison of the effects of N-acetyl-cysteine & ginseng in prevention of noise induced hearing loss in male textile workers. Noise Health 16(71):223-7, 2014

FELDMAN L, SHERMAN RA, WEISSGARTEN J. *N-acetylcysteine use for amelioration of aminoglycoside-induced ototoxicity in dialysis patients.* Semin Dial 25(5):491-4, 2012

FUERTES E, BRAUER M, MACINTYRE E ET AL. *Childhood allergic rinitis, traffic-related air pollution, & variability in the GSTP1, TNF, TLR2, & TLR4 genes:* results from the TAG Study. J Allergy Clin Immunol 132(2):342-52, 2013

GABAIZADEH R, STAECKER H, LIU W, VAN DE WATER TR. *BDNF protection of auditory neurons from cisplatin involves changes in intracellular levels of both reactive oxygen species & glutathione.* Brain Res. Mol. Brain Res. 50: 71-78, 1997

GARETZ SL, ALTSHULER RA, SCHACHT J. *Attenuation of gentamycin ototoxicity by glutathione in the guinea pig in vivo.* Hearing Research 77: 81-87, 1994

GERBASE MVV, KEIDEL D, IMBODEN M. *Effect modification of immunoglobulin E-mediated atopy & rhinitis by glutathione S-transferase genotypes in passive smokers.* Clin Exp Allergy 41(11):1579-86, 2011

GERVASI PG, LONGO V, NALDI F, ET AL. *Xenobiotic-metabolizing enzymes in human respiratory nasal mucosa.* Biochem. Pharmacol. 41: 177-184, 1991

GURBUZIER L, SOGUT E, KOC S ET AL. *Manganese-superoxide dismutase & glutathione peroxidase 1 polymorphisms in recurrent tonsillitis & tonsillar hypertrophy.* Int J Pediatr Otorhinolaryngol 76(9):1270-3, 2012

HAMAGUCHI Y, JUHN SK, SAKAKURA Y. *Recurrence of antigen-induced otitis media by thiol compound.* American J. Otolaryngol. 9: 111-116, 1988

HENDERSON D, MCFADDEN SL, LIU CC ET AL. *The role of antioxidants in protection from impulse noise.* Ann N Y Acad Sci 884:368-80, 1999

HIGHT NG, MCFADDEN SL, HENDERSON D, BURKARD RF, NICOTERA T. *Noise-induced hearing loss in chinchillas pre-treated with glutathione monoethylester & R-PIA.* Hear Res 179(1-2):21-32, 2003

HOFFMAN DW, WHITWORTH CA, JONES KL, RYBAK LP. *Nutritional status, glutathione levels, & ototoxicity of loop diuretics & aminoglycoside antibiotics.* Hearing Research 31: 217-222, 1987

HOFFMAN DW, WHITWORTH CA, JONES KL, RYBAK LP. *Potentiation of ototoxicity by glutathione depletion.* Ann. Otol. Laryngol. 97: 36-41, 1988

HONKURA Y, MATSUO H, MURAKAMI S ET AL. *NRF2 Is a Key Target for Prevention of Noise-Induced Hearing Loss by Reducing Oxidative Damage of Cochlea.* Sci Rep 6:19329, 2016

JACONO AA, HU B, KOPKE RD, ET AL. *Changes in cochlear antioxidant enzyme activity after sound conditioning & noise exposure in the chinchilla.* Hearing Research 117: 31-38, 1998

KALAYCI A ET AL. *Superoxide dismutase & glutathione peroxidase enzyme activities in larynx carcinoma.* Acta Otolaryngol 125(3):312-5, 2005

KEINER S, ZIMMERMANN U. *Glutathione-SH as protection from cytotoxic side effects of gentamycin. Studies with isolated outer hair cells.* HNO 43: 492-497, 1995

KOPKE RD, COLEMAN JK LIU J ET AL. *Candidate's thesis: enhancing intrinsic cochlear stress defenses to reduce noise-induced hearing loss.* Laryngoscope 112(9):1515-32, 2002

KOPKE R, SLADE MD, JACKSON R ET AL. *Efficacy & safety of N-acetylcysteine in prevention of noise induced hearing loss: a randomized clinical trial.* Hear Res 323:40-50, 2015

KRANZER K, ELAMIN WF, COX H ET AL. *A systematic review & meta-analysis of the efficacy & safety of N-acetylcysteine in preventing aminoglycoside-induced ototoxicity:* implications for the treatment of multidrug-resistant TB. Thorax 70(11):1070-7, 2015

KOCYIGIT I, VURAL A, UNAL A ET AL. *Preventing amikacin related ototoxicity with N-acetylcysteine in patients undergoing peritoneal dialysis.* Eur Arch Otorhinolaryngol 272(10):2611-20, 2015

KRISHNA NS, GETCHALL TV, DHOOPER N, ET AL. *Age- & gender-related trends in the expression of glutathione S-transferases in human nasal mucosa.* Ann. Otol. Rhinol. Laryngol. 104: 812-822, 1995

LAUTERMANN J, MCLAREN J, SCHACHT J. *Glutathione protection against gentamycin ototoxicity depends on nutritional status.* Hearing Research 86: 15-24, 1995

LI Q, LIU M. *Glutathione S-transferase T1 null genotype & laryngeal cancer risk: a meta-analysis.* Tumour Biol 35(9):8781-5, 2014

LIN CY, WU JL, SHIH TS ET AL. *Glutathione S-transferase M1, T1, & P1 polymorphisms as susceptibility factors for noise-induced temporary threshold shift.* Hear Res 257(1-2):8-15, 2009

LIN CY ET AL. *N-Acetyl-cysteine against noise-induced temporary threshold shift in male workers.* Hear Res 269(1-2):42-7, 2010

LINDBLAD AC, ROSENHALL U, OLOFSSON A, HAGERMAN B. *The efficacy of N-acetylcysteine to protect the human cochlea from subclinical hearing loss caused by impulse noise: a controlled trial.* Noise Health 13(55):392-401, 2011

LORITO G, GIORDANO P, PETRUCCELLI J ET AL. *Different strategies in treating noiseinduced hearing loss with N-acetylcysteine.* Med Sci Monit 14(8):BR 159-64, 2008

MACCI A, TERRANOVA P, CASTELNUOVO

P. *Recurrent acute rhinosinusitis: a single blind clinical study of N-acetylcysteine vs ambroxol associated to corticosteroid therapy.* Int J Immunopathol Pharmacol 25(1):207-17, 2012

MANCHE SK, JANGALA M, PUTTA P, KORALLA RM, AKKA J. *Association of oxidative stress gene polymorphisms with presbycusis.* Gene 593(2):277-83, 2016

MCFADDEN SL, OHLEMILLER KK, DING D ET AL. *The Influence of Superoxide Dismutase & Glutathione Peroxidase Deficiencies on Noise-Induced Hearing Loss in Mice.* Noise Health 3(11):49-64, 2001

MAURIZI CP. *Could antioxidant therapy reduce the incidence of deafness following bacterial meningitis?* Med. Hypotheses 52: 85-87, 1999

MISCHLEY LK, VESPIGNANI MF, FINNELL JS. *Safety survey of intranasal glutathione.* J Altern Complement Med 19(5):459-63, 2013

MROWICKA M ET AL. *Evaluation of oxidative DNA damage & antioxidant defense in patients with nasal polyps.* Redox Rep 20(4):177-83, 2015

NISHIDA I, TAKUMIDA M. *Attenuation of aminoglycoside ototoxicity by glutathione. ORL J Otorhinolaryngol.* Relat. Spec. 58: 68-73, 1996

OHINATA Y, YAMASOBA T, SCHACHT UJ, MILLER JM. *Glutathione limits noise-induced hearing loss.* Hear Res 146(1-2):28-34, 2000

OKUR E, KILINC M, YILDIRIM I ET AL. *Effect of N-acetylcysteine on carboplatin-induced ototoxicity & nitric oxide levels in a rat model.* Laryngoscope 117(12):2183-6, 2007

OVESEN T, FELDING JU, TOMMERUP B ET AL. *Effect of N-acetylcysteine on the incidence of recurrence of otitis media with effusion & re-insertion of ventilation tubes.* Acta Otolaryngol Suppl 543:79-81, 2000

OVESEN T, PAASKE PB, ELBROEND O. *Local application of n-acetylcysteine in secretory otitis media in rabbits.* Clin. Otolaryngol. 17: 327-331, 1992

OZCAN C, TAMER L, ATES NA, GORUR K. *The glutathione-S-transferase gene polymorphisms (Gstt1, Gstm1, & Gstp1) in patients with non-allergic nasal polyposis.* Eur Arch Otorhinolaryngol 267(2):227-32, 2010

PALODETTO B, POSTAL M, GRIGNOLI CR ET AL. *Influence of glutathione s-transferase on the ototoxicity caused by aminoglycosides.* Bran J Otorhinolaryngol 76(3):306-9, 2010

PARKS RR, HUANG CC, HADDAD J JR. *Middle ear catalase distribution in an animal model of otitis media.* Eur. Arch. Otorhinolaryngol. 253: 445-449, 1996

PINTUCCI JP, CORNO S, GAROTTA M. *Biofilms & infections of the upper respiratory tract.* Eur Rev Med Pharmacol Sci 14(8):683-90, 2010

POTTER DW, FINCH L, UDINSKY JR. *Glutathione content & turnover in rat nasal epithelia.* Toxicol. appl. Pharmacol. 135: 185-191, 1995

RAPONI G, ALPINE D, VOLONTE S ET AL. *The role of free radicals & plasmatic antioxidant in Meniere's syndrome.* Int Tinnitus J 9(2):104-8, 2003

RAVI R, SOMANI SM, RYBAK LP. *Mechanism of cisplatin ototoxicity: antioxidant system.* Pharmacol. Toxicol. 76: 386-394, 1995

RHEE CS, MAJIMA Y, CHO JS, ET AL. *Effects of mucokinetic drugs on rheological properties of reconstituted human nasal mucus.* Arch. Otolaryngol. Head Neck Surg. 125: 101-105, 1999

RIGA MG, CHELIS L ET AL. *Transtympanic injections of N-acetylcysteine for the prevention of cisplatin-induced ototoxicity: a feasible method with promising efficacy.* Am J Clin Oncol 36(1):1-6, 2013

RUIZ JW, GUZMAN J. POLAK M ET AL. *Glutathione ester protects against hydroxynonenal-induced loss of auditory hair cells.* Otolaryngol Head Neck Surg 135(5):792-7, 2006

SCANNAPIECO FA, PAPANDONATOS GD, DUNFORD RG. *Associations between oral conditions & respiratory disease in a national sample survey population.* Ann. Periodontol. 3: 251-256, 1998

SHA SH, SCHACHT J. *Emerging therapeutic interventions against noise-induced hearing loss.* Expert Opin Invest Drugs 26(1):85-96, 2017

SHEN H, HUO X, LIU K ET AL. *Genetic variation in GSTM1 is associated with susceptibility to noise-induced hearing loss in a Chinese population.* J Occup Environ Med 54(9):1157-62, 2012

TAYSI S, USLU C, YILMAZ A ET AL. *Lipid peroxidation & some antioxidant enzymes in nasal polyp tissue.* Cell Biochem Funct 25(5):461-5, 2006

TEPEL M. *N-Acetylcysteine in the prevention of ototoxicity.* Kidney Int 72(3):231-2, 2007

TESTA D, GUERRA G, MARCUCCIO G ET AL. *Oxidative stress in chronic otitis media with effusion.* Acta Otolaryngol 132(8):834-7, 2012

TESTA B, TESTA D, MESOLELLA M ET AL. *Management of chronic otitis media with effusion:* the role of glutathione. Laryngoscope 111(8):1486-9, 2001

TESTA B, MESOLELLA M, TEATA D, ET AL. *Glutathione in the upper respiratory tract.* Ann. Otol. Rhinol. Laryngol. 104: 117-119, 1995

TILLINGER JA, GUPTA C, ILA K ET AL. *I-N-acetylcysteine protects outer hair cells against TNFa initiated ototoxicity in vitro.* Acta Otolaryngol 138(8):676-684, 2018

VAN DER VILET A, O'NEIL CA, CROSS CE, ET AL. *Determination of low-molecular mass antioxidant concentrations in human respiratory tract lining fluids.* American J. Physiol. 276(2 Pt 1): L289-L296, 1999

WESTERVELD GJ, DEKKER I, VOSS HP, ET

AL. *Antioxidant levels in the nasal mucosa of patients with chronic sinusitis & healthy controls.* Arch. Otolaryngol. Head Neck Surg. 123: 201-204, 1997

WESTERVELD GJ, DEKKER I, VOSS HP ET AL. *Antioxidant levels in the nasal mucosa of patients with chronic sinusitis & healthy controls.* Arch Otolaryngol Head Neck Surg 123(2):201-4, 1997

WU HP, HSU CJ, CHENG TJ, GUO YL. *N-acetylcysteine attenuates noise-induced permanent hearing loss in diabetic rats.* Hear Res 267(1-2):71-7, 2010

YAMASOBA T, HARRIS C, SHOJI F ET AL. *Influence of intense sound exposure on glutathione synthesis in the cochlea.* Brain Res 804(1):72-78, 1998

YAMASOBA T, NUTTALL AL, HARRIS C. *Role of glutathione in protection against noise-induced hearing loss.* Brain Research 784: 82-90, 1998

YARIKTAS M, DONER F, DOGRU H ET AL. *The role of free oxygen radicals on the development of otitis media with effusion.* Int J Pediatr Otorhinolaryngol 68(7):889-94, 2004

YILMAZ T, KOCAN EG, BESLER HT. *The role of oxidants & antioxidants in chronic tonsillitis & adenoid hypertrophy in children.* Int J Pediatr Otorhinolaryngol 68(8):1053-8, 2004

YILMAZ T, KOCAN EG, BESLER HT ET AL. *The role of oxidants & antioxidants in otitis media with effusion in children.* Otolaryngol Head Neck Surg 131(6):797-803, 2004

ZHOU S, WANG R, ZHOU J ET AL. *[Association of GSTM1 & GSTT1 polymorphisms with noise-induced hearing loss: a meta-analysis].* Zhonghua Lao Dong Wei Sheng Zhi Ye Bing Za Zhi 32(2):123-5, 2014

ZEIGER RS. *Prospects for ancillary treatment of sinusitis in the 1990's.* J. Allergy Immunol. 90: 478-495, 1992

16
Dentistry & Periodontology

A FACT LITTLE KNOWN by doctors but common knowledge to dentists is that tooth (dental) and gum (periodontal) disease are the most common illnesses in America. More importantly, periodontal disease has recently been linked to more serious systemic diseases that may be enabled by poor oral hygiene. Robert Genco, editor-in-chief of the Journal of Periodontology has said, "It seems clear that gum disease, far from being just an oral health problem, actually represents a significant health risk to millions of people."

It goes beyond unsightly smiles and bad breath. Infections and toxins in the mouth have been linked to heart disease, stroke, bacteremia, prosthetic device infection, diabetes, pulmonary disease, impairment of fetal growth and other systemic diseases. Dr. Charles Mayo, founder of the Mayo Clinic is purported to have said, "Preventive dentistry can extend your life expectancy ten years."

One of the most impressive of all studies is the Veteran Administration's Normative Aging Study in Boston. It followed the medical history of over one thousand outwardly healthy men, starting in the 1960's. Those who began with any sign of gum disease suffered about twice the death rate—mostly due to cardiovascular disease—of those with healthy gums. At a conference on the subject, Dr. Raul Garcia, one of the researchers, stated, "Gum disease kills. Floss or die!"

Links have been made between the infective and inflammatory[1] processes of periodontitis and free radicals. Research clearly shows that elevated glutathione levels combat the formation of free radicals and bolster the immune system's defenses.

Glutathione in Periodontal Disease

In an article entitled The Antioxidant Master Glutathione and Periodontal Health, authors Bains & Bains make the statement that glutathione, "is the most-important redox regulator that controls inflammatory processes, and thus damage to the periodontium." In simpler words, they acknowledge that the antioxidant defense system in the mouth relies most heavily on glutathione, and that without it, our gums and teeth would be

[1] *infections* from invading microorganisms versus *inflammation*: the body's response to irritants

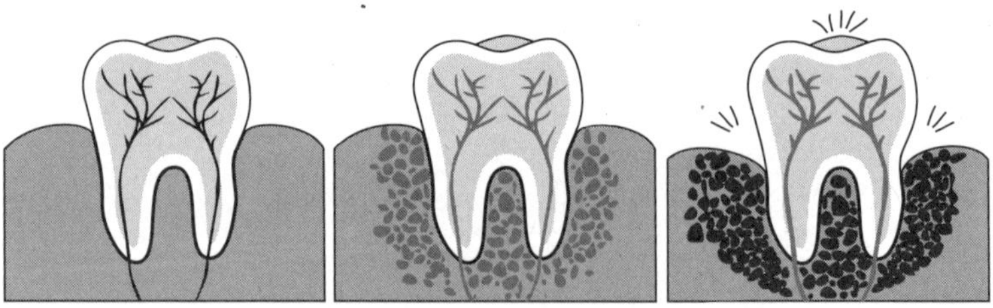

FIGURE 36: Gums in health and sickness

damaged by unrestrained inflammation.

It has repeatedly been shown that glutathione levels in the saliva are lower in patients suffering from gum disease and periodontitis. More interestingly, after adequate treatment of periodontal disease, glutathione levels often reset back to normal. Saliva is normally rich in glutathione and this offers not only antioxidant protection but also higher white blood cell activity in the mouth, to combat bacteria and other microbes.

Periodontal disease doesn't only deplete GSH in the mouth. Several researchers have shown that patients with gum disease also have lower than normal blood levels of GSH.

In a recent issue of the Journal of Periodontology, Villa-Correa and his colleagues suggested that measures of salivary glutathione could be strong, independent markers for both chronic periodontal and aggressive periodontal disease. This has been confirmed by many other research teams.

Glutathione in Dental Disease

Extensive research has been reviewed on the critical role of glutathione in supporting the immune system (see Chapter 3). This includes the many bacteria that enter via the mouth and cause dental caries (cavities). Increased oxidative stress anywhere in the body enables pathogens to flourish. This includes cariogenic (cavity-causing) microorganisms.

Brazilian researchers examined young adults (average age 20 years), comparing dental health on the DMFT index (Decayed, Missing, or Filled Teeth) with salivary glutathione levels. They found those with higher glutathione levels were in much better dental health. Similar findings have been demonstrated in schoolchildren as well.

A fascinating Italian study looked at the effect of cigarettes on oral health. Smokers not only have a higher incidence of oral cancer, but also a higher level of periodontal disease and dental cavities. Astonishingly, a single cigarette was enough to weaken defenses against these problems. The correlation between smoking and decreased glutathione levels in the mouth is well documented.

Glutathione in Dental Toxicology

The controversial area of dental amalgams causing systemic toxicity through mercury and other heavy metals is covered in Chapter 2: GSH & Detoxification. Quite apart from this, restorative dentistry employs many chemical agents to enhance and repair teeth and the underlying bone. These include glues and resins, bonding agents and inorganic bone substitutes. Like so many medical treatments, there are potentially toxic side effects.

Resins such as PMMA (poly-methyl methacrylate), HEMA (hydroxy-methyl acrylate), and TEGDMA (triethylene glycol dimethacrylate) are some of the most commonly-used materials in dental practice and are used to repair the damage of cavities, erosions or fractures. These resins release breakdown products into surrounding tissues that may cause local and systemic problems, including impaired immune function.

Several studies have investigated the use of either glutathione or N-acetylcysteine (a potent GSH precursor) in combination with these resins. This led to a reversal of cytotoxicity (cellular toxin damage) and restoration of osteoblasts (bone-forming cells), with an overall protective effect.

Raising Glutathione in Dental Infection

Pathogenic bacteria of all sorts invade the mouth, causing both dental and gum infection. Chinese research into some of the most common microorganisms concluded

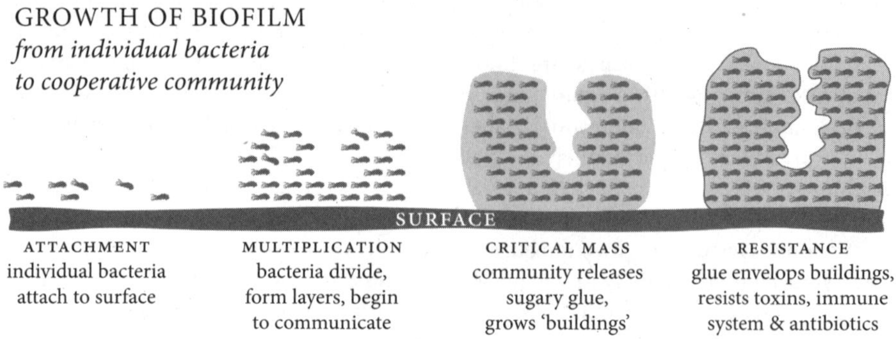

FIGURE 37: From individual bacteria to the cooperative community

that the glutathione precursor NAC provided excellent antibacterial activity against endodontic (tooth infection) pathogens, and suggested that NAC be used as an alternative medication within root canals.

Individual bacteria are easy to combat, but bacteria can group together into more resilient 'biofilms.' These multiple layers of bacteria are often made up of several different species that grow thick and gluey over certain tissues (see Figure 36). They are particularly active in the mouth. NAC has shown great promise experimentally to break down and destroy the microbes that form them. Rasmussen and his team put forward the idea that NAC, "Has the potential to be used as a long-term, anti-plaque bacteriostatic agent for managing chronic dental decay." More studies are ongoing.

Conclusion

Dentistry's importance in total health care is now acknowledged. Periodontal disease is considered a risk factor for heart disease, stroke and other systemic diseases. Glutathione levels are well documented to be lower in dental and gum tissues as well as in the saliva of periodontal patients. Enhancing glutathione levels should be part of a good oral hygiene program.

DENTISTRY & PERIODONTOLOGY

REFERENCES

BAINS VK, BAINS R. *The antioxidant master glutathione & periodontal health.* Dent Res J (Isfahan) 12(5): 389-405, 2015

BIJU T, SHABEER MM, AMITHA R, RAJENDRA BP, SUCHETHA K. *Comparative evaluation of serum superoxide dismutase & glutathione levels in periodontally diseased patients: an interventional study.* Indian J Dent Res. 25(5) 613-6, 2014

BUDUNELI N, KARDESLER L, ISIK H, WILLIS CS3RD, HAWKINS SI, KINANE DF, SCOTT DA. *Effects of smoking & gingival inflammation on salivary antioxidant capacity.* J Clin Periodontol. 33(3):159-64, 2006

CHAPPLE IL, BROCK G, EFTIMIADI C, MATTHEWS JB. *Glutathione in gingival crevicular fluid & its relation to local antioxidant capacity in periodontal health & disease.* Mol Pathol. 55(6) :367-73, 2002

CHOI YS, KIM C, MOON JH, LEE JY. *Removal & killing of multispecies endodontic biofilms by N-acetylcysteine.* Braz J Microbiol S-1517-8382(16)30347-1, 2017

D'AIUTO F, NIBALI L, PARKAR M, PATEL K, SUVAN J, DONOS N. *Oxidative stress, systemic inflammation, & severe periodontitis.* J Dent Res 89(11):1241-6, 2010

DIAS IH, CHAPPLE IL, MILWARD M, GRANT MM, HILL E, BROWN J, GRIFFITHS HR. *Sulforaphane restores cellular glutathione levels & reduces chronic periodontitis neutrophil hyperactivity in vitro.* PLoS One 8(6):e66407, 2013

Garcia RI, Krall EA, Vokonas PS. Periodontal disease & mortality from all causes in the VA Dental Longitudinal Study. *Ann. Periodontol. 3: 339-349, 1998*

Garg N, Singh R, Dixit J, Jain A, Tewari V. *Levels of lipid peroxides & antioxidants in smokers & nonsmokers.* J Periodontal Res 41(5):405-10, 2006

Grant MM, Brock GR, Matthews JB, Chapple IL. *Crevicular fluid glutathione levels in periodontitis & the effect of non-surgical therapy.* J Clin Periodontol 37(1):17-23, 2010

Greabu M, Totan A, Battino M, Mohora M, Didilescu A, Total C, Spinu T. *Cigarette smoke effect on total salivary antioxidant capacity, salivary glutathione peroxidase & gamma-glutamyltransferase activity.* Biofactors 33(2):129-36, 2008

Garcia RI, Krall EA, Vokonas PS. *Periodontal disease & mortality from all causes in the VA Dental Longitudinal Study.* Ann. Periodontol. 3: 339-349, 1998

Hand DH, Kim MJ, Jun EJ, Kim JB. *The role of glutathione metabolism in cariogenic bacterial growth & caries in Korean children.* Arch Oral Biol. 58(5):493-9, 2013

Jeeva JS, Sunitha J, Ananthalakshmi R, Rajkumari S, Ramesh M, Krishnan R. *Enzymatic antioxidants & its role in oral diseases.* J Pharm Bioallied Sci 7(Suppl 2):S331-3, 2015

Jiao Y, Ma S, Wang Y et al. *N-Acetyl Cysteine Depletes Reactive Oxygen Species & Prevents Dental Monomer-Induced Intrinsic Mitochondrial Apoptosis in Vitro in Human Dental Pulp Cells.* PLoS One 11(1):e0147858, 2016

Kojima N, Yamada M, Paranjpe A, Tsukimura N, Kubo K, Jewett A, Ogawa T. *Restored viability & function of dental pulp cells on polymethlmethacrylate (PMMA)-based dental resin supplemented with N-acetyl cysteine (NAC).* Dent Mater 24(12):1686-93, 2008

Krifka S, Spagnuolo G, Schmalz G, Schweiki H. *A review of adaptive mechanisms in cell responses towards oxidative stress caused by dental resin monomers.* Biomaterials 34(19):4555-63, 2013

Kim NR, Park HC, Kim I, Lim BS, Yang HC. *In vitro cytocompatibility of N-acetylcysteine-supplemented dentin bonding agents.* J Endod 36(11):1844-50, 2010

Marton IJ, Balla G, Hegedus C, et al. *The role of reactive oxygen intermediates in the pathogenesis of chronic apical periodontitis.* Oral Microbiol Immunol 8(4):254-7, 1993

Mendez MV, Scott T, LaMorte W, et al. *An association between periodontal disease & peripheral vascular disease.* American J. Surgery 176: 153-157, 1998

Moon JH, Choi YS, Lee HW, et al. *Antibacterial effects of N-acetylcysteine against endodontic pathogens.* J Microbiol 54(4):322-9, 2016

Mendez MV, Scott T, LaMorte W, et al. *An association between periodontal disease & peripheral vascular disease.* American J. Surgery 176: 153-157, 1998

Nassar M, Hiraishi N, Islam MS, et al. *The effect of glutathione on 2-hydroxyethylmethacrylate cytotoxicity & on resin-dentine bond strength.* Int Endod J 47(7):652-8, 2014

Novakovic N, Todorovic T, Rakic M, et al. *Salivary antioxidants as periodontal biomarkers in evaluation of tissue status & treatment outcome.* J Periodontal Res 49(1):129-36, 2014

Oztürk LK, et al. *Association between dental-oral health in young adults & salivary glutathione, lipid peroxidation & sialic acid levels & carbonic anhydrase activity.* Braz J Med Biol Res 41(11):956-9, 2008

Patel SP, Pradeep AR, Chowdhry S. *Crevicular fluid levels of plasma glutathione peroxidase (eGPx) in periodontal health & disease.* Arch Oral Biol 54(6):543-8, 2009

Patel SP, Rao NS, Pradeep AR. *Effect of nonsurgical periodontal therapy on crevicular fluid & serum glutathione peroxidase levels.* Dis Markers 32(1):1-7, 2012

Rasmussen K, Mikrad J, Reilly C, Li Y, Jones RS. *N-Acetyl-l-cysteine effects on multi-species oral biofilm formation & bacterial ecology.* Lett Appl Microbiol 62(1):30-8, 2016

Savita AM, Sarun E, Arora S, Krishnan S. *Evaluation of glutathione level in gingival crevicular fluid in periodontal health, in chronic periodontitis & after nonsurgical periodontal therapy: A clinicobiochemical study.* Contemp Clin Dent 6(2):206-10, 2015

Scannapieco FA. *American Academy of Periodontology, Position Paper Periodontal disease as a potential risk factor for systemic diseases.* J. Periodontol. 69: 841-850, 1998

Scannapieco FA, Papandonatos GD, Dunford RG. *Associations between oral conditions & respiratory disease in a national sample survey population.* Ann. Periodontol. 3: 251-256, 1998

Sculley DV, Langley-Evans SC. *Salivary antioxidants & periodontal disease status.* Proc Nutr Soc. 61(1):137-43, 2002

Sculley DV, Langley-Evans SC. *Periodontal disease is associated with lower antioxidant capacity in whole saliva & evidence of increased protein oxidation.* Clin Sci (Lond) 105(2):167-72, 2003

Sweeney MP, Bagg J, Fell GS, Yip B. *The relationship between micronutrient depletion & oral health in geriatrics.* J. Oral Pathol. Med. 23: 168-171,

1994

Toker H, Ozdemir H, Eren K, Ozer H, Sahin G. *N-acetylcysteine, a thiol antioxidant, decreases alveolar bone loss in experimental periodontitis in rats.* J Periodontol 80(4):672-8, 2009

Trivedi S, Lal N, Mahdi AA, Singh B, Pandey S. *Association of salivary lipid peroxidation levels, antioxidant enzymes, & chronic periodontitis.* Int J Periodontics Restorative Dent. 35(2):e14-9, 2015

Tsukimura N, Yamada M, Aita H, et al. *N-acetyl cysteine (NAC)-mediated detoxification & functionalization of poly (methyl methacrylate) bone cement.* Biomaterials 30(20):3378-89, 2009

Ueno T, Yamada M, Igarashi Y, Ogawa T. *N-acetyl cysteine protects osteoblastic function from oxidative stress.* J Biomed Mater Res A 99(4):523-31, 2011

Villa-Correa YA, Isaza-Guzmán DM, Tobón-Arroyave SI. *Influence of Periodontal Clinical Status on Salivary Levels of Glutathione Reductase.* J Periodontol 87(6):716-24, 2016

Waddington RJ, Moseley R, Embery G. *Reactive oxygen species: a potential role in the pathogenesis of periodontal diseases.* Oral Dis 6(3):138-51, 2000

Wang Y, Andrukhov O, Rausch-Fan X. *Oxidative Stress & Antioxidant System in Periodontitis.* Front Physiol, 8:910, 2017

Wei PF, Ho KY, et al. *The investigation of glutathione peroxidase, lactoferrin, myeloperoxidase & interleukin-1beta in gingival crevicular fluid:* implications for oxidative stress in human periodontal diseases. J Periodontal Res 39(5):287-93, 2004

Yamada M, Kojima N, et al. *N-acetyl cysteine (NAC)-assisted detoxification of PMMA resin.* J Dent Res 87(4):372-7, 2008

Yamada M, Kojima N, et al. *N-Acetyl cysteine restores viability & function of rat odontoblast-like cells impaired by polymethylmethacrylate dental resin extract.* Redox Rep 14(1):1-22, 2009

Yamada M, Ueno T, et al. *N-acetyl cysteine alleviates cytotoxicity of bone substitute.* J Dent Res 89(4):411-6, 2010

Zappacosta B, Persichilli S, Mordente A, et al. *Inhibition of salivary enzymes by cigarette smoke & the protective role of glutathione.* Hum Exp Toxicol 21(1):7-11, 2002

17

Eyes and Vision

Of all our senses, the most cherished is usually vision. Given the intricacy and extremely sensitive tissues involved in eyesight, it's no surprise that glutathione plays a major role. Ophthalmologists, the medical specialists who treat the eye, were among the first to outline the importance of glutathione to our health. Some of the earliest studies with GSH focused on its role in preventing cataracts. A huge number of articles were published on this topic as far back as the 1930s.

Many different eye diseases have been associated with glutathione impairment (see Table 29). This chapter will focus on the role of glutathione in cataracts, glaucoma, macular degeneration and pterygium.

Cataracts

The lens of the eye is the only organ in the body that does not shed or lose cells. Nutrients required by the lens are delivered through the liquid lying adjacent to it rather than through blood vessels. For this reason, higher antioxidant levels than usual are required to ensure adequate protection.

Cataract is a clouding (opacification) of the lens of the eye. It is the leading cause of poor health and functional impairment among the elderly and leads to more than one million operations per year in the United States.

The lens consists of deceptively simple tissue. This entirely transparent part of the eye is tasked with focusing light on the retina, which it does by changing shape to adjust its focal length. Scientists believe that any damage to the lens, no matter how small, contributes to opacification. This usually results from physical injury, repeated exposure to ionizing radiation (such as sunlight) or from any number of different illnesses. Over time the damage accumulates and the clouding becomes noticeable.

Oxidative stress contributes to aging of the lens, so antioxidants are an important defense against cataracts. The Russian researcher Babizhaev tracked the development of cataracts by measuring the breakdown products of lipid peroxidation. He found that, as cataracts worsened, oxidative stress increased. An Italian team at the University of Bari went one step further and demonstrated that the GSH levels of people with cataracts actually fall as oxidative breakdown products increase.

It is known that cataracts in humans are usually marked by extensive oxidation of lens proteins. In search of a solution, researchers tried stimulating cataract defenses with

Cataracts	Conjunctivitis
Macular Degeneration	Diabetic Retinopathy
Glaucoma	Radiation Exposure
Pterygium	Keratitis

Table 29: *Eye diseases associated with low glutathione*

various biochemicals. They showed that cataracts could be delayed or even prevented by products that raise GSH levels. This demonstrates emphatically that glutathione is the key defense against oxidation in the lens.

The legendary GSH expert, Alton Meister and a team at Cornell University in New York, used the drug BSO to deplete glutathione levels in the eyes of laboratory animals. The animals subsequently developed cataracts. Meister's team was then able to prevent cataract formation by reestablishing glutathione levels with GSH monoester. They suggested that this strategy could be an effective way to delay cataract formation.

As genetic testing advances the state of medicine, it is becoming easier to identify individuals with inherited glutathione enzyme abnormalities. There is abundant evidence that this population is prone to cataracts. Identifying such people sooner rather than later would give them an opportunity to protect their long-term health.

Diabetics develop more cataracts than non-diabetics. Altomare's team in Italy measured glutathione status in the lens of four groups of patients: diabetics with and without cataracts and non-diabetics with and without cataracts. As expected, both cataract groups showed impaired glutathione defenses, but the diabetic groups always fared worse. This highlights the fact that in addition to diabetic retinopathy and glaucoma (see below), people with diabetes need to be concerned about a higher rate of cataracts as well.

Eye drops with glutathione-related agents have been used in the past and are still being investigated in the treatment and prevention of cataracts. The use of oral glutathione boosters such as N-acetylcysteine also shows promise. An interesting observation published in the journal Clinical Experimental Optometry showed that maternal malnutrition leading to glutathione depletion increased the risk that mothers would give birth to children prone to childhood cataracts.

Case study

Edgar loved to paint. Now retired, he could pursue his hobby full-time. In recent years his wife had commented that the colors in his landscapes were too "loud." He didn't at first believe his technique had changed, but a side-by-side comparison with earlier works proved him wrong. However, he now felt the colors in previous paintings were "weak." A routine check revealed that he was developing cataracts. One eye required surgery, the other was "not yet ripe" for it. Following surgery he recovered excellent vision, but only after experiencing post-operative complications, so he was wary of operating on the other eye. His wife did some homework and, learning about glutathione and cataracts, supplemented his dietary intake with selenium and alpha-lipoic acid. One year later, his ophthalmologist saw that the cataract was less dense, and was baffled.

Macular degeneration

Macular degeneration is progressive loss of sight due to breakdown of the macula—the part of the retina that enabling fine vision. Figure 37 shows its location in the back of the eye.

Age-related macular degeneration (ARMD) is a leading cause of visual loss in people over 65. Although susceptibility to this disease may be predominantly genetic, it can be worsened by contributing factors such as smoking and atherosclerosis. This disease is thought to result from free radical damage over time, primarily by exposure to ultraviolet (UV) sunlight, but also to other sources of oxidative stress.

Elderly people generally have low GSH levels and so are predisposed to oxidative damage. Researchers have shown that low GSH levels go along with poor eye health in ARMD patients compared to normal control

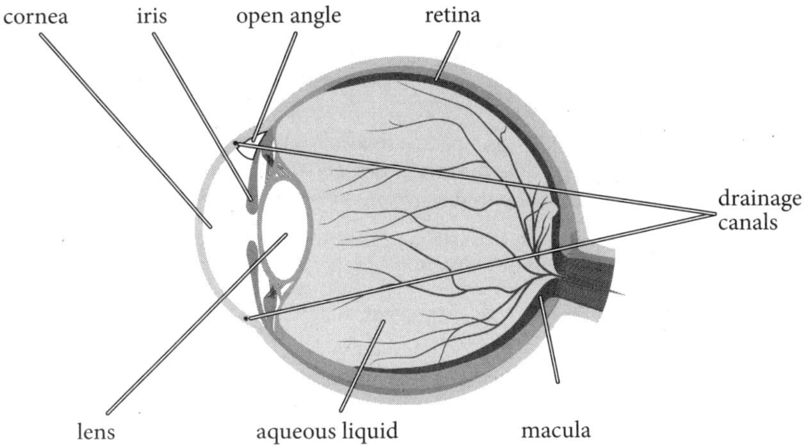

Figure 38: The Eye

groups. Patients with macular degeneration were examined to record glutathione's antioxidant function, both in the whole body and specifically in the eyes. Cohen and his team at the University of California (Davis) found significantly altered GSH activity in the blood of macular degeneration patients. It appears that high GSH levels are a feature of healthy eyes and suggests a possible role for GSH in protection against or delay of this disease.

Abnormally low glutathione levels have been found even in the early stages of ARMD. Blood levels of people exhibiting early ARMD showed higher levels of oxidative stress and lower active glutathione levels than healthy individuals of the same age. This suggests that such blood tests might be a way of diagnosing ARMD.

Intervention with antioxidants including glutathione precursors have provoked hope of a novel approach to regaining retinal function in age-related macular degeneration.

Glaucoma

Glaucoma is a serious condition caused by rising fluid pressure within the eye. Internal pressure is needed to maintain the shape of the eyeball—but only a certain amount. Too much, and the small blood vessels within the eye become compressed, cutting off blood flow and damaging surrounding areas—most importantly the optic nerve.

Glaucoma is one of the leading causes of visual loss. We become more susceptible as we age. It also runs in some families, and often strikes along with diabetes, hypertension (high blood pressure) and severe myopia (nearsightedness). Traditional therapy aims to relieve the pressure in the eye either surgically or with drugs.

Glutathione's presence in the fluid of the inner eye not only detoxifies the aqueous liquid but has also been shown to improve the circulation and outflow of this fluid. Researchers have demonstrated that glutathione depletion and oxidative stress in the eye's drainage system is correlated with an increased likelihood of progression to glaucoma.

The Russians Bunin, Filina and Erichev measured GSH levels in the aqueous fluid of hundreds of patients undergoing various sorts of eye surgery. The lowest GSH levels were found among cataract patients and in patients with open angle glaucoma[1]. They noticed they were low even at the earliest stages of the disease, and suggested that raising glutathione levels might prevent or delay this process. They used the nutritional supplement lipoic acid to test their theory (see Chapter 4).

A Harvard University group tried various GSH-related compounds to help reduce internal pressure by improving the drainage of fluid from the eye. In combination with the topical form of ethacrynic acid (a diuretic drug) they found that cysteine, glutathione and N-acetylcysteine all helped. In fact, they also lessened the drug's side-effects.

A genetic screening test enables us to identify people with glutathione-enzyme defects. It's been shown that such people are at greater risk of developing glaucoma—another newly-identified risk factor.

Pterygium

Although you may not have heard of pterygium before, you may have seen and described it as a "red eye." A pterygium is a growth of superficial tissue over the cornea (the white part of the eye). It's pink or red because it's full of blood vessels. It grows slowly and does not pose a great danger to vision. It can be treated medically or surgically.

A pterygium is more likely in people exposed to a combination of wind, sand and sun. For this reason, it's been called "surfer's eye," and is more common in people from coastal or island environments.

Investigations into pterygium have shown that its tissue displays high levels of oxidative stress, free-radical damage and glutathione depletion. In addition, individuals with abnormal glutathione enzyme genetics are more prone to developing pterygium.

Conclusion

Scientists studying the eye have long recognized glutathione's importance as an ocular antioxidant. Practical applications are now available for the prevention and treatment of cataract, glaucoma, macular degeneration and other eye disorders.

---

[1] In open-angle glaucoma, the angle in the eye where the iris meets the cornea is as wide and open as it should be, but the eye's drainage canals are clogged. This increases internal eye pressure and damages the optic nerve.

EYES & VISION

REFERENCES

ALTOMARE E, VENDEMIALE G, GRATTAGLIANO I, ET AL. *Human diabetic cataract: role of lipid peroxidation.* Diabetes Metab. 21: 173-179, 1995

AYDIN B, YAGCI R, YILMAZ FM ET AL. *Prevention of selenite-induced cataractogenesis by N-acetylcysteine in rats.* Curr Eye Res 34(3):196-201, 2009

BABIZHAYEV MA. *New concept in nutrition for the maintenance of the aging eye redox regulation & therapeutic treatment of cataract disease; synergism of natural antioxidant imidazole-containing amino acid-based compounds, chaperone, & glutathione boosting agents: a systemic perspective on aging & longevity emerged from studies in humans.* Am J Ther 17(4):373-89, 2010

BABIZHAEV MA. *Accumulation of lipid peroxidation products in the human lens during cataract maturation.* Vopr. Med. Khim. 31: 100-104, 1985

BABIZHAEV MA, SHVEDOVA AA, ARKHIPENKO IV, KAGAN VE. *Accumulation of lipid peroxidation products in cataractous lenses.* Biull. Eksp. Biol. Med. 100: 299-301, 1985

BALCI M, SAHIN S, MUTLU FM ET AL. *Investigation of oxidative stress in pterygium tissue.* Mol Vis 17:443-7, 2011

BARBOSA AM, FRARE AB, COSTA NB ET AL.

GSTM1 polymorphism in patients with primary open-angle glaucoma. Genet Mol Res 11(3):3256-62, 2012

Bunin AI, Filina AA, Erichev VP. *A glutathione deficiency in open-angle glaucoma & the approaches to its correction.* Vestn. Oftalmol. 108: 13-15, 1992

Campbell DA. *Glutathione in the blood in senile cataract & other ocular conditions.* Br J Ophthalmol 20(1):33-8, 1936

Cejik SK, Aras N, Yildirim O et al. *Glutathione S-transferase GSTM1, null genotype may be associated with susceptibility to age-related cataract.* Ady Clin Exp Med 24(1):113-9, 2015

Cohen SM, Olin KL, Feuer WJ, et al. *Low glutathione reductase & peroxidase activity in age-related macular degeneration.* Br. J. Ophthalmol. 78: 791-794, 1994

De La Paz MA, Zhang J, Fridovitch I. *Antioxidant enzymes of the human retina: effect of age on enzyme activity of macula & periphery.* Curr. Eye Res. 15: 273-278, 1996

Epstein DL, Hooshmand LB, Eptein MP. *Thiol adducts of ethacrynic acid increase outflow facility in enucleated calf eyes.* Curr. Eye Res. 11:253-258, 1992

Fan X, Monnier VM, Whitson J. *Lens glutathione homeostasis: Discrepancies & gaps in knowledge standing in the way of novel therapeutic approaches.* Exp Eye Res 156:103-111, 2017

Filina AA, Davydova NG, Kolomoitseva EM. *The effect of lipoic acid on the components of the glutathione system in the lachrymal fluid of patients with open-angle glaucoma.* Vestn. Oftalmol. 109: 5-7, 1993

Ganea E, Harding JJ. *Glutathione-related enzymes & the eye.* Curr Eye Res 31(1):1-11, 2006

Gherghel D, Griffiths HR, Hilton EJ et al. *Systemic reduction in glutathione levels occurs in patients with primary open-angle glaucoma.* Invest Ophthalmol Vis Sci 46(3):877-83, 2005

Gherghel D, Mroczkowska S, Quin L. *Reduction in blood glutathione levels occurs similarly in patients with primary-open angle or normal tension glaucoma.* Invest Ophthalmol Vis Sci 54(5):3333-9, 2013

Giblin FJ. *Glutathione: a vital lens antioxidant.* J Ocul Pharmacol Ther. 16(2):121-35, 2000

Gukasyan HJ, Kim KJ, Lee VH, Kannan R. *Glutathione & its transporters in ocular surface defense.* Ocul Surf 5(4):269-79, 2007

Huang W, Wan W, Zhou M et al. *Association of glutathione S-transferase polymorphisms (GSTM1 & GSTT1) with primary open-angle glaucoma: an evidence-based meta-analysis.* Gene 526(2):80-6, 2013

Karadag R, Bayram N, Oguztuzun S, Bozer B et al. *Investigation of Glutathione S-Transferase Isoenzyme Protein Expression in Patients With Pterygium.* Cornea 35(8):1089-92, 2016

Kilic F, Handelman GJ, Traber K et al. *Modeling cortical cataractogenesis 22. In vitro effect of alpha-lipoic acid on glutathione concentrations in lens in model diabetic cataractogenesis. Biochem. Mol. Biol. Int. 46: 585-595, 1998*

Kormanovski A, Parra F, Jarillo-Luna A et al. *Oxidant/antioxidant state in tissue of prymary & recurrent ptergium.* BMC Ophthalmol 14:149, 2014

Kumar D, Lim JC, Donaldson PJ. *A link between maternal malnutrition & depletion of glutathione in the developing lens: a possible explanation for idiopathic childhood cataract?* Clin Exp Optom 96(6):523-8, 2013

Linetsky M, Ranson N, Ortwerth BJ. *The aggregation in human lens proteins blocks the scavenging of UVA-generated singlet oxygen by ascorbic acid & glutathione.* Arch. Biochem. Biophys. 351: 180-188, 1998

Maddirala Y, Tobwala S, Karacal H, Ercal N. *Prevention & reversal of selenite-induced cataracts by N-acetylcysteine amide in Wistar rats.* BMC Ophthalmol 17(1):54-, 2017

Martensson J, Steinherz R, Jain A, Meister A. *Glutathione ester prevents buthionine sulfoxamine-induced cataracts & lens epithelial cell damage.* Proc. Natl. Acad. Sci. USA 86: 8727-8731, 1989

Megaw JM. *Glutathione & ocular photobiology.* Curr Eye Res 3(1):83-7, 1984

Micelli-Ferrari T, Vendemiale G, Grattagliano I, et al. *Role of lipid peroxidation in the pathogenesis of myopic & senile cataract.* Br. J. Ophthalmol. 80: 840-843, 1996

Moriarty-Craige SE et al. *Antioxidant supplements prevent oxidation of cysteine/cystine redox in patients with age-related macular degeneration.* Am J Ophthalmol 140(6):1020-6, 2005

Othman H, Gholampour AR, Saadat I et al. *Age-related macular degeneration & genetic polymorphisms of glutathione S-transferases M1 (GSTM1) & T1 (GSTT1).* Mol Biol Rep. 2012 Mar; 39(3):3299-303, 2012

Pau H, Graf P, Sies H. *Glutathione levels in human lens: regional distribution in different forms of cataract.* Exp. Eye Res. 50: 17-20, 1990

Plestina-Borjan I, Katusic D, Medvidovic-Grubisic M et al. *Association of age-related macular degeneration with erythrocyte antioxidant enzymes activity & serum total antioxidant status.* Oxid Med Cell Logev 2015:804054, 2015

Prashar S, Pandav SS, Gupta A, Nath R. *Antioxidant enzymes in RBC's as a biological index of age-related macula degeneration.* Acta. Ophthalmol. (Copnh) 71: 214-218, 1993

Quin L et al. *Patients with early age-related macular degeneration exhibit signs of macro- & micro-vascular disease & abnormal blood glutathione levels.* Graefes Arch Clin Exp Ophthalmol 252(1):23-30, 2014

Rao GN, Sadasivudu B, Cotlier E. *Studies on glutathione S-transferases, glutathione peroxidase & glutathione reductase in human normal & cataractous lenses.* Ophthalmic Res. 15: 173-179, 1983

Saadat I, Ahmadi Z, Farvardin-Jahromi M, Saadat M. *Association between cataract & genetic polymorphisms of GSTM1, GSTT1, & GSTO2 with respect of work place.* Mol Vis 18:1996-2000, 2012

Samiec PS et al. *Glutathione in human plasma: decline in association with aging, age-related macular degeneration, & diabetes.* Free Radic Biol Med 24(5):699-704, 1998

Schimel AM, Abraham L, Cox D et al. *N-acetylcysteine amide (NACA) prevents retinal degeneration by upregulating reduced glutathione production & reversing lipid peroxidation.* Am J Pathol 178(5):2032-43, 2011

Sireesha R, Laxmi SG, Mamata M et al. *Total activity of glutathione-S-transferase (GST) & polymorphisms of GSTM1 & GSTT1 genes conferring risk for the development of age-related cataracts.* Exp Eye Res 98:67-74, 2012

Simonelli F, Nesti A, Pensa M, et al. *Lipid peroxidation & human cataractogenesis in diabetics & severe myopia.* Exp. Eye Res. 49: 181-187, 1989

Stamenkovic M, Radic T, Stefanovic I et al. *Glutathione S-transferase omega-2 polymorphism Asn142Asp modifies the risk of age-related cataract in smokers & subjects exposed to ultraviolet irradiation.* Clin Exp Ophthalmol 42(3):277-83, 2014

Sun W, Su L, Sheng Y et al. *Is there association between Glutathione S Transferases polymorphisms & cataract risk: a meta-analysis?* BMC-Opthalmol 15:84, 2016

Tsai YY, Cheng YW, Lee H et al. *Oxidative DNA damage in pterygium.* Mol Vis 11:71-5, 2005

Tsai YY, Lee H, Tseng SH et al. *Null type of glutathione S-transferase M1 polymorphism is associated with early onset pterygium.* Mol Vis 10:458-61, 2004

Tingey DP, Schroeder A, Epstein MP, Epstein DL. *Effects of topical ethacrynic acid adducts on intraoccular pressure in rabbits & monkeys.* Arch. Ophthalmol. 110: 699-702, 1992

Tuzcu EA, Tuzcu K, Basarslan F et al. *Protective effects of N-acetylcysteine on triamcinolone acetonide-induced lens damage in rats.* Cutan Ocul Toxicol 33(4):294-8, 2014

Wei Z, Caty J, Whitson J et al. *Reduced Glutathione Level Promotes Epithelial-Mesenchymal Transition in Lens Epithelial Cells via a Wnt/β-Catenin-Mediated Pathway: Relevance for Cataract Theraphy.* Am J Pathol 187(11):2399-2412, 2017

Weil M, Xing KY, Fan YC et al. *Loss of thiol repair systems in human cataractous lenses.* Invest Ophthalmol Vis Sci 56(1):598-605, 2014

Yu, Weng Y, Guo J et al. *Association of glutathione S transferases polymorphisms with glaucoma: a meta-analysis.* PLoS One 8(1):e54037, 2013

Zafrilla P, Losada M, Perez A et al. *Biomarkers of oxidative stress in patients with wet age-related macular degeneration.* J Nutr Health Aging 17(3):219-22, 2013

Zhang S, Chai FY, Yan H et al. *Effects of N-acetylcysteine & glutathione ethyl ester drops on streptozotocin-induced diabetic cataract in rats.* Mol Vis 14:862-70, 2008

Zhao C, Shichi H. *Prevention of acetaminophen-induced cataract by a combination of diallyl disulfide & N-acetylcysteine.* J Ocul Pharmacol Ther 14(4):345-55, 1998

18
Pregnancy, Lactation & Childbirth

PREGNANCY IS FRAUGHT with hazards and potential complications. Women undergo drastic physiological changes—more so than at any other time except during their own birth. Mother and child are at the mercy of their genetic makeup, which may be the main cause of some of these challenges. However, they are also susceptible to the environment—mainly the air, food and liquids they consume. It is especially important to avoid or limit exposure to toxins and teratogens (substances causing birth defects). Good general health and nutrition are important for both mother and child. Vitamins and antioxidants naturally have an important role to play. Glutathione wears several hats in this scenario, some of them crucial.

The list of pregnancy-related illnesses is very long and we cannot describe them all in this chapter. We will cover those in which the role of GSH has particular relevance. Since the newborn's GSH levels greatly depend on the mother's glutathione status, we will also discuss the brief but eventful stages of childbirth and the neonatal period (from birth to six weeks).

Pre-eclampsia, eclampsia & hypertension of pregnancy

It's not unusual for pregnant women to experience hypertension (high blood pressure). This is caused by hormonal shifts and changes in blood volume and circulation. Some women are always hypertensive, while some experience this problem only during pregnancy. About one in twenty has a more serious condition called pre-eclampsia.

Symptoms of pre-eclampsia are hypertension, proteinurea (protein in the urine) and edema—accumulation of water in the tissues leading to swelling, particularly of the hands, feet and face. It usually occurs between the 20th week of gestation and the week following birth. Its exact cause is unknown but most obstetricians (pregnancy and delivery doctors) consider it a vascular disease. It most often shows up in first-time pregnancies and in women who already have high blood pressure. It is also more common at each end of the age spectrum—in women who become pregnant at a particularly young

Eclampsia	Oligohydraminos
Pre-eclampsia	Abruptio Placentae
Gestational Hypertension	Congenital Abnormalities
Gestational Diabetes	Spontaneous Abortion/miscarriage
Premature Delivery	Premature Rupture of Membranes

TABLE 30: Complications of pregnancy resulting from increased oxidative stress, free radical damage and low glutathione

or particularly old age.

If left unchecked, one in 200 cases of pre-eclampsia turns into full-blown eclampsia—a very serious condition producing convulsive seizures and coma. If not addressed promptly, eclampsia is usually fatal, so it must be treated aggressively. Another major complication of pre-eclampsia is the threefold HELLP syndrome: Hemolysis (red blood cell breakdown), Elevated Liver enzymes (indicator of liver damage), and Low Platelet count (impaired blood clotting).

The treatment for mild cases of pre-eclampsia includes bed rest, increased fluid intake and nutritional support. Attempts to stimulate urination and stabilize fluid levels with diuretics and salt restriction have little effect. Blood pressure and neurological symptoms are best controlled with intravenous magnesium sulfate and hydralazine. The definitive remedy for eclampsia patients is childbirth, which is often induced or by cesarean delivery.

Pre-eclampsia and GSH

The first study reporting abnormally low levels of glutathione in pre-eclampsia patients (according to most search engines) dates back to 1958—over 60 years ago! Since then, dozens of research teams have noticed that whenever pregnancy is complicated by pre-eclampsia, there is a precipitous fall in the patient's antioxidant function. Moreover, it has been discovered that the severity of the condition corresponds directly to the level of glutathione deficiency. Also noted was that the increased risk of pre-eclampsia with age is probably a reflection of the normal drop in glutathione status that accompanies aging. Many researchers have suggested that the measure of glutathione could be a marker for risk assessment, providing the time needed to properly correct glutathione and antioxidant function.

The falling costs and increased accuracy of genetic testing have greatly improved our ability to predict future risks for patients, and to protect them. One area of great interest is genetic testing for glutathione enzyme abnormalities. There is much evidence that women with a variety of glutathione enzyme defects are significantly more likely to develop eclampsia and pre-eclampsia. Given the benefit of predictive testing, doctors can monitor these issues and address them earlier, hopefully pre-empting their complications.

GSH deficiency has been linked to the oxidation of circulating fats (lipid peroxidation) which damages the sensitive endothelium (lining of the blood vessels—see Chapter 7). Subsequent constriction of muscles in the artery wall leads to narrowed passageways, decreasing blood flow. Combined with the demands of gestation, this triggers a cascade of events leading to full-blown eclampsia.

Chen and his team at the University of Glasgow believe this depletion might account for some of the important symptoms of pregnancy-induced hypertension—excess calcium in cells, reduced elasticity of red blood cells and damaged blood vessels. Branch's team at the University of Utah believe that the lipid peroxidation that follows may be part of the disease process that begins when foam cells[1] form in the decidua[2] of pre-eclamptic placentas.

The HELLP[3] syndrome is a serious complication of pre-eclampsia. Patients suffer liver damage, breakdown of red blood cells and loss of blood-clotting cells. GSH loss is particularly pronounced. Researchers have established a threefold correlation—severity of the pre-eclampsia, cell fragility and the level of GSH oxidation.

---

[1] Fat-laden immune cells that form in the early stages of atherosclerosis.

[2] The mucosal lining of the uterus when modified in preparation for pregnancy.

[3] Hemolysis (red blood cell breakdown), Elevated Liver enzymes (indicator of liver damage), and Low Platelet count (impaired blood clotting).

Teams around the world have applied antioxidants to pre-eclampsia with mixed results relating to the size and makeup of these trials. N-acetylcyteine has also shown some promise but no definitive large studies have yet confirmed its usefulness. Trials with the GSH peroxidase booster selenium showed more promise, and double-blind, randomized controlled studies are underway looking at a variety of glutathione-enhancing strategies.

For example, Lees' obstetrical team in London attempted to control symptoms in a group of pre-eclampsia patients. Women with severe cases that had stopped responding to traditional therapy were given S-nitroso-glutathione. Arterial pressure, platelet activation, and uterine artery resistance all improved, with no adverse affects on the fetus. In other words, it safely slowed or reversed the symptoms of the disorder.

Gestational diabetes & diabetes in pregnancy

Some women become pregnant following a long history of diabetes, while others suffer the disease's high blood-sugar levels only when pregnant. This is called 'gestational diabetes' and occurs in one to three percent of pregnancies. A number of gestational diabetics will go on to develop true diabetes later in life.

The main cause of death among newborn children of diabetic pregnancies is abnormal development of the child in the uterus (congenital malformation). Causes can be traced to inadequate control of the mother's diabetes during pregnancy. Diabetic mothers run the risk of larger babies and tougher deliveries. As a result, if birth hasn't occurred by week forty-two it's usually induced. Aside from developmental defects, these babies are also at higher risk of jaundice, respiratory difficulties, blood sugar abnormalities, low blood calcium and other metabolic abnormalities.

Many articles have studied glutathione levels in diabetic pregnancies, confirming that diabetics who become pregnant, expectant mothers who develop diabetes, and prediabetic women who become pregnant are all prone to increased oxidative stress, free radical damage and low glutathione levels. In other words, glutathione depletion is apparent in all stages of pregnancy.

GSH and diabetes in pregnancy

All diabetic patients are subject to higher levels of free radical production and lipid peroxidation (see Chapter 8). In the wombs of diabetic mothers, embryos are more prone to malformations and developmental problems—a phenomenon called "embryotoxicity." The exact mechanism of embryotoxicity in diabetes is not yet entirely clear, but it is known that oxidative damage to cells plays an important role. Low GSH levels in these patients' embryos put the fetus at the mercy of free radicals.

Wender-Ozegwska definitively wrote in the journal Free Radical Research, "…oxidative stress is one of several important factors contributing to unfavorable outcome of human diabetic pregnancy." In Oxidative Medicine and Cell Longevity, Al-Shelby and Masour state that, "Alterations in antioxidant and prooxoidant components…may be regarded as an increased risk factor for pregnant women as well as the fetus." More specifically, Japanese researchers have reported in the journal Diabetes, "Our results indicate that GSH depletion and impaired responsiveness of GSH-synthesizing enzyme to oxidative stress during organogenesis may have important roles in the development of embryonic malformations in diabetes."

A link between low glutathione levels in the pregnant mother and low glutathione levels in the developing child has also been established. In the journal Placenta, Biri and his team described the low GSH levels found in both the umbilical cord blood and the placentas of gestational diabetics.

An indirect link between impaired glutathione status and gestational diabetes can be established with newer genetic testing for abnormal glutathione genes. Testing of various genetic GSH abnormalities has shown a direct correlation with the incidence of diabetic pregnancies.

Clinicians are naturally interested in these theoretical findings, but they are even more interested in ways to better manage gestational diabetes. A number of journals—including Nutrition, the Journal of Maternal and Fetal Neonatal Medicine, Diabetes, Clinical Biochemistry and others—have published suggestions that oxidative stress and glutathione levels must be monitored, and that antioxidant therapy should be provided to pregnant mothers with diabetes.

A Japanese study confirmed that restoring GSH status in embryo cultures normalized any retardation or malformation of embryos in untreated mothers. A Swedish group shared similar, positive results after treating embryo cultures with NAC (N-acetylcysteine), a potent GSH-enhancing precursor.

Toxins and teratogens in pregnancy

Teratogens are substances that disturb the development of an embryo or fetus, often leading to birth defects. Those of us over 50 years of age will recall the disastrous consequences of giving the drug Thalidomide to pregnant women. Thalidomide was very effective for nausea—especially the morning sickness associated with pregnancy—and so was initially popular. But tragedy stepped in as a whole new population of physically deformed babies was born. It turned out that Thalidomide was a potent teratogen, leaving many children with misshapen arms and legs. I mention this story here because it was discovered in retrospect that what resistance the body does mount against Thalidomide-induced birth defects is through glutathione detoxification. It may well be that the individuals who suffered the worst of these unexpected deformities were born to mothers with relative glutathione deficiency.

We're all exposed to toxins from our environment. They come in the food we eat, the water we drink, the air we breathe, the medications we take and the jobs we hold, along with bad habits like drinking and smoking. In pregnancy, the embryo is exposed to the same toxins as the mother, but the fundamental complexity of fetal growth and development makes it much more susceptible to defects.

Consequences range from low birth weight to malformations or even death of the fetus. Some consequences may not appear for years; for example, diminished IQ scores in later childhood. The mother is the only one in a position to minimize these risks. Above all, she must ensure that her built-in detoxification processes are well supplied and in working order.

Oxidative stress is a well-known mechanism of teratogenesis.[4] Many toxins that cause birth abnormalities act by increasing free radical damage. It goes without saying that the protective effects of glutathione are very much in play here. Any factor that lowers glutathione levels may potentially increase the likelihood of defects.

In the journal Toxicological Science, Wells and his team write, "A better understanding of the developmental effects of ROS (reactive oxygen species) may provide insights for risk assessment and the reduction of adverse postnatal consequences." In Reproductive Toxicology, Hansen and Harris state that studying oxidative stress during pregnancy is, "important to identify potential teratogens and develop therapeutic interventions for attenuation of harmful chemical effects in utero following exposure." In other words,

4 Development of birth defects.

the way to reduce congenital defects in our population is first to recognize the toxins that increase free radicals, and then either avoid them or counter them with antioxidants.

GSH and toxicology in pregnancy

According to recent research, the fetus itself is low in antioxidant defenses. It presumably depends on the mother's good health for protection, so anything that depresses the mother's antioxidant levels also compromises fetal development. The fetus grows from the embryo, and GSH levels are very high in the embryo's conceptual tissue. Conceptual tissue is the undefined mass of cells that differentiates and grows into the organs and systems of a human fetus. The process of organ development (organogenesis) is extremely sensitive, but at this stage is especially well protected by higher glutathione levels. Researchers in toxicology are studying the possibility that elevated GSH levels may protect unborn children from foreign substances (xenobiotics). If this proves so, measuring glutathione in early pregnancy may also be a way to identify possible risks of toxicity.

A recent article in the Journal of Internal Medicine Research studied glutathione levels in the amniotic fluid of pregnant mothers. Ultrasound imaging identified fetuses with congenital neurological defects, who were compared to those with normal ultrasound results. Glutathione in the amniotic fluid of those with defects was significantly lower than those without.

Some pediatric researchers have tried to match low levels of antioxidant defense systems to the frequency and severity of birth defects. Graf and his associates at the University of Washington successfully correlated the frequency of neural tube defects with low GSH enzyme levels. Following the Chernobyl nuclear disaster, a very significant study was conducted in the Ukraine. Scientists collected the placentas of women affected to a greater or lesser extent by radioactive pollution. As expected, the placentas from those living in most polluted areas had the lowest GSH levels. They were simply depleted by the overwhelming demands of ongoing radiation. This study showed that placentas with low GSH levels experienced more difficult pregnancies, harder deliveries and poorer postnatal health. They concluded that "glutathione status [is] a prerequisite of the detoxifying activity of the feto-placental barrier." In other words, without placental GSH the fetus is largely unprotected from toxins and other xenobiotics.

The two most common toxins found in pregnancy are alcohol and tobacco. Although most pregnant women can and do choose to avoid them, abuse of these drugs is not uncommon. The mother may have a habitual dependence on these drugs or may simply be exposed to second-hand smoke. In either case, glutathione plays an important role in protecting mother and child against such toxic threats.

Alcohol and tobacco

Most drug-induced malformations of the fetus result from alcohol abuse during pregnancy. Fetal alcohol syndrome is a clinical condition leading to a long list of possible abnormalities, the most serious being severe mental retardation. In tests on laboratory mammals, alcohol drained GSH from the liver much more quickly in the fetus than in the mother. Other studies combined alcohol with cocaine, which further precipitated the fall of GSH levels. At the University of New Mexico, researchers gave test animals GSH-depleting drugs, increasing the severity of fetal alcohol syndrome. On a more positive note, Henderson and his team at the University of Texas used antioxidants on test animals, showing that much of the damage of fetal alcohol exposure could be avoided by maintaining adequate glutathione levels.

Women who smoke during pregnancy risk many complications, including early labor, rupture of membranes and premature delivery. Researchers demonstrated that cigarette smoke interferes with signals between certain white blood cells and blood platelets, thus interfering with normal blood clotting. The same researchers successfully put an end to this interference by raising glutathione levels.

Polish researchers led by Chelchowska and her team have looked extensively into glutathione levels in pregnant women who smoked. They found low GSH in the mothers-to-be, and also in the umbilical cords of their infants. These children were "glutathione starved" during pregnancy.

A dramatic finding in children born to women who smoked while pregnant is decreased cognitive functioning. The children did more poorly than expected in school and on the psychosocial scale. In the International Journal of Epidemiology, Morales and his team wrote that the children of mothers with genetic glutathione abnormalities were prone to cognitive issues later in life. They continued, "GSTM1[5] deficiency increases the adverse effects of active maternal smoking during pregnancy on cognition in preschoolers, suggesting a biological interaction between child metabolic genes and tobacco smoke components in [the] detoxification process during foetal neurodevelopment." In other words, the child's genes are caught up in the war waged by the body on the tobacco products in it. The increased sophistication of genetic testing has revealed that tobacco abuse during pregnancy can actually exert epigenetic pressure on the unborn child, triggering new genetic abnormalities.

More detailed discussions on smoking can be found in chapter 12 (lung) and chapter 2.

Other toxins

Many other studies have shown that antioxidant defenses—notably the glutathione system—play an indispensable role in detoxifying the newborn child. They remove numerous xenobiotics, including heavy metals such as mercury, lead, cadmium and arsenic, as well as drugs such as hydantoin, phenytoin, and various poisons. In the lab, GSH enhancing drugs like NAC actually diminish the toxic effects of mercury that can lead to congenital abnormalities and death. NAC is in fact recommended as an emergency measure for pregnant women who have overdosed on acetaminophen.

GSH, childbirth, and the perinatal period

One of the major complications around childbirth (the perinatal period) is insufficient oxygen supply to the baby (hypoxia). Before the separation, the baby draws its oxygen from umbilical supplies, but this can be compromised during delivery. Also, a variety of different factors might lead the baby into respiratory difficulties. In either case, the consequences of insufficient oxygen are serious. Every effort is made to avoid it.

When the baby is oxygen deprived individual cells are also deprived and unable to maintain energy levels. This leads to hypoxic damage. GSH can be considered anti-hypoxic because it stimulates the production of ATP (adenosine triphosphate), which carries energy from the power generators (mitochondria) of individual cells. Another complication of the hypoxic child is lipid peroxidation, which is also addressed by GSH. And there is every reason to believe it would also help infants suffering from diminished liver function and jaundice.

A less dramatic situation is the condition

[5] A GSH gene

described as "Small for Gestational Age," when babies are born at the very low end of the weight scale. This is not strictly speaking a "disease," but it is associated with complications to the placenta and mother's health, as well as the child's. Franco and others have shown that babies born small for gestational age generally suffer increased oxidative damage. Researchers led by Franco, Gupta, Delee and other teams have shown that they suffer from low GSH levels too.

Oxygen—source of life & oxidative stress

It is not uncommon for premature infants to need oxygen therapy. This raises energy production, but along with that comes additional oxidative stress. This may cause visual problems in premature infants. A condition called retrolental fibroplasia (or retinopathy of prematurity) causes tissues in the retina that have not yet matured to shut down the blood vessels supplying the eye, resulting in serious consequences including retinal detachment. Antioxidants may be an antidote to this side effect of oxygen therapy. Papp from Hungary suggests that it might be avoided by giving mothers sulfur-containing amino acids that sustain GSH levels.

Other problems resulting from high oxygen levels include developmental changes to the nervous system and oxidative lung injury. Newborn animals depleted[6] of glutathione experienced a dramatic increase in damage like this. Sastre and his group from Spain conducted laboratory tests to show that NAC administered to mothers lessened oxidative stress in newborns. Brown of Emory University in Atlanta successfully prevented oxygen-induced lung injury in mammals using GSH supplementation. It is believed that elevated GSH levels in the mother counteract the negative effects of many perinatal complications.

GSH and lactation

Lactation and breast-feeding are usually discussed alongside pregnancy and childbirth. In this context, glutathione is particularly interesting. You could say it plays the starring role.

It's impossible to overstate the benefits of mother's milk on the health and development of newborns—especially its long-term effects on the immune system. Compared with bottle-fed children, those who are breast-fed suffer from fewer infectious diseases (especially ear infections and pneumonia), fewer problems with allergies, and fewer cases of childhood cancer, including leukemia, lymphoma, bone tumors and brain tumors.

Compared to the milk of other mammals, human milk has the lowest proportion of all proteins. The make-up is also very different. The two main proteins in milk are whey and casein, and in human milk the ratio of whey to casein is much higher. These whey proteins contain the critical precursors of glutathione—including beta-lactoglobulin, alpha-lactalbumin, serum albumin, and lactoferrin. They're high in sulfur-containing amino acids such as cysteine and cystine. Their structure too is important. Cysteine and cystine, integrated into these larger proteins, can survive the rigors of digestion and arrive intact in the infants' cells, where they form glutathione. Breast-feeding therefore profoundly affects the baby's immune function by providing high levels of glutathione precursors.

These proteins are available in cow's milk too, but the way milk is normally pasteurized and handled degrades them into a form that is biologically inactive. This doesn't affect the milk's food value, but does prevent the GSH precursors from reaching individual cells and

6 With BSO (a GSH inhibitor).

stimulating GSH production. New technologies have been developed to extract these proteins from mammalian milk without denaturing them. You might call it mother's milk protein for adults—a natural way to raise glutathione levels.

Conclusion

Glutathione's role in embryonic, fetal and placental development is critical. It is constantly working to scavenge free radicals and detoxify dozens of foreign substances and toxins. Without GSH, these harmful substances accumulate, pushing the child towards an unnerving variety of developmental and health problems. Once past the stage of organogenesis,[7] the unborn child's principal GSH protection comes from its environment—the placenta. There is an interesting similarity between the placenta and the liver. Among their many other functions, both carry high levels of glutathione. It is no coincidence. It must be stressed that the healthy functioning of placenta directly correlates with the child's birth and health, both of which can be compromised by glutathione abnormalities.

Many common complications of pregnancy—including high blood pressure, pre-eclampsia and gestational diabetes—coincide with low glutathione levels. Decreased GSH can cause many difficulties in pregnancy. A great deal of research is being carried out with GSH-enhancing strategies to combat these problems. There is some success and great optimism.

Congenital nervous system anomalies associated with glutathione abnormalities include anencephaly, acrania, neural tube defects, encephalocele, and iniencephaly.

[7] the phase of embryonic development when primitive cells differentiate into various tissues and organs

PREGNANCY, LACTATION & CHILDBIRTH

REFERENCES

Addolorato G, Gasparinin A, Marcoccia S, et al. *Prenatal exposure to ethanol in rats: effects on liver energy level & antioxidant status in mothers, fetuses, & newborns.* Alcohol 14: 569-573, 1997

Afifi NM, Abdel-Rahman MS, Nassar AM. *Effect of alcohol &/or cocaine on blood glutathione & the ultrastructure of the liver of pregnant CF-1 mice.* Toxicol. Lett. 98: 1-12, 1998

Al-Shebly MM, Mansour MA. *Evaluation of oxidative stress & antioxidant status in diabetic & hypertensive women during labor.* Oxid Med Cell Longev. doi: 10.1155/2012/329743, 2012

Anvar Z, Saadat I, Namavar-Jahromi B, et al. *Genetic polymorphisms of glutathione S-transferase M1 (GSTM1) & T1 (GSTT1) & susceptibility to pre-eclampsia: a case-control study & a meta-analysis.* EXCLI J. 10: 44-51, 2011

Arribas L, Almansa I, Miranda M, et al. *Serum Malondialdehyde Concentration & Glutathione Peroxidase Activity in a Longitudinal Study of Gestational Diabetes.* PLoS One 11:e0155353, 2016

Asemi Z, Jamilian M, Mesdaghinia E, et al. *Effects of selenium supplementation on glucose homeostasis, inflammation, & oxidative stress in gestational diabetes: a randomized, double-blind, placebo-controlled trial.* Nutrition. 31: 1235-1242, 2015

Aydin A, Sayal A, Isimir A. *Plasma glutathione peroxidase activity & selenium levels of newborns with jaundice.* Biol. Trace Elem. Res. 58: 85-90, 1997

Aydogan U, Durmaz E, Ercan CM, et al. *Effects of smoking during pregnancy on DNA damage & ROS level consequences in maternal & newborns' blood.* Arh Hig Rada Toksikol. 64: 35-46, 2013

Bannon M, Halliday HL, McMaster D. *Glutathione peroxidase activity in cord blood: effects of fetal sex & maternal smoking.* Biol Neonate. 50: 274-277, 1986

Biri A, Onan A, Devrim E, et al. *Oxidant status in maternal & cord plasma & placental tissue in gestational diabetes.* Placenta 27: 327-332, 2006

Bisseling TM, Maria Roes E, Raijmakers MT, et al. *N-acetylcysteine restores nitric oxide-mediated effects in the fetoplacental circulation of preeclamptic patients.* Am J Obstet Gynecol. 191: 328-333, 2004

Bizon A, Milnerowicz-Nabzdyk E, et al. *Changes in pro/antioxidant balance in smoking*

& non-smoking pregnant women with intrauterine growth restriction. Reprod Toxicol. 32: 360-367, 2011

BOHLES H. *Antioxidative vitamins in prematurely & maturely born infants. Int. J. Vitamin Nutr.* Res. 67: 321-328. 1997

BOUNOUS G, KONGSHAVN PAL, TAVEROFF A, GOLD P. *Evolutionary traits in human milk proteins.* Medical Hypothesis 27: 133-140, 1988

BOUTET M, ROLAND L, THOMAS N, ET AL. *Specific systemic antioxidant response to preeclampsia in late pregnancy: the study of intracellular glutathione peroxidases in maternal & fetal blood.* Am J Obstet Gynecol. 200: 530.e1-7, 2009

BRANCH DW, MITCHELL MD, MILLER E, ET AL. *Pre-eclampsia & serum antibodies to oxidized low-density lipoprotein.* Lancet 343; 645-646, 1994

BROWN LA, PEREZ JA, HARRIS FL, CLARK RH. *Glutathione supplements protect pre-term rabbits from oxidative lung injury.* American J. Physiol. 270(3 Pt 1): L446-L451, 1996

CHANDRA RK. *Prospective studies of the effect of breast-feeding on incidence of infection & allergy.* Acta. Paed. Scand. 68:691, 1987

CHAMY VM, LEPE J, CATALAN A, ET AL. *Oxidative stress is closely related to clinical severity of pre-eclampsia.* Biol Res. 39: 229-236, 2006

CHELCHOWSKA M, LASKOWSKA-KLITA T, LEIBSCHANG J. *[Activities of superoxide dismutase, catalase, glutathione peroxidase & reductase in umbilical cord blood of newborns from mothers smoking during pregnancy].* Przegl Lek 63: 970-973, 2006

CHELCHOWSKA M, LASKOWSKA-KLITA T, NIEMIEC KT. *[Activites of superoxide dismutase, glutathione peroxidase & catalase in erythrocytes of women smoking during pregnancy].* Przegl Lek 62: 1039-1042, 2005

CHEN G, WILSON R, CUMMING G, ET AL. *Intracellular & extracellular antioxidant buffering levels in erythrocytes from pregnancy-induced hypertension.* J. Human Hypertension 8: 37-42, 1994

CIM N, TOLUNAY HE, KARAMAN E, ET AL. *Amniotic fluid oxidant-antioxidant status in foetal congenital nervous system anomalies.* J Int Med Res. 46:1146-1152, 2018

CORAL-VAZQUEZ RM, ROMERO ARAUZ JF, CANIZALES-QUINTEROS S, ET AL. *Analysis of polymorphisms & haplotypes in genes associated with vascular tone, hypertension & oxidative stress in Mexican-Mestizo women with severe preeclampsia.* Clin Biochem. 46: 627-632, 2013

COUGHLAN MT, VERVAART PP, PERMEZEL M, ET AL. *Altered placental oxidative stress status in gestational diabetes mellitus.* Placenta 25: 78-84, 2004

DATTA K, ROY SK, MITRA AK, ET AL. *Glutathione S-transferase mediated detoxification & bioactivation of xenobiotics during early human pregnancy.* Early Human Development 37: 167-174, 1994

DAVIDGE ST, HUBEL CA, BRAYDEN RD, ET AL. *Sera antioxidant activity in uncomplicated & preeclamptic pregnancies.* Obstetrics & Gynecology 79: 897-901, 1992

DELLEE U, TOBIAS S, LI H, ET AL. *Expression of NO synthases & redox enzymes in umbilical arteries from newborns born small, appropriate, & large for gestational age.* Pediatr Res. 73: 146-146, 2013

DEWANTININGRUM J, HAFIZ A. *The role of glutathione peroxidase maternal serum level in late onset of severe preeclampsia.* Hypertens Pregnancy. 35: 483-489, 2016

DJORDJEVIC A, SPASIC S, JOVANOVIC-GALOVIC A, ET AL. *Oxidative stress in diabetic pregnancy: SOD, CAT & GSH-Px activity & lipid peroxidation products.* J Matern Fetal Neonatal Med. 16: 367-372, 2004

D'SOUZA V, RANI A, PATIL V, ET AL. *Increased oxidative stress from early pregnancy in women who develop preeclampsia.* Clin Exp Hypertens. 38: 225-232, 2016

DUNCAN B, EY J, HOLBERG CJ, ET AL. *Exclusive breast-feeding for at least 4 months protects against otitis media.* Paediatrics 91: 867-872, 1993

ERMIS B, ORS R, YILDIRIM A, ET AL. *Influence of smoking on maternal & neonatal serum malondialdehyde, superoxide dismutase, & glutathione peroxidase levels.* Ann Clin Lab Sci. 34: 405-409, 2004

EVERETT TR, WILKINSON IB, LEES CC. *Pre-eclampsia: the Potential of GSNO Reductase Inhibitors.* Curr Hypertens Rep. 19: 20. doi:10.1007/s11906-017-0717-2

EVERETT TR, WILKINSON IB, MAHENDRU AA, ET AL. *S-Nitrosoglutathione improves haemodynamics in early-onset preeclampsia.* Br J Clin Pharmacol. 78 :660-669, 2014

FRANCO MC, KAWAMOTO EM, GORJAO R, ET AL. *Biomarkers of oxidative stress & antioxidant status in children born small for gestational age: evidence of lipid peroxidation.* Pediatr Res. 62: 204-208 2007

FRANK AL, TABER LN, GLEZEN WP, ET AL. *Breast-feeding & respiratory virus infection.* Paediatrics 70: 239-245, 1982

GAO H, LIU C, LIN P, ET AL. *Effects of GSTP1 & GPX1 Polymorphisms on the Risk of Preeclampsia in Chinese Han Women.* Cell Physiol Biochem. 39: 2025-2032, 2016

GOHIL JT, PATEL PK, GUPTA P. *Evaluation of oxidative stress & antioxidant defence in subjects of preeclampsia.* J Obstet Gynaecol India. 61: 638-640, 2011

GRAF WD, OLEINUK OE, PIPPENGER CE, ET AL. *Comparison of erythrocyte antioxidant activi-*

ties & embryologic level of neural tube defects. Eur. J. Pediatr. Surg. 5(Suppl 1): 8-11, 1995

Gupta P, Narang M, Banerjee BD, et al. *Oxidative stress in term small for gestational age neonates born to undernourished mothers: a case control study.* BMC Pediatr. 20;4:14, 2004

Gupta A, Gupta A, Shukla GS. *Development of brain free radical scavenging system & lipid peroxidation under the influence of gestational & lactational cadmium exposure.* Human Exp. Toxicol. 14: 428-433, 1995

Hansen JM. *Oxidative stress as a mechanism of teratogenesis.* Birth Defects Res C Embryo Today. 78: 293-307, 2006

Hansen JM, Harris C. *Redox control of teratogenesis.* Reprod Toxicol. 35: 165-179, 2013

Haque SK, Siddiqui MU, Islam N, et al. *Erythrocyte markers of oxidative stress in higher age-group preeclamptic & normal pregnant mothers.* Hypertens Pregnancy 29: 69-81, 2010

Henderson GI, Devi BG, Perez A, Schenker S. *In utero ethanol exposure elicits oxidative stress in the rat fetus.* Alcohol Clin. Exp. Res. 19: 714-720, 1995

Infante-Rivard C, Weinberg CR, Guiguet M. *Xenobiotic-metabolizing genes & small-for-gestational-age births: interaction with maternal smoking.* Epidemiology 17: 38-46. 2006

Kamrin MA, Carney EW, Chou K, Cummings A, et al. *Female reproductive & developmental toxicology: overview & current approaches.* Toxicol. Lett. 74: 99-119, 1994

Kharb S. *Low whole blood glutathione levels in pregnancies complicated by preeclampsia & diabetes.* Clin Chim Acta. 294:179-183, 2000

Knapen MF, Mulder TP, Van Rooij IA, et al. *Low whole blood glutathione levels in pregnancies complicated by preeclampsia or the hemolysis, elevated liver enzymes, low platelets syndrome.* Obstetrics & Gynecology 92: 1012-1015, 1998

Knobloch J, Reimann K, Klotz LO, et al. *Thalidomide resistance is based on the capacity of the glutathione-dependent antioxidant defense.* Mol Pharm 5: 1138-1144, 2008

Korneev AA, Komissarova IA, Nartissov IR. *The use of glutathione as a protector agent in hypoxic exposure. Biull. Eksp. Biol.* Med. 116: 261-263, 1993

Langley SC, Kelly FJ. *N-acetylcysteine ameliorates hyperoxic lung injury in the preterm guinea pig.* Biochem. Pharmacol. 45: 841-846, 1993

Lees C, Langford E, Brown AS, et al. *The effects of S-nitrosoglutathione on platelet activation, hypertension, & uterine & fetal doppler in severe preeclampsia.* Obstetrics & Gynecology 88: 14-19, 1996

Li Y, Li S, Zhai Q, Hai J, et al. *Association of GSTs polymorphisms with risk of gestational diabetes mellitus.* Int J Clin Exp Pathol. 8: 15191-15197, 2015

Li H, Yin Q, Li N, et al. *Plasma Markers of Oxidative Stress in Patients with Gestational Diabetes Mellitus in the Second & Third Trimester.* Obstet Gynecol Int. 3865454, 2016

Liu CS, Wu HM, Kao SH, Wei YH. *Phenytoin-mediated oxidative stress in serum of female epileptics: a possible pathogenesis in the fetal hydantoin syndrome.* Human Exp. Toxicol. 16: 177-181, 1997

Lopez-Tinoco C, Roca M, García-Valero A, et al. *Oxidative stress & antioxidant status in patients with late-onset gestational diabetes mellitus.* Acta Diabetol. 50: 201-208, 2013

Maged AM, Torky H, Fouad MA, et al. *Role of antioxidants in gestational diabetes mellitus & relation to fetal outcome: a randomized controlled trial.* J Matern Fetal Neonatal Med. 29: 4049-4054, 2016

Mather G, Gupta N, Mather S, et al. *Breastfeeding & childhood cancer.* Ind. Paediatrics 30: 652-657, 1993

Menegola E, Broccia ML, Prati M, et al. *Glutathione status in diabetes-induced embryopathies.* Biol. Neonate 69: 293-297, 1996

Mihailovic M, Cvetkovic M, Ljubic A, et al. *Selenium & malondialdehyde content & glutathione peroxidase activity in maternal & umbilical cord blood & amniotic fluid.* Biol Trace Elem Res. 73: 47-54, 2000

Miranda Guisado ML, Vallejo-Vaz AJ, Garcia Junco PS, et al. *Abnormal levels of antioxidant defenses in a large sample of patients with hypertensive disorders of pregnancy.* Hypertens Res. 35: 274-278, 2012

Mistry HD, Wilson V, Ramsay MM, et al. *Reduced selenium concentrations & glutathione peroxidase activity in preeclamptic pregnancies.* Hypertension. 52: 881-888, 2008

Morales E, Sunyer J, Julvez J, et al. *GSTM1 polymorphisms modify the effect of maternal smoking during pregnancy on cognitive functioning in preschoolers.* Int J Epidemiol. 38:690-697, 2009

Mukherji S, Banerjee S. *Blood glutathione & ascorbic acid in normal pregnancy & in pre-eclamptic toxaemia.* Indian J Psychol. 2: 501-504, 1958

Narahara H, Johnston JM. *Smoking & preterm labor: effect of cigarette smoke extract on the secretion of platelet activating factor-acetylhydrolase by human decidual macrophages.* American J. Obstet. Gynecol. 169: 1321-1326, 1993

Nemeth I, Orvos H, Boda D. *Blood glutathione redox status in gestational hypertension.* Free Radic Biol Med. 30:715-721, 2001

Obolenskaya MY, Tschaikovskaya TL, et al. *Glutathione status of placentae from differently polluted regions of Ukraine.* Eur. J. Obstet. Gynecol. Reprod. Biol. 71: 23-30, 1997

Obolenskaya MY, Chaikovska TL, et al. *Detoxicating function of the placenta of childbearing women from ecologically unfavorable regions of the Ukraine.* Ukr. Biokhim. Zh. 70: 89-97, 1998

Orhan H, Onderoglu L, Yücel A, et al. *Circulating biomarkers of oxidative stress in complicated pregnancies.* Arch Gynecol Obstet. 267:189-195, 2003

Ornaghi F, Ferrini S, Prati M, Giavini E. *The protective effects of n-acetylcysteine against methyl mercury embryotoxicity in mice.* Fundam. Appl. Toxicol. 20: 437-445, 1993

Papp A, Nemeth I, Pelle Z, Tekulic P. *Prospective biochemical study of the antioxidant defense capacity in retinopathy of prematurity.* Orv. Hetil. 138: 201-205, 1997

Patil SB, Kodliwadmath MV, Kodliwadmath SM. *Role of lipid peroxidation & enzymatic antioxidants in pregnancy-induced hypertension.* Clin Exp Obstet Gynecol. 34: 239-241, 2007

Perkins AV. *Placental oxidative stress, selenium & preeclampsia.* Pregnancy Hypertens. 1: 95-99, 2011

Peuchant E, Brun JL, Rigalleau V, et al. *Oxidative & antioxidative status in pregnant women with either gestational or type 1 diabetes.* Clin Biochem. 37: 293-298, 2004

Qui YH, Xu YL, Zhang WH. *Effect of GSTM1, GSTT1, & GSTP1 lle105Val polymorphisms on susceptibility to gestational diabetes mellitus.* Genet Mol Res. 15: doi: 10.4238/gmr. 15027711. 2016

Raijmakers MT, Roes EM, Zusterzeel PL, et al. *Thiol status & antioxidant capacity in women with a history of severe pre-eclampsia.* BJOG. 111: 207-212, 2004

Rajdl D, Racek J, Steinerova A, et al. *Markers of oxidative stress in diabetic mothers & their infants during delivery.* Physiol Res. 54: 429-436, 2005

Rani N, Dhingra R, Arya DS, et al. *Role of oxidative stress markers & antioxidants in the placenta of preeclamptic patients.* J Obstet Gynaecol Res. 36: 1189-1194, 2010

Rayman MP, Searle E, Kelly L, et al. *Effect of selenium on markers of risk of pre-eclampsia in UK pregnant women: a randomised, controlled pilot trial.* Br J Nutr. 112: 99-111, 2014

Reyes E, Ott S. *Effects of buthionine sulfoxamine on the outcome of the in utero administration of alcohol on fetal development.* Alcohol Clin. Exp. Res. 20: 1243-1251, 1996

Riggs BS, Bronstein AC, Kulig K, et al. *Acute acetaminophen overdose during pregnancy. Obstet.* Gynecol. 74: 247-253, 1989

Rumiris D, Purwosunu Y, Wibowo N, et al. *Lower rate of preeclampsia after antioxidant supplementation in pregnant women with low antioxidant status.* Hypertens Pregnancy. 25: 241-253, 2006

Sakamaki H, Akazawa S, Ishibashi M, et al. *Significance of glutathione-dependent antioxidant system in diabetes-induced embryonic malformations.* Diabetes. 48: 1138-1144, 1999

Sandoval-Carrillo A, Aguilar-Duran M, Vazquez-Alaniz F, et al. *Polymorphisms in the GSTT1 & GSTM1 genes are associated with increased risk of preeclampsia in the Mexican mestizo population.* Genet Mol Res 13: 2160-2165, 2014

Sastre J, Aseni M, Rodrigo F, et al. *Antioxidant administration to the mother prevents oxidative stress associated with birth in the neonatal rat.* Life Science 54: 2055-2059, 1994

Schmidt H, Gruner T, Muller R, et al. *Increased levels of lipid peroxidation products malondialdehyde & 4-hydroxynonenal after perinatal hypoxia.* Pediatr. Res. 40: 15-20, 1996

Shang M, Zhao J, Yang L, et al. *Oxidative stress & antioxidant status in women with gestational diabetes mellitus diagnosed by IADPSG criteria.* Diabetes Res Clin Pract. 109 : 404-410, 2015

Sharma JB, Sharma A, Bahadur A, et al. *Oxidative stress markers & antioxidant levels in normal pregnancy & pre-eclampsia.* Int J Gynaecol Obstet. 94: 23-27, 2006

Siddiqui IA, Jaleel A, Al'Kadri HM, et al. *Biomarkers of oxidative stress in women with pre-eclampsia.* Biomark Med. 7: 229-234, 2013

Simsek M, Naziroglu M, Simsek H, et al. *Blood plasma levels of lipoperoxides, glutathione peroxidase, beta carotene, vitamin A & E in women with habitual abortion.Cell. Biochem. Funct. 16: 227-231, 1998*

Spickett CM, Reglinski J, Smith WE, et al. *Erythrocyte glutathione balance & membrane stability during preeclampsia.* Free Radic. Biol. Med. 24: 1049-1055, 1998

Sudharshana Murthy KA, Bhandiwada A, Chandan SL, et al. *Evaluation of Oxidative Stress & Proinflammatory Cytokines in Gestational Diabetes Mellitus & Their Correlation with Pregnancy Outcome.* Indian J Endocrinol Metab. 22: 79-84, 2018

Tabacova S, Baird DD, Balabaeva L, et al. *Placental arsenic & cadmium in relation to lipid peroxides & glutathione levels in maternal-infant pairs from a copper smelter area.Placenta 15: 873-881, 1994*

Tabacova S, Balabaeva L, Little RE. *Maternal exposure to exogenous nitrogen compounds & complications of pregnancy.Arch. Environ.* Health 52: 341-347, 1997

Tabacova S, Little RE, Balabaeva L. *Complications of pregnancy in relation to maternal lipid peroxides, glutathione, & exposure to metals.* Reprod.

Toxicol. 8: 217-224, 1994

Taglialatela G, Perez-Polo JR, Rassin DK. *Induction of apoptosis in the CNS during development by the combination of hyperoxia & inhibition of glutathione synthesis.* Free Radic. Biol. Med. 25: 936-942, 1998

Tenório MB, Ferreira RC, Moura FA, et al. *Oral antioxidant therapy for prevention & treatment of preeclampsia: Meta-analysis of randomized controlled trials.* Nutr Metab Cardiovasc Dis. 28: 865-876, 2018

Tortiadze M, Kintraia N, Parkauli M, et al. *[Blood antioxidant enzyme activity during physiological & preeclampsia syndrome complicated pregnancy].* Georgian Med News. 215: 12-6, 2013

Trocino RA, Akazawa S, Ishibashi M, et al. *Significance of glutathione depletion & oxidative stress in early embryogenesis in glucose-induced rat embryo culture.* Diabetes 44: 992-998, 1995

Uotila JT, Tuimala RJ, Aarnio TM, et al. *Findings on lipid peroxidation & antioxidant function in hypertensive complications of pregnancy.* Br. J. Obstet. Gynaecol. 100: 270-276, 1993

Uotila JT, Tuimala RJ, Pyykko K. *Erythrocyte glutathione peroxidase activity in hypertensive complications of pregnancy.* Gynecol. Obstet. Invest. 29: 259-262, 1990

Viskova H, Vesela K, Janosikova B, et al. *Plasma cysteine concentrations in uncomplicated pregnancies.* Fetal Diagn Ther. 22: 254-258, 2007

Wagner PD, Mathieu-Costello O, Bebout DE, et al. *Protection against pulmonary O2 toxicity by n-acetylcysteine.* Eur. Respir. J. 2: 116-126, 1989

Walsh SW, Wang Y. *Deficient glutathione peroxidase activity in preeclampsia is associated with increased placental production of thromboxane & lipid peroxidases.American J. Obstet. Gynecol. 169: 1456-1461, 1993*

Warshaw JB, Wilson CW, Saito K, Prough RA. *The responses of glutathione & antioxidant enzymes to hyperoxia in the developing lung.* Pediatr. Res. 8: 819-823, 1985

Wdowiak A, Brzozowski I, Bojar I. *Superoxide dismutase & glutathione peroxidase activity in pregnancy complicated by diabetes.* Ann Agric Environ Med. 22: 297-300, 2015

Wells PG, McCallum GP, Chen CS, et al. *Oxidative stress in developmental origins of disease: teratogenesis, neurodevelopmental deficits, & cancer.* Toxicol Sci. 108: 4-18, 2009

Wender-Ozegowska E, Koźlik J, Biczysko R, et al. *Changes of oxidative stress parameters in diabetic pregnancy.* Free Radic Res. 38: 795-803, 2004

Wentzel P, Thunberg L, Eriksson UJ. *Teratogenic effect of diabetic serum is prevented by supplementation of superoxide dismutase & n-acetylcysteine in rat embryo culture.* Diabetologia 40: 7-14, 1997

Wibowo N, Purwosunu Y, Sekizawa A, et al. *Antioxidant supplementation in pregnant women with low antioxidant status.* J Obstet Gynaecol Res. 38: 1152-1161, 2012

Woods JR Jr, Plessinger MA, Fantel A. *An introduction to reactive oxygen species & their possible roles in substance abuse.* Obstet. Gynecol. Clin. North America 25:219-236, 1998

Yamazaki H, Suemizu H, Shimizu M, et al. *In vivo formation of dehydroxylated & glutathione conjugate metabolites derived from thalidomide & 5-Hydroxythalidomide in humanized TK-NOG mice.* Chem Res Toxicol 25: 274-276, 2012

Zhang Y, Gu Y, Lewis DF, et al. *Reduced cellular glutathione reductase activity & increased adhesion molecule expression in endothelial cells cultured with maternal plasma from women with preeclampsia.* J Soc Gynecol Investig. 13: 412-417, 2006

Zhao W, Mosley BS, Cleves MA, et al. *Neural tube defects & maternal biomarkers of folate, homocysteine, & glutathione metabolism.* Birth Defects Res A Clin Mol Teratol. 76: 230-236, 2006

19

Women's Health

For millennia the major cause of death of men was trauma. For women, it was childbirth. In today's world we expect a longer life span overlaid by a completely different spectrum of problems, with different causes of mortality. Although most health conditions are shared by women and men, many affect women differently and others are unique to them. This includes breast cancer, cervical and ovarian cancer, menopause, pregnancy and more. A good example of a disease that is shared by men but is expressed differently in women would be osteoporosis, which occurs both more frequently and earlier in women. Urinary tract infections are more common in women and sexually transmitted diseases tend to harm women more seriously. There is discrepancy even with heart attacks, which are less likely to be predicted or diagnosed in females.

This chapter focuses on a few of these unique challenges: infertility, uterine problems, PCO (polycystic ovaries), menopausal issues, osteoporosis and benign uterine tumors like polyps and fibroids. Cancer is covered in Chapter 5, and pregnancy in Chapter 18.

Female infertility

Female infertility has several definitions. It is customarily defined as the inability to get pregnant after one year of trying. Or, a woman is unable to remain pregnant and consistently miscarries. Regardless of the definition, female infertility rates reach 10% in the USA and more in poorer countries.

The most common cause of infertility results from problems with ovulation—the production and release of a normal egg (ova) for fertilization. This can be interrupted by hormonal irregularities, toxins, infection and more, but one of the most frequently seen problems is polycystic ovarian syndrome (PCOS), discussed separately later on. Another common cause is primary ovarian

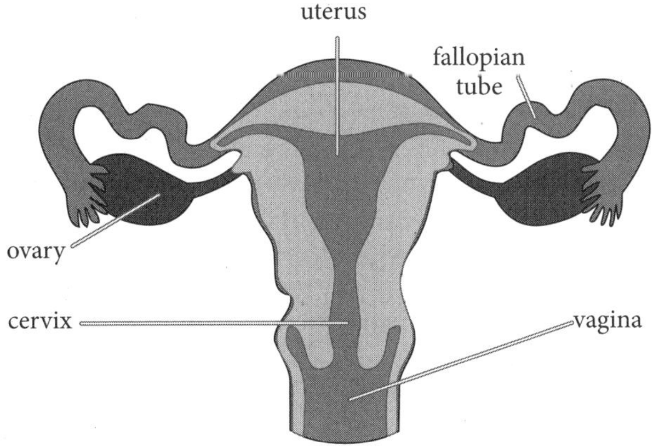

Figure 39: The female reproductive system, showing uterus, ovaries and fallopian tubes

insufficiency (POI), in which the ovaries prematurely stop working. Many cases of infertility are classified as "idiopathic," which is how doctors say, "We don't know why."

Lifestyle contributes to infertility as well. Smoking, alcohol consumption, severe weight loss and overtraining can all result in failure to produce normal ova—even losing menstrual periods altogether. Other causes include blocked fallopian tubes, possibly due to infection—PID (pelvic inflammatory disease), endometriosis, trauma or ectopic pregnancy (pregnancy that takes root in the tubes rather than the uterus). Other anatomical features contributing to infertility are abnormalities of the uterus and the growth of uterine fibroids.

Glutathione & infertility[1]

When examining the role of glutathione in female infertility, the first thing to determine is whether oxidative stress and glutathione insufficiency levels are, in fact, more prevalent among infertile women. Studies have repeatedly confirmed this. In the journal Reproductive Biomedicine Online, Spanish investigators documented oxidative stress markers and glutathione enzyme levels in patients treated at a fertility clinic. Women who responded successfully to treatment were compared to ones who failed. Clear and significant differences were evident in free radical formation and glutathione depression between the two groups. Similar findings have emerged from studies in China, the USA, India and Europe.

Another way to demonstrate the value of GSH in fertility would be to determine whether genetic errors in GSH enzymes result in lower fertility rates. Genetic abnormalities are now easy to identify with DNA testing.

With in-vitro fertilization (IVF), even a viable ova (egg) is sometimes unable to "stick" to the lining of the uterus. This is called implantation failure. Karimio and his team compared successful cases with failed ones. The results were remarkable: one quarter of the failures featured abnormal glutathione genes, but none of the successful cases did.

Delving deeper into the role of glutathione as a detoxification agent (see also Chapter 2), researchers including the Scandinavians Knapen et al., showed that fertility decreases when the body is unable to clear toxins and free radicals properly due to abnormal GSH-related genes. Focusing on glutathione's role in the immune system, the Serbian researcher Tosic-Pajic and her team demonstrated significant glutathione deficiency in patients who were infertile after infection by chlamydia.[2]

An extensive review article on glutathione and infertility was published in 2018 in the journal JBRA Assisted Reproduction. It covers topics such as oxidative stress and infertility, polycystic ovary syndrome, endometriosis, essential infertility and other areas where glutathione deficiency contributes to this troubling problem.

Polycystic ovary syndrome (PCOS)

Polycystic ovary syndrome (PCOS) is a condition that produces higher than normal amounts of male hormones in women, causing them to skip menstrual periods and making it harder to get pregnant.

Women typically have two ovaries, each the size of a ping-pong ball. These reproductive organs produce "ova" (eggs) that are released into the uterus each month, ready to be fertilized. Examination of the ovaries in PCOS patients revealed multiple cysts, hence the name poly (many) cyst (sac). It is called a "syndrome" because it comes with a combination of signs and symptoms unique to each patient.

Generally caused by a hormonal

---

[1] Male infertility is covered in chapter 20; glutathione has been shown to play a clear role.

[2] A common sexually transmitted disease.

imbalance, PCOS is quite common, affecting about one in ten women of childbearing age. Not only is this one of the most common causes of infertility, it causes other problems too, including metabolic alterations and changes in physical appearance. There is a tendency for PCOS to run in families.

Aside from infertility, signs and symptoms of polycystic ovary syndrome may include: irregular menstrual cycles, excessive body and facial hair, persistent acne, thinning of scalp hair; obesity, darkening of skin around the groin, under the breasts or along neck creases, and skin tags around the neck or armpits.

Two hormones are usually the culprits—excess androgens (male hormones) and high insulin levels. The androgens cause "male" features such as increased body hair, decreased head hair and acne. High insulin levels trigger weight gain and, of course, diabetes.

Other health issues that result from PCOS include high blood pressure, high cholesterol levels, sleep apnea, depression and anxiety, as well as higher rates of uterine cancer.

Glutathione and PCOS

Many studies have established that PCOS comes with higher levels of oxidative stress and free radical damage. This is mirrored by the expected fall in glutathione levels. Moreover, many authors have correlated the fall of glutathione with an expanding waist size, heart disease, insulin resistance, abdominal fat, DNA damage, elevated homocysteine levels and hirsuitism (hairiness).

Since it's clear that high oxidative stress and low glutathione levels are directly associated with polycystic ovary syndrome, many authors have suggested that measuring GSH and oxidation would be a useful way to follow these patients and predict their risk. As described in the journal Human Reproduction Update, Murri and his team believe that changes in these parameters can occur even in the absence of clinical weight gain, implying that glutathione measurements might be a sensitive screening tool.

What do all these findings imply on a practical level? Clinicians certainly would want to know whether raising glutathione is a useful way to address PCOS. To find out, doctors and researchers have used the glutathione precursor NAC (N-acetylcysteine) as a treatment.

Put simply, NAC has been proven many times to lower oxidative stress in polycystic ovary syndrome. In addition, NAC was shown to improve the problem of insulin resistance in the same patient group. This is a welcome first step towards further study that would establish actual clinical results.

In a 2015 publication in Obstetrics and Gynecology International, Thakker's group concluded that "NAC showed significant improvement in pregnancy and ovulation rate as compared to placebo." This is good news for women who are infertile due to PCOS.

Doctors have used other medications to treat polycystic ovary syndrome, both to control insulin regulation and to improve fertility rates. These include the common medication Metformin (used by non-insulin-dependent diabetics), and Clomiphene or Letrozole (used in infertility). Several studies have used a combination of NAC with several of the drugs mentioned above, resulting in improved ovulation and pregnancy rates.

Even more dramatically, scientists have compared NAC head-to-head with these drugs to see which were more effective. Oner's team states, "Metformin and NAC appear to have comparable effects on hyperandrogenism, hyperinsulinemia, and menstrual irregularity in women with PCOS." Cheraghi's paper concludes, "NAC improves oocyte and embryo quality and could be administered as an alternative to Metformin." Javanmanesh goes further: "NAC can improve lipid profile and fasting blood sugar better than Metformin."

Experimental studies raising GSH levels in women with polycystic ovary syndrome have shown improvements in fertility rates and insulin function as well as cholesterol levels, sugar levels and masculinization effects, along with other clinical benefits.

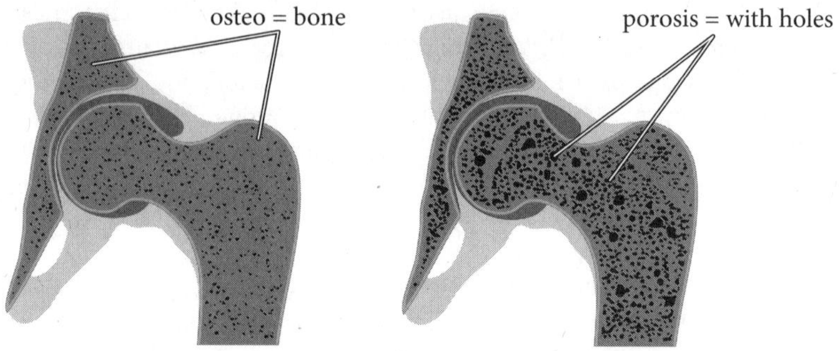

FIGURE 40: Bone is living tissue with a honeycomb-like structure that loses density in late adulthood and can become osteoporotic (porous bones)

Osteoporosis

Osteoporosis appears in both men and women. However, it is more prevalent in women, and appears earlier too. The rate of osteoporosis in men starts to catch up after age 70 years.

Osteoporosis is a loss of bone mass, such that bones are more prone to breaking. The earliest stage of osteoporosis is called "osteopenia" (thinning of the bones). This is when weakened bone density can be identified for the first time by radiographs and other sensitive medical equipment. It often progresses to full-blown osteoporosis (osteo = bone, porosis = with holes). The early stages of osteoporosis are symptom-free. Too often, first diagnosis is made only when the patient goes to the emergency department after breaking a bone.

Osteoporosis is extremely common. In the USA about one in six people have osteoporosis and one-half of women and one-quarter of men will break a bone as a result.

Many factors lead to osteoporosis, but the most common includes genetics (family history), lack of exercise, low body weight, inadequate dietary calcium and vitamin D, and use of alcohol, tobacco and other drugs or medications.

Treatments for osteoporosis include dietary improvements, exercise and other lifestyle changes. Calcium and vitamin D both remain a mainstay treatment, although recent research has questioned their efficacy. Many pharmaceutical alternatives have been developed for the treatment of osteoporosis.

Osteoporosis and glutathione

Research into oxidative stress and free radicals as contributing factors to osteoporosis goes back many years. An Italian study in 1991 showed that patients with low bone density had significantly lower levels of glutathione when compared to normal subjects. Subsequent studies over many years have confirmed that both free radical formation and glutathione depletion are a critical part of the development of this disease.

Mexican researchers led by Sanchez-Rodriguez suggest that oxidative stress and glutathione deficiency are independent risk factors for osteoporosis—in other words, women with depleted GSH are at greater risk. A large systematic review and meta-analysis of scientific writings on this subject by Chinese researchers was published in the journal Disease Markers. They proposed that measuring these parameters would be a useful tool in the treatment and management of patients who develop osteoporosis.

An indirect approach to studying glutathione deficiency in osteoporosis was taken by scientists working with genetics that include glutathione metabolism errors. Milakar and his Slovenian team were instrumental in correlating abnormal GSH genes with increased osteopenia and osteoporosis.

These findings beg the question—can we help combat osteoporosis by increasing glutathione and reducing oxidative stress? Many papers have shown improvements with the use of common antioxidants. Researchers are now looking specifically at GSH-enhancing strategies. Early research in laboratory animals with the GSH precursor NAC have shown promise. It seems that glutathione acts in osteoblasts[3] to reduce bone breakdown and promote growth, meaning that cells that weaken bones are inhibited, while those that make new bone are stimulated to produce more.

Australian researchers Sanders, Kotowicz and Nicholson conducted a pilot study called "Potential role of the antioxidant N-acetyl-cysteine in slowing bone resorption in early post-menopausal women." Compared to untreated women, they showed that those given NAC benefited from increased bone density and a lower threat of osteoporosis.

Menstruation

Historically and culturally, the moon has long been associated with women, presumably because both follow an approximate 28-day period. Each month, a woman's body prepares for pregnancy by releasing an ova ("egg") from the ovaries, which passes through the fallopian tubes and into the uterus. Unfertilized eggs, along with the lining of the uterus, are shed during the menstrual period through the vagina.

Periods start at the age of fertility—generally from age 11 to 14. In the Western world, the average has fallen in recent decades. Menstruations normally stop around age 50 years, when the ovaries run out of eggs. This cessation is called "menopause." The years in and around this time are called "peri-menopause," during which woman's bodies adjust to profound physical and hormonal changes. When the changes are complete, women are said to be in a "post-menopause" phase. Each of these different life phases carries its own set of health issues and challenges.t

It's interesting to note that glutathione levels fluctuate during the menstrual cycle. Generally, they peak during the ovulation phase, coinciding with the estrogen peak. The physiological reasons why are still unknown, but there is reason to surmise that high GSH levels at this time promote fertility.

Menopause

Surprisingly, women are born with a fixed number of eggs in their ovaries. More eggs are not produced during their lifetime. If a woman lives long enough, she will run out of eggs, sparking a cascade of events that results in altered production of the sex hormones estrogen and progesterone. The cessation of menstruation is just the beginning of menopause. A long list of physical changes take place, with far-reaching implications.

Perimenopause typically begins a few years before complete menopause. The production of female hormones diminishes, and symptoms begin (see Table 32).

Even more concerning than the symptoms accompanying menopause are the consequences for women's health, affecting their quality of life and even raising their risk of death. Some are listed in Table 31.

There are many treatment options, the most common being hormone-replacement therapy. Antidepressants and neuromodulators are commonly used, as well as disease-specific drugs for hypertension (high blood pressure), osteoporosis, and more.

---

3 Cells that form new bone.

Osteoporosis	Heart disease	Alzheimer's Disease
Cataracts	Macular Degeneration	Wrinkling Skin
Autoimmune Disease	Neurodegeneration	Hormonal Cancers

TABLE 31: Some long-term health issues after menopause

Menopause and glutathione

To verify glutathione's importance in menopause, it is first necessary to establish that perimenopausal and postmenopausal women suffer from higher levels of oxidative stress and free radical damage, along with diminished GSH levels. In an aptly-titled article, "Antioxidant status and reproductive hormones in women during reproductive, perimenopausal and postmenopausal phases of life," the answer is clear. GSH levels are highest in young fertile women. They start falling in perimenopause, and reach their lowest levels after menopause. These findings have been established in numerous human clinical studies, and documented not only in serum (blood) samples but also in uterine and endometrial tissues.

Researchers have long observed that both antioxidant levels and glutathione levels are affected by estrogen levels. Estrogen appears to improve both antioxidant and glutathione functioning, suggesting that that the decline of estrogen with menopause would tax all antioxidants—not just glutathione.

As far back as 2001, Bednarek and her team examined premenopausal (before menopause) and postmenopausal (after menopause) women. They clearly demonstrated a negative correlation of estrogen with free radical damage, and a positive correlation with glutathione levels. In other words, the higher the estrogen levels, the more these women of differing age groups were protected.

Spanish investigators looked beyond the mere association of estrogen and good GSH function. Examining biochemical markers for inflammatory agents, they concluded that general inflammation results from estrogen deprivation and diminished glutathione.

This justifies exploring the possibility that hormone replacement therapy would decrease antioxidant damage and improve GSH levels. Bellanti's Italian group and others have all demonstrated that estrogen therapy does counteract oxidative stress and improve the gene expression of various endogenous antioxidants, including catalase, superoxide dismutase and of course, glutathione.

Again, to the clinician and even to the patient, these laboratory findings may be fascinating—but do they have a practical application? A clinical study entitled "Effect of hormone therapy with estrogens on oxidative stress and quality of life in postmenopausal women," resulted in a resounding, "Yes." This trial enrolled more than a hundred Mexican women. It showed a clear association between estrogen supplementation and GSH status. More importantly it improved their quality-of-life measurements.

Looking at some of the more serious medical problems that arise during the menopausal years reveals some interesting facts. The incidence of heart disease in post-menopausal women begins to approach that of men. Investigators have found that as antioxidants and glutathione levels fall

Insomnia	Mood swings	Decreased sex drive
Fatigue	Depression	Vaginal dryness
Irritability	Palpitations	Bladder control problems
Headaches	Aches & pains	Hot flashes

TABLE 32: Some symptoms of menopause

in menopause, coronary artery disease increases. Furthermore, GSH deficiencies are even worse in menopausal women with active heart disease.

Further aggravating heart disease is sleep disturbance, including apnea (see Chapter 33), where GSH plays an important role. Menopausal women with sleep difficulties are at significantly higher risk of developing cardiac problems. In the journal "Menopause" Mexican scientists showed how estrogen depletion led to decreased antioxidant/GSH levels and even more insomnia.

Other metabolic disturbances associated with menopause include obesity and metabolic syndrome (comprising increased abdominal fat, high blood pressure, high blood sugar and cholesterol levels). As expected, all of these were associated with abnormal glutathione activity. Further health issues in this vein include memory problems, hair loss, osteoporosis, increased cancer risk and other challenges to the aging female.

Simpler and safer than hormone replacement therapy in menopause is the use of oral antioxidants. They are less effective, but suitable for the many women who cannot or choose not to take hormone supplements. In the journal "Archives of Gerontology and Geriatrics," Spanish researchers state that additional dietary antioxidants have, "favorable effects on the health and quality of life of women, especially those who cannot be treated with hormone-replacement therapy, (and who) suffer high levels of oxygen stress...."

Endometriosis, fibroids and polyps

The uterus (womb) lies in the pelvis, and hosts pregnancy. It is a hollow, muscular organ with a fragile lining and elevated blood supply. Other than abnormal bleeding or issues with menstruation, the uterus can develop a number of other problems, including cancer, nonmalignant growths such as fibroids and polyps, infection and inflammation.

Endometriosis

Some women develop uterine tissue outside the uterus—on the ovaries, fallopian tubes, bowels, bladder or elsewhere—causing problems. This is endometriosis.

Its main symptom is pain—it could be in the back, the abdomen, the pelvis and through menstrual cramps. Endometriosis tends to produce heavy periods; bleeding between periods may also occur.

There is no definitive cure, but treatments include pain relievers, hormone therapy and even surgery to remove the excess tissue.

Glutathione and endometriosis

In all the conditions described above, high levels of oxidative stress and low levels of glutathione have been clearly demonstrated. In the journal "Fertility and Sterility," Szczepanska reports that low GSH levels play a role in the development of endometriosis. A year later in this same journal, Foyouzi stated that women with endometriosis had increased free radical damage compared to ones without, and that their condition could be positively treated with the glutathione precursor N-acetylcysteine.

While attempting to correlate genetic abnormalities in GSH enzymes with susceptibility to endometriosis, Chinese, Brazilian, Indian and other researchers across the world established clear evidence that women with genetic GSH errors are at greater risk.

A Mexican team led by Mier-Cabrera published the results of a series of interventions in endometriosis, using glutathione. Many of the parameters that marked endometriosis improved. Several European research bodies looked specifically at raising glutathione levels using NAC. Improvements were reported—including pain reduction.

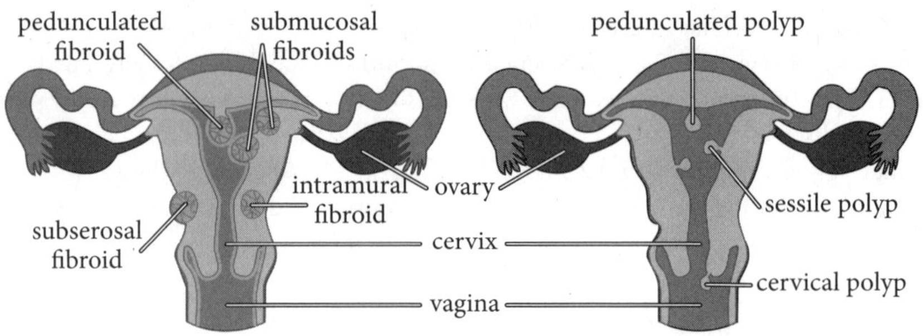

FIGURE 41: Difference between a uterine polyp and a fibroid

Uterine fibroids and polyps

The uterus can overgrow and result in both malignant (cancerous) and non-malignant masses. Overgrowth of the lining of the uterus can produce "polyps," balls of tissue connected by a "stalk" or "stem." Besides their tendency to cause heavier periods, polyps carry the risk of becoming cancerous themselves.

Overgrowth of the muscular wall of the uterus may lead to the formation of "fibroids," referred to medically as, "leiomyoma" or "myoma." Fibroids can range in size from pea-sized to large masses. They can be single or multiple, and commonly cause heavy periods. Fibroids are exceedingly common and most women will have some by age 50 years.

Polyps and fibroids are often left untouched. Because polyps are potentially malignant however, doctors tend to take a more aggressive approach. If fibroids become overly problematic, the usual approach is local surgery, and sometimes a full hysterectomy (removal of uterus).

Uterine fibroids, polyps and glutathione

Uterine polyps are connected with abnormal antioxidant status and glutathione levels. Glutathione depletion increases as polyps become increasingly malignant. (Glutathione in cancer has been covered in Chapter 5.)

Fibroids are found more commonly in women with abnormal glutathione genetics. Fibroids examined under a microscope reveal increased free radical damage and decreased glutathione levels. In an article in the journal, "Clinical and Experimental Obstetrics and Gynecology," Markowska concluded that oxidative stress and glutathione dysregulation play a part in the development of fibroids. Active intervention using glutathione precursors has yet to be studied.

Conclusion

Women face a whole different spectrum of health issues from men. In many cases—including infertility, polycystic ovary syndrome, osteoporosis, menopause and uterine fibroids—the common thread of GSH deficiency is well recognized. Treatment options which improve glutathione status have shown promise in many human clinical trials.

WOMEN'S HEALTH

REFERENCES

ENDOMETRIOSIS, FIBROIDS AND POLYPS

AGOSTINIS C, ZORZET S, DE LEO R, ET AL. *The combination of N-acetyl cysteine, alpha-lipoic acid, & bromelain shows high anti-inflammatory properties in novel in vivo & in vitro models of endometriosis.* Mediators Inflamm. doi: 10.1155/2015/918089

Andrisiani A, Donà G, Brunati AM, et al. *Increased oxidation-related glutathionylation & carbonic anhydrase activity in endometriosis.* Reprod Biomed Online 28: 773-779, 2014

Chen XP, Xu DF, Xu WH, et al. *Glutathione-S-transferases M1/T1 gene polymorphisms & endometriosis: a meta-analysis in Chinese populations.* Gynecol Endocrinol. 31: 840-845, 2015

Chiou JF, Hu ML. *Elevated lipid peroxidation & disturbed antioxidant enzyme activities in plasma & erythrocytes of patients with uterine cervicitis & myoma.* Clin Biochem. 32: 189-192, 1999

Foyouzi N, Berkkanoglu M, Arici A, et al. *Effects of oxidants & antioxidants on proliferation of endometrial stromal cells.* Fertil Steril. 82: 1019-1022, 2004

Kubiszeski EH, de Medeiros SF, da Silva Seidel JA, et al. *Glutathione S-transferase M1 & T1 gene polymorphisms in Brazilian women with endometriosis.* J Assist Reprod Genet. 32: 1531-1535, 2015

Lete I, Mendoza N, de la Viuda E, et al. *Effectiveness of an antioxidant preparation with N-acetyl cysteine, alpha lipoic acid & bromelain in the treatment of endometriosis-associated pelvic pain: LEAP study.* Eur J Obstet Gynecol Reprod Biol. 228: 221-224, 2018

Li H, Zhang Y. *Glutathione S-transferase M1 polymorphism & endometriosis susceptibility: a meta analysis.* J Gynecol Obstet Biol Reprod (Paris). 44: 136-144, ;2015

Markowska A, Mardas M, Gajdzik E, et al. *Oxidative stress markers in uterine fibroids tissue in pre- & postmenopausal women.* Clin Exp Obstet Gynecol. 42: 725-729, 2015

Mier-Cabrera J, Aburto-Soto T, Burrola-Méndez S, et al. *Women with endometriosis improved their peripheral antioxidant markers after the application of a high antioxidant diet.* Reprod Biol Endocrinol. doi: 10.1186/1477-7827-7-54, 2009

Mier-Cabrera J, Jiménez-Zamudio L, Garcia-Latorre E, et al. *Quantitative & qualitative peritoneal immune profiles, T-cell apoptosis & oxidative stress-associated characteristics in women with minimal & mild endometriosis.* BJOG 118: 6-16, 2011

Mostafavi SS, Ebrahimi A, Sadat SM, et al. *Impact of null genotypes of GSTT1 & GSTM1 with uterine leiomyoma risk in Iranian population.* J Obstet Gynaecol Res. 42: 434-439, 2016

Oner-Iyidoğan Y, Koçak H, Gürdöl F, et al. *Indices of oxidative stress in eutopic & ectopic endometria of women with endometriosis.* Gynecol Obstet Invest. 57: 214-217, 2004

Pejić S, Kasapović J, Todorović A, et al. *Lipid peroxidation & antioxidant status in blood of patients with uterine myoma, endometrial polypus, hyperplastic & malignant endometrium.* Biol Res. 39: 619-629, 2006

Pejić SA, Kasapović JD, Todorović AU, et al. *Antioxidant enzymes in women with endometrial polyps: relation with sex hormones.* Eur J Obstet Gynecol Reprod Biol. 170: 241-246, 2013

Pejić S, Todorović A, Stojiljković V, et al. *Antioxidant status & sex hormones in women with complex endometrial hyperplasia.* Cell Mol biol. 62: 51-56, 2016

Roya R, Baludu GS, Reddy BS. *Possible aggravating impact of gene polymorphism in women with endometriosis.* Indian J Med Res. 129: 395-400, 2009

Szczepańska M, Koźlik J, Skrzypczak J, et al. *Oxidative stress may be a piece in the endometriosis puzzle.* Fertil Steril. 79: 1288-1293, 2003

Fertility

Adeoye O, Olawumi J, Opeyemi A, et al. *Review on the role of glutathione on oxidative stress & infertility.* JBRA Assist Reprod. 22:61-66, 2018

Babuška V, Cedíková M, Rajdl D, et al. *Comparison of selective oxidative stress parameters in the follicular fluid of infertile women & healthy fertile oocyte donors. Ceska Gynekol. 77:543-548, 2012*

Choi YS, Cho S, Seo SK, et al. *Alteration in intrafollicular thiol-redox system in infertile women with endometriosis.* Reproduction. 149: 155-162, 2015

Ebisch IM, Thomas CM, Peters WH, et al. *The importance of folate, zinc & antioxidants in the pathogenesis & prevention of subfertility. Hum Reprod Update. 13:1 163-174, 2007*

Ito M, Muraki M, Takahashi Y, et al. *Glutathione S-transferase theta 1 expressed in granulosa cells as a biomarker for oocyte quality in age-related infertility.* Fertil Steril. 90: 1026-1035 2008

Karimlo FK, Mashayekhi F, Sorouri ZZ, et al. *Association of GSTM1 & GSTT1 gene polymorphisms & in-vitro fertilisation outcome in a population in northern Iran.* J Obstet Gynaecol. 35: 46-48, 2015

Knapen MF, Zusterzeel PL, Peters WH, et al. *Glutathione & glutathione-related enzymes in reproduction.* A review. Eur J Obstet Gynecol Reprod Biol. 82: 171-184, 1999

Nuñez-Calonge R, Cortés S, Gutierrez Gonzales LM, et al. *Oxidative stress in follicular fluid of young women with low response compared with fertile oocyte donors.* Reprod Biomed Online. 32: 446-456, 2016

Paszkowski T, Traub AI, Robinson SY, et al. *Selenium dependent glutathione peroxidase activity in human follicular fluid. Clin Chim Acta. 236: 173-180, 1995*

Pieczyńska J, Grajeta H. *The role of selenium in*

human conception & pregnancy. J Trace Elem Med Biol. 29: 31-38, 2015

Polak G, Koziol-Montewka M, Tarkowski R, et al. *Glutathione peroxidase concentration in the peritoneal fluid from infertile women.* (Article in Polish). Ginekol Pol. 71:1017-1021, 2000

Singh AK, Chattopadhyay R, Chakravarty B, et al. *Markers of oxidative stress in follicular fluid of women with endometriosis & tubal infertility undergoing IVF.* Reprod toxicol. 42: 116-124, 2013

Tošić-Pajić J, Šeklić D, Radenković J, et al. *Augmented oxidative stress in infertile women with persistent chlamydial infection. Reprod Biol. 17: 120-125, 2017*

Younis A, Clower C, Nelsen D, et al. *The relationship between pregnancy & oxidative stress markers on patients undergoing ovarian stimulations.* J Assist Reprod Genet. 29: 1083-1089, 2012

Menopausia

Ansar S, Alhefdhi T, Aleem AM. *Status of trace elements & antioxidants in premenopausal & postmenopausal phase of life: a comparative study.* Int J Clin Exp Med. 8: 19486-19490

Baeza I, Fdez-Tresguerres J, Ariznavarreta C, et al. *Effects of growth hormone, melatonin, oestrogens & phytoestrogens on the oxidized glutathione (GSSG)/reduced glutathione (GSH) ratio & lipid peroxidation in aged ovariectomized rats.* Biogerontology 11: 687-701, 2010

Bednarek-Tupikowska G, Bohdanowicz-Pawlak A, Bidzińska B, et al. *Serum lipid peroxide levels & erythrocyte glutathione peroxidase & superoxide dismutase activity in premenopausal & postmenopausal women.* Gynecol Endocrinol. 15 : 298-303, 2001

Bellanti F, Matteo M, Rollo T, et al. *Sex hormones modulate circulating antioxidant enzymes: impact of estrogen therapy.* Redox Biol. 1 :340-346, 2013

Gökkusu C, Özbek Z, Tata G. *Hormone replacement therapy: relation to homocysteine & prooxidant-antioxidant status in healthy postmenopausal women.* Arch Gynecol Obstet. 285: 733-739, 2012

Gürdöl F, Oner-Yyidothan Y, Yalçýn O, et al. *Changes in enzymatic antioxidant defense system in blood & endometrial tissues of women after menopause.* Res Commun Mol Pathol Pharmacol. 97: 38-46, 1997

Ha EJ, Smith AM. *Plasma selenium & plasma & erythrocyte glutathione peroxidase activity increase with estrogen during the menstrual cycle.* J Am Coll Nutr. 22: 43-51, 2003

Ha EJ, Smith AM. *Selenium-dependent glutathione peroxidase activity is increased in healthy post-menopausal women.* Biol Trace Elem Res. 131: 90-95, 2009

Hachul de Campos H, Brandão LC, D'Almeida V, et al. *Sleep disturbances, oxidative stress & cardiovascular risk parameters in postmenopausal women complaining of insomnia.* Climacteric. 9: 312-319, 2006

Klisic A, Kotur-Stevuljevic J, Kavaric N, et al. *The association between follicle stimulating hormone & glutathione peroxidase activity is dependent on abdominal obesity in postmenopausal women.* Eat Weight Disord. 23: 133-141, 2018

Kolesnikova L, Semenova N, Madaeva I, et al. *Antioxidant status in peri- & postmenopausal women.* Maturitas 81: 83-87, 2015

Krstevska M, Dzhekova-Stojkova S, Bosilkova G. *Menopause, coronary artery disease & antioxidants.* Clin Chem Lab Med. 39: 641-644, 2001

Lutoslawska G. Tkaczyk J, Panczenko-Kresowska B, et al. *Plasma TBARS, blood GSH concentrations, & erythrocyte antioxidant enzyme activities in regularly menstruating women with ovulatory & anovulatory menstrual cycles.* Clin Chim Acta 331: 159-163. 2003

Madeddu C, Gramignano G, Floris C, et al. *Role of inflammation & oxidative stress in post-menopausal oestrogen-dependent breast cancer.* J Cell Mol Med. 18: 2519-2529, 2014

Markowska A, Mardas M, Gajdzik E, et al. *Oxidative stress markers in uterine fibroids tissue in pre- & postmenopausal women.* Clin Exp Obstet Gynecol. 42: 725-729, 2015

Miguel J, Ramirez-Boscá A, Ramirez-Bosca JV, et al. *Menopause : A review on the role of oxygen stress & favorable effects of dietary antioxidants.* Arch Gerontol Geriatr. 42: 289-306, 2006

Massafra C, Gioia D, De Felice C, et al. *Effects of estrogens & androgens on erythrocyte antioxidant superoxide dismutase, catalase & glutathione peroxidase activities during the menstrual cycle.* J Endocrinol. 167: 447-452, 2000

Priyanka HP, Sharma U, Gopinath S, et al. *Menstrual cycle & reproductive aging alters immune reactivity, NGF expression, antioxidant enzyme activities, & intracellular signaling pathways in the peripheral blood mononuclear cells of healthy women. Brain Behav Immun 32: 131-143, 2013*

Ogunro PS, Bolarinde AA, Owa OO, et al. *Antioxidant status & reproductive hormones in women during reproductive, perimenopausal & postmenopausal phase.* Afr J Med Med Sci, 43: 49-57, 2014

Palasuwan A, Margaritis I, Soogarun S, et al. *Dietary intakes & antioxidant status in mind-body exercising pre- & postmenopausal women.* J Nutr Health Aging. 15: 577-584, 2011

Sánchez-Rodriguez MA, Zacarias-Flores M, Arronte-Rosales A, et al. *Menopause as risk factor for oxidative stress.* Menopause. 19 :

361-367, 2012

Sánchez Rodrigues MA, Zacarias Flores M, Arronte Rosales A, et al. *Effect of hormone therapy with estrogens on oxidative stress & quality of life in postmenopausal women.* Ginecol Obstet Mex. 81: 11-22, 2013

Sánchez-Rodriguez MA, Zacarias-Flores M, Castrejón-Delgado L, et al. *Effects of Hormone Therapy on Oxidative Stress in Postmenopausal Women with Metabolic Syndrome.* Int J Mol Sci. 17: pii: E1388. doi: 10.3390-ijms17091388, 2016

Shafin N, Zakaria R, Hussain NH, et al. *Association of oxidative stress & memory performance in postmenopausal women receiving estrogen-progestin therapy.* Menopause. 20: 661-666, 2013

Unfer TC, Figueiredo CG, Zanchi MM, et al. *Estrogen plus progestin increase superoxide dismutase & total antioxidant capacity in postmenopausal women.* Climacteric. 18: 379-388, 2015

Viña J, Gambini J, Garcia-Garcia FJ, et al. *Role of oestrogens on oxidative stress & inflammation in ageing. Horm Mol B.iol Clin Investig. 16: 65-72, 2013*

Osteoporosis

Avitabile M, Campagna NE, Magri GA, et al. *Correlation between serum glutathione reductases & bone densitometry values.* Boll Soc Ital Biol Sper. 67: 931-937, 1991

Jun JH, Lee SH, Kwak HB, et al. *N-acetylcysteine stimulates osteoblastic differentiation of mouse calvarial cells.* J Cell Biochem. 103: 1246-1255, 2008

Jurkovic Mlakar S, Prezelj J, Osredkar J, et al. *BMD values & GSTM3 gene polymorphisms in combination with GSTT1/GSTM1 genes: a genetic association study in Slovenian elderly.* Gerontology. 58: 238-248, 2012

Mata-Granados JM, Cuenca-Acebedo R, Luque de Castro MD, et al. *Lower vitamin E serum levels are associated with osteoporosis in early postmenopausal women: a cross-sectional study.* J Bone Miner Metab. 31: 455-460, 2013

Mlakar SJ, Osredkar J, Prezelj J, et al. *The antioxidant enzyme GPX1 gene polymorphisms are associated with low BMD & increased bone turnover markers.* Dis Markers. 29: 71-80, 2010

Mlakar SJ, Osredkar J, Prezelj J, et al. *Antioxidant enzymes GSR, SOD1, SOD2, & CAT gene variants & bone mineral density values in postmenopausal women: a genetic association analysis.* Menopause 19: 368-376, 2012

Mlakar SJ, Prezelj J, Marc J. *Testing GSTP1 genotypes & haplotypes interactions in Slovenian post-/pre-menopausal women: novel involvement of glutathione S-transferases in bone remodeling process.* Maturitas 71: 180-187, 2012

Maggio D, Barabani M, Pierandrei M, et al. *Marked decrease in plasma antioxidants in aged osteoporotic women: results of a cross-sectional study.* J clin Endocrinol Metab 88: 1523-1527, 2003

Muhammad N, Luke DA, Shuid AN, et al. *Tocotrienol supplementation in postmenopausal osteoporosis: evidence from a laboratory study.* Clinics (Sao Paulo) 68: 1338-1343, 2013

Ozgocmen S, Kaya H, Fadillioglu E, et al. *role of antioxidant systems, lipid peroxidation, & nitric oxide in postmenopausal osteoporosis.* Mol Cell Biochem. 295: 45-52, 2007

Sánchez-Rodriguez MA, Ruiz-Ramos M, Correa-Muñoz E, et al. *Oxidative stress as a risk factor for osteoporosis in elderly Mexicans as characterized by antioxidant enzymes.* BMC Musculoskelet Disord. 8: 124, 2007

Sanders KM, Kotowicz MA, Nicholson GC. *Potential role of the antioxidant N-acetylcysteine in slowing bone resorption in early post-menopausal women: a pilot study.* Transl Res. 150: 215, 2007

Sendur OF,Turan Y, Tastaban E, et al. *Antioxidant status in patients with osteoporosis: a controlled study.* Joint Bone Spine. 76: 514-518, 2009

Zhou Q, Zhu L, Zhang D, et al. *Oxidative Stress-Related biomarkers in Postmenopausal Osteoporosis: A Systematic Review & Meta-Analyses.* Dis Markers. 2016: 7067984. Doi: 10.1155/2016/7067984

Zinnuroglu M, Dincel AS, Kosova F, et al. *Prospective evaluation of free radicals & antioxidant activity following 6-month risedronate treatment in patients with postmenopausal osteoporosis.* Rheumatol Int. 32: 875-880, 2012

Polycystic ovary syndrome

Badawy A, State O, Abdelgawad S. *N-Acetyl cysteine & clomiphene citrate for induction of ovulation in polycystic ovary syndrome: a cross-over trial.* Acta Obstet Gynecol Scand. 86: 218-222, 2007

Baskol G, Aygen E, Erdem F, et al. *Assessment of paraoxonase 1, xanthine oxidase & glutathione peroxidase activities, nitric oxide & thiol levels in women with polycystic ovary syndrome.* Acta Obstet Gynecol Scand. 91: 326-330, 2012

Chen L, Xu WM, Zhang D. *Association of abdominal obesity, insulin resistance, & oxidative stress in adipose tissue in women with polycystic ovary syndrome.* Fertil Steril. 102: 1167-1174, 2014

Cheraghi E, Mehranjani MS, Shariatzadeh MA, et al. *N-Acetylcysteine improves oocyte & embryo quality in polycystic ovary syndrome patients undergoing intracytoplasmic sperm injection.* Reprod Fertil Dev. 28: 723-731, 2016

Dincer Y, Ozen E, Kadioglu P, et al. *Effect of sex hormones on lipid peroxidative in women with polycystic ovary syndrome, healthy womenm & men.* Endocr Res. 27: 309-316, 2001

Dinger Y, Akcay T, Erdem T, et al. *DNA damage, DNA susceptibility to oxidation & glutathione level in women with polycystic ovary syndrome.* Scand J Clin Lab Invest. 65: 721-728, 2005

Donà G, Sabbadin C, Fiore C, et al. *Inositol administration reduces oxidative stress in erythrocytes of patients with polycystic ovary syndrome.* Eur J Endocrinol. 166:703-710, 2012

Dong F, Deng D, chen H, et al. *Serum metabolomics study of polycystic ovary syndrome based on UPLC-QTOF-MS coupled with a pattern recognition approach.* Anal Bioanal Chem. 407: 4683-4695, 2015

Enli Y, Fenkci SM, Fenkci V, et al. *Serum Fetuin-A levels, insulin resistance & oxidative stress in women with polycystic ovary syndrome.* Gynecol Endocrinol. 29: 1036-1039, 2013

Flughesu AM, Ciampelli M, Muzj G, et al. *N-acetyl-cysteine treatment improves insulin sensitivity in women with polycystic ovary syndrome.* Fertil Steril. 77: 1128-1135, 2002

Javanmanesh F, Kashanian M, Rahimi M, et al. *A comparison between the effects of metformin & N-acetylcysteine (NAC) on some metabolic & endocrine characteristics of women with polycystic ovary syndrome.* Gynecol Endocrinol. 32: 285-289, 2016

Kilic-Okman T, Kucuk M. *N-acetyl-cysteine treatment for polycystic ovary syndrome.* Int J Gynaecol Obstet. 85: 296-297, 2004

Köse SA, Naziroğlu M. *NAC reduces oxidative toxicity, apoptosis, & calcium entry through TRPV1 channels in neutrophils of patients with polycystic ovary syndrome.* Free Radic Res. 49: 338-346, 2015

Köse SA, Naziroğlu M. *Selenium reduces oxidative stress & calcium entry through TRPV1 channels in the neutrophils of patients with polycystic ovary syndrome.* Biol Trace Elem Res. 158: 136-142, 2014

Kurdoglu Z, Ozkol H, Tuluce Y, et al. *Oxidative status & its relation with insulin resistance in young non-obese women with polycystic ovary syndrome.* J Endocrinol Invest. 35: 317-321, 2012

Macut D, Simic T, Lissounov A, et al. *Insulin resistance in non-obese women with polycystic ovary syndrome: relation to byproducts of oxidative stress.* Exp Clin Endocrinol Diabetes. 119: 451-455, 2011

Macut D, Bjekić-Macut J, Savić-Radojević A. *Dyslipidemia & oxidative stress in PCOS.* Front Horm Res. 40: 51-63, 2013

Masha A, Manieri C, Dinatale S, et al. *Prolonged treatment with N-acetylcysteine & L-arginine restores gonadal function in patients with polycystic ovary syndrome.* J Endocrinol Invest. 32: 870-872, 2009

Mostajeran F, Tehrani HG, Rahbary B. *N-Acetylcysteine as an Adjuvant to Letrozole for Induction of Ovulation in Infertile Patients with Polycystic Ovary Syndrome.* Adv Biomed Res. Jun 25; 7:100. doi: 10.4103/abr.abr_157_17. eCollection 2018.

Murri M, Luque-Ramirez M, Insenser M, et al. *Circulating markers of oxidative stress & polycystic ovary syndrome (PCOS): a systematic review & meta-analysis.* Hum Reprod Update. 19: 268-288, 2013

Oner G, Muderris II. *Clinical, endocrine & metabolic effects of metformin vs N-acetyl-cysteine in women with polycystic ovary syndrome.* Eur J Obstet Gynecol Reprod Biol. 159: 127-131, 2011

Öser A, Bakacak M, Kiran H, et al. *Increased oxidative stress is associated with insulin resistance & infertility in polycystic ovary syndrome.* Ginekol Pol. 87: 733-738, 2016

Rodrigues JK, Dib LA, Ferriani RA, et al. *Serum markers of oxidative stress & assisted reproduction procedures results in infertile patients with polycystic ovary syndrome & controls.* Rev Bras Ginecol Obstet. 32: 118-125, 2010

Sabuncu T, Vural H, Harma M, et al. *Oxidative stress in polycystic ovary syndrome & its contribution to the risk of cardiovascular disease.* Clin Biochem. 34: 407-413, 2001

Salehpour S, Sene AA, Saharkhiz N, et al. *N-Acetylcysteine as an adjuvant to clomiphene citrate for successful induction of ovulation in infertile patients with polycystic ovary syndrome.* J Obstet Gynaecol Res. 38: 1182-1186, 2012

Thakker D, Raval A, Patel I, et al. *N-acetylcysteine for polycystic ovary syndrome: a systematic review & meta-analysis of randomized controlled clinical trials.* Obstet Gynecol Int. 2015:817849. doi: 10.1155/2015/817849

Victor VM, Rocha M, Bañuls C, et al. *Induction of oxidative stress & human leukocyte/endothelial cell interactions in polycystic ovary syndrome patients with insulin resistance.* J Clin Endocrinol Metab. 96: 3115-3122, 2011

Vrbiková J, Tallová J, Biciková M, et al. *Plasma thiols & androgen levels in polycystic ovary syndrome.* Clin Chem Lab Med. 41: 216-221, 2003

Zagrodzki P, Krzyczkowska-Sendrakowska M, Nicol F, et al. *Selenium status parameters in patients with polycystic ovary syndrome.* J Trace Elem Med Biol. 44: 241-246, 2017

20
Glutathione in Men

In this chapter we discuss issues unique to the human male, including prostate hypertrophy, prostate cancer, male infertility, male pattern baldness and erectile dysfunction.

Prostate problems

Of the hundreds of animal species with a prostate gland, only humans and dogs are known to suffer from prostate cancer and prostatic hypertrophy (overgrowth of prostate tissue). The prostate is a walnut-sized gland that encircles the urethra, the tube through the penis that drains the bladder (see Figure 40). It produces the fluid that carries sperm during ejaculation. Other problems include both acute and chronic infections called prostatitis. The majority of men will experience some sort of prostate problem in their lifetimes.

Prostatic hypertrophy (enlarged prostate gland)

Not all hypertrophy (enlargement) of the prostate is cancer. Usually it isn't. Benign (non-cancerous) swelling can be caused by enlargement of the cells in the gland, whereas cancer grows by multiplying the number of cells. This condition is age-related and increases from an incidence of 8% in 30 to 40 year olds, to over 80% in men over 80. Enlargement of the prostate may "squeeze" the urethra, obstructing flow from the bladder. Symptoms are frequent and difficult urination, a weak urinary stream, straining, dribbling, incomplete emptying and recurrent urinary infections.

Traditional treatments include surgical removal of all or part of the prostate, widening of the urethral passage by scraping or laser surgery, and a number of drugs that either relax the muscles at the neck of the bladder or actually shrink the prostate. Saw palmetto is an herbal therapy greatly valued by alternative practitioners that is now also gaining acceptance by conventional doctors as an adjunct[1] to help shrink prostatic tissues.

In prostatic hypertrophy as well as in prostate cancer, the prostate overgrows for several reasons. Male hormones (androgens) play a large part in this growth, and physicians may prescribe anti-androgens as an antidote.

Low GSH levels are expected in older men. Biopsies of those with benign prostatic hypertrophy (BPH) show even lower levels, as well as specific GSH deficiencies. One is in the enzyme[2] glutathione S-transferase, which has several subtypes. The relative proportions of these sub-types vary according to whether the prostate tissue is normal, hypertrophic or cancerous. Researchers propose that such deficiencies contribute to prostate enlargement and carcinogenesis. Since genetic GSH-enzyme abnormalities are commonly found in enlarged prostates and in prostate cancer, Kumar and his team wrote in the journal Disease Markers that measurement of GSH enzymes could be a potential screening test.

---

[1] An addition to (not replacement of) conventional treatment

[2] Protein molecules in cells that work as catalysts (enable chemical reactions without being consumed)

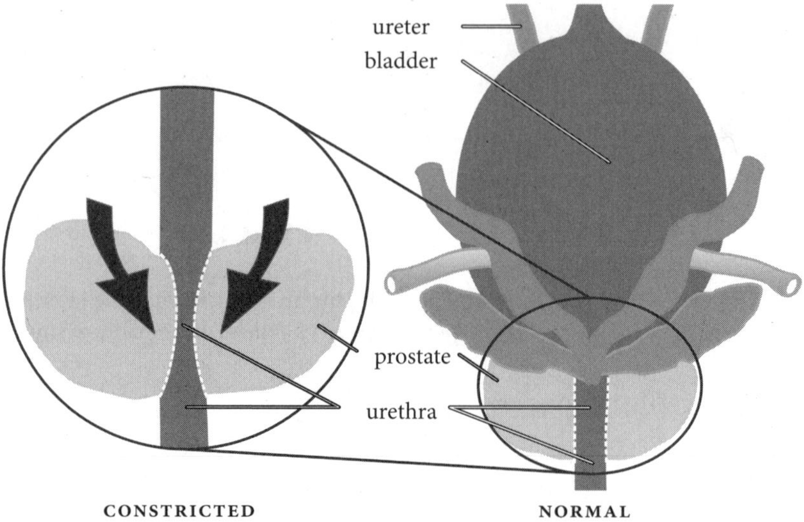

FIGURE 42: The urethra passes through the donut-shaped prostate gland and is easily constricted by swelling of the prostate

Prostate cancer

Well-known nutritional specialist Bonnie Liebman writes about "Death, taxes…and prostate cancer…," a poignant comment on the prevalence of prostate cancer in our population. When researchers include in their statistics individuals with pre-cancerous cells, they claim that more than three-quarters of men over the age of 80 show evidence of cancer in their prostate glands. Some scientists opine that any man who lives long enough will eventually get prostate cancer. By this definition, prostate cancer is definitely a disease of aging (see Chapter 6).

Nevertheless, the vast majority of men outlive prostate cancer, and may not even suffer significant symptoms. Most are diagnosed around age 72, but its origin is usually a slow-growing tumor that may have begun thirty or forty years earlier. Although it is by far the most common type of cancer in men, it kills less frequently than the two most deadly cancers—of the lung and of the colon.

Screening for prostate cancer is aggressive, usually starting with a digital rectal exam, ultrasonography, or a prostate specific antigen (PSA) blood test. Rectal exams are an easy way to check for swelling and sensitivity. PSA levels rise in the presence of prostate cancer and are a good screening tool. They also reveal how anti-cancer treatments are doing. Traditional treatments include surgical removal, heat therapy, laser therapy, radiotherapy, chemotherapy and hormonal therapy. When interventions are more intrusive than they're worth, benign neglect is appropriate.

Alternative therapy focuses on slowing down the process rather than curing it. Diet is one important factor. Prostatic cancer has been linked to high-fat, low-fiber diets. The use of antioxidants such as vitamin A or selenium is popular for reasons described below. A carotenoid[3] called lycopene gives certain fruits and vegetables their rich color and has been linked to the prevention of prostate cancer. It seems that men who eat lycopene-rich foods (tomato sauces, dark grapes) have lower rates of prostatic disease. This theory is still under investigation.

One of the more significant series of papers to be published on glutathione and

[3] Any of a class of mainly yellow, orange, or red fat-soluble pigments

prostate cancer comes from the University of Wisconsin. Researchers there describe male hormones (androgens) as a source of oxidative stress—particularly in cancerous prostate cells. An article in the Journal of the National Cancer Institute claims that androgens stimulate free radical damage while also depleting glutathione. Given the natural decline of glutathione levels in ageing males, the article suggests that "unopposed androgen pro-oxidant stress" contributes to prostate cancer and that natural defenses against oxidative stress are weakened by the decline of GSH enzymes. This is an interesting new way to regard the development of prostate cancer.

Another finding links prostate cancer to a loss of glutathione activity. The function of a particular glutathione enzyme—glutathione-S-transferase-pi-1 (GSTP1)—is almost always turned off early in the development of pre-cancerous and cancerous prostate cells. Many studies have remarked on the connection between GSTP1 function and other genetic GSH anomalies in the cancerous transformation of prostatic tissues.

Medical discoveries are often a matter of chance. A very large study undertaken by the National Cancer Institute (USA) was meant to determine whether selenium could bring down the rate of skin cancer—notoriously caused by strong exposure to sunlight. Researchers Clarke and Combs from Cornell University and the University of Arizona already knew of selenium's ability to raise glutathione levels (see Chapter 4) and to oppose cancer-causing free radical damage from ultraviolet light. As it turned out, selenium supplementation did not affect the incidence of skin cancer, but did surprisingly and dramatically diminish the incidence of prostate cancer in the selenium-supplemented group.

A study at Harvard University confirmed that higher selenium levels come with a lower risk of prostate cancer. It measured selenium levels in the toenail clippings of over 51,000 male health professionals between 40 and 75 years of age. Those with the highest selenium levels were least likely to get advanced prostate cancer. What is of special interest is that selenium is generally only biologically active—and only expresses its positive health benefits—when part of the enzyme glutathione peroxidase (see Chapter 4).

An article published by the Department of Human Nutrition at Ohio State University showed that selenium supplementation in middle-aged men both increased glutathione peroxidase levels and significantly decreased PSA readings on their blood tests.

Studies that raise GSH with undenatured whey protein isolates have been conducted at several research centers, including McGill and Harvard Universities, to evaluate its usefulness in the treatment of prostate cancer.

Case study

Franklin was a semi-retired general practitioner who at age 68 scored a PSA reading of over 8 micrograms/liter on a routine screening exam, strongly suggesting prostate cancer. A urologist took a cystoscopic biopsy[4] and confirmed the diagnosis. Four out of the six sites sampled in the biopsy tested positive for high-grade tumor. For personal and practical reasons, Franklin delayed aggressive treatment and opted to take 30 grams/day of a specially-prepared whey-protein isolate designed to raise glutathione levels. Bimonthly testing of PSA levels showed a gradual decline, his latest reading being 3.8 u/L. He is still being closely monitored by his urologist, and all chemotherapy, radiotherapy or surgery is on hold, unless his PSA levels rise again.

Male infertility

Infertility affects about one fifth of American couples, and many complicated factors play a role. Ovulatory dysfunction accounts for 20% of cases, tubal dysfunction for 30% and

[4] A flexible tube and viewing device (cystoscope) is passed through the urethra

abnormal cervical mucus for 5%. These are all female problems. However, sperm (male) disorders explain the infertility in 35% of the cases. The problem may be low sperm count or another abnormality of the sperm, such as impaired motility (ability to swim).

A growing body of evidence implies that oxidative stress causes sperm cells to lose their function. Because they are highly active, they generate excessive levels of reactive oxygen molecules that can damage their own cell walls through lipid peroxidation (oxidation of fatty substances), leading to poor motility and impaired ability to fuse with the female's ova (egg). This evidence opens the door to innovative treatments of male infertility.

Patients with idiopathic[5] male infertility were compared to fertile volunteers by measuring oxidative stress, antioxidant activity and glutathione levels. The Urologist Alkan and his team found significant differences among all parameters of both groups, supporting the idea that oxidation may cause infertility. Similar studies conducted by Ochsendorf at the Center of Dermatology and Andrology in Germany also support these findings. Researchers have even measured glutathione activity in semen and seminal fluid, demonstrating significant differences between fertile and infertile men.

There is also good reason to divide infertile males into subgroups. Several studies have reported that overweight infertile men have particularly low GSH levels. Glutathione deficiency has already been well documented in overweight individuals, and infertility in the obese may have this common link.

As we get better at deciphering the human genome, genetic abnormalities in GSH enzyme activity are easier to identify. Several of these are strongly correlated to male infertility, adding strength to the GSH-infertility connection.

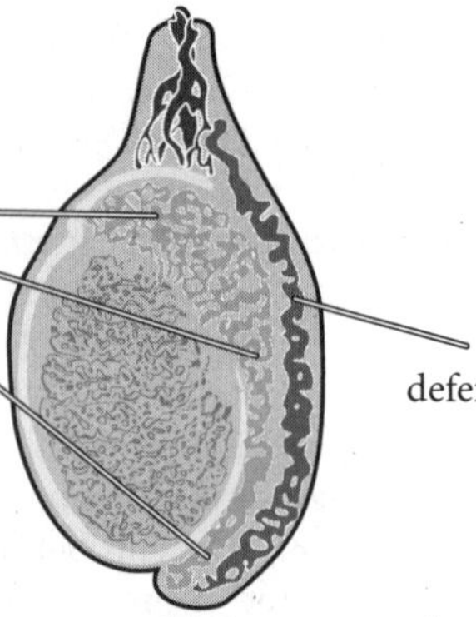

FIGURE 43: Adult human testicle

In Scotland, a group of reproductive biology scientists led by the Edinburgh-based researcher Irvine is raising GSH levels in infertile male patients. In his paper, "Glutathione for male infertility," he says that GSH seems to act at the epididymis (see Figure 41) and during sperm formation, and also improves the function of ejaculated spermatozoa. A German team headed by Oeda experimented with NAC (N-acetylcysteine), showing that it reduced oxidative stress and improved impaired sperm function.

Lenzi's team at the University Laboratory of Seminology and Reproduction in Rome has published many papers on the use of injectable GSH in a variety of infertile males. These were human, double-blind, cross-over studies and the therapy had consistently positive effects on sperm motility, morphology (structure), and semen quality.

Writing in the journal Urology, Ciftci's team reported improved semen parameters using the glutathione precursor NAC. Beneficial results were seen in the volume, motility and viscosity of the subjects' ejaculate.

Balding & hair loss

Human hair varies widely in texture, color, thickness and distribution. It is a sensitive tissue, prone to loss or balding (alopecia). Alopecia universalis is a rare autoimmune condition of total body hair loss. Alopecia areata is loss of hair in patches. Toxic

[5] "Cause unknown"

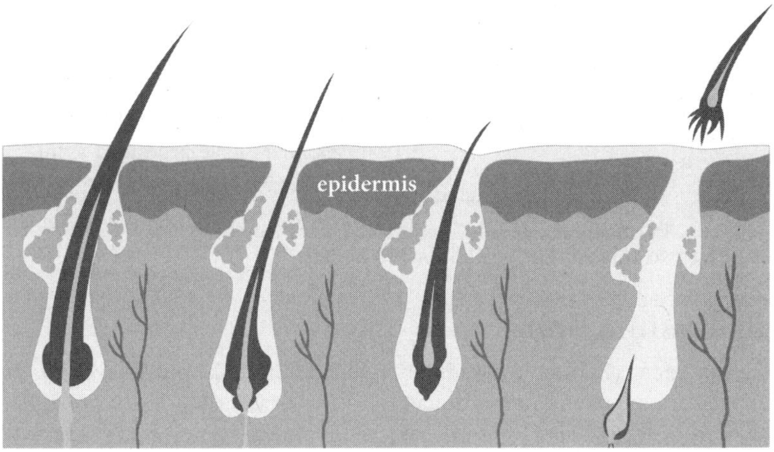

FIGURE 44: *The four phases of hair growth*

alopecia, a common cause of hair loss, is usually temporary, triggered by serious illness, fever, pregnancy, various drugs (especially those used in chemotherapy) or overdoses of vitamin A. The most common cause of hair loss is male-pattern baldness (androgenic alopecia), which varies in pattern and severity.

Normal hair grows in cycles. Anagen is the active growing phase, catagen is a brief phase of slow growth, and telogen is a resting dormant phase, where hair falls out—hopefully to be replaced in the next anagen phase. See Figure 42.

Close examination of blood samples as well as scalp tissue has shown that oxidative stress contributes to various forms of hair loss, including male pattern baldness. Abnormalities have even been found in hair progenitor[6] cells of bald men, which seem less able than their hairier counterparts to handle oxidative stress.

Testing the theory that free radical formation contributes to male pattern baldness, researchers have shown a positive correlation between GSH content and the percentage of anagen hairs in a scalp sample, concluding that glutathione helps maintain the hair growth cycle. Balding skin revealed twice as many breakdown products of oxidative stress, while hairy skin contained three times as much glutathione.

In male-pattern baldness, androgens (male hormones) target hair follicles. Upon reaching them, they're converted into even stronger hormones. The unfortunate result is that hair growth slows or stops. The researcher Sawaya at the University of Miami showed that the conversion of these hormones can be influenced by glutathione, suggesting that GSH could play a protective role.

Age-related GSH decline in human hair follicles is part of the total body glutathione depletion described in Chapter 6 (Aging). Working at the L'Oréal Research Laboratory in France, Kermici and his team measured follicular GSH activity in men and women ranging in age from 19 to 102 years. They found a significant decline up until about age seventy, followed by a slower, second decline.

For cancer patients, a distressing side effect of chemotherapy is hair loss. The cells of hair follicles (like those of the intestinal lining)

[6] Cells destined to become hair cells, but not yet hair.

are fast-growing and highly sensitive to the chemo-toxins that trigger rapid hair loss and also cause diarrhea and cramps. Elevated GSH levels help protect these cells from chemotherapeutic agents and diminish their side-effects.

For example, the action of the drug doxorubicin, a skin-cancer treatment, is aided in at least two ways by the glutathione precursor NAC. This enhances the tumor-killing effectiveness of the drug, and also completely prevents the hair loss that normally accompanies this treatment. Other researchers have produced similar hair-protective effects using NAC with cyclophosphamide and cytarabine, two other anti-cancer agents.

Erectile Dysfunction

Erectile dysfunction (ED) is a condition making an erection impossible or inadequate for intercourse. It is also known as "impotence."

Occasional ED is quite common, and can result from a number of psychological and physiological factors. However, recurrent or chronic ED warrants medical investigation for underlying causes. Medical problems leading to erectile dysfunction include high blood pressure, cardiovascular disease, high cholesterol levels, diabetes, alcohol abuse, obesity and more. All these preconditions are amenable to medical treatment. Also, drugs such as Viagra have revolutionized ED treatment. These generally act by increasing blood flow to the organ involved.

The relationship between oxidative stress and erectile dysfunction has been under investigation since the turn of the century. Indicators of oxidative stress—including GSH deficiency—are commonly found in this condition.

In the aptly titled article, "Oxygen free radicals and the penis," Jones and his group review existing literature and conclude that antioxidants may benefit both short-term and long-term ED patients. Portuguese researchers led by Castel have gone as far as placing patients on NAC, as a way to improve certain parameters found in ED.

Conclusion

Oxidative damage and low glutathione levels have been implicated in the onset and development of many prostate problems, including cancer. GSH supplementation may provide protection against carcinogenesis in this gland, or at least slow down its growth. Male infertility is associated with increased oxidative stress and low GSH levels. Elevated GSH levels may enhance the quality of sperm and increase fertility. Glutathione also feeds hair follicles and may prevent or delay hair loss, especially that suffered as a side-effect of chemotherapy. Erectile dysfunction too is marked by oxidative stress and glutathione deficiency, and may be helped by elevated glutathione levels.

GLUTATHIONE IN MEN

REFERENCES

AITKEN RJ. *A free radical theory of male infertility.* Reprod. Fertil. Dev. 6: 19-23, 1994

AKAR A, ARCA E, ERBIL H, ET AL. *Antioxidant enzymes & lipid peroxidation in the scalp of patients with alopecia areata.* J Dermatol Sci. 29: 85-90, 2002

ALDEMIR M, OKULU E, NESELIOGLU S, ET AL. *Evaluation of serum oxidative & antioxidative status in patients with erectile dysfunction.* Andrologia 44: 266-271, 2012

ALKAN I, SIMSEK F, HAKLAR G, ET AL. *Reactive oxygen species production by the spermatozoa of patients with idiopathic infertility: relationship to seminal plasma antioxidants.* J. Urology 157: 140-143, 1997

Avdin A, Arsova-Sarafinovska Z, Sayal A, et al. *Oxidative stress & antioxidant status in non-metastatic prostate cancer & benign prostatic hyperplasia.* Clin Biochem. 39 : 176-179, 2006

Bell DA, Taylor JA, Paulson DF, et al. *Genetic risk & carcinogen exposure: a common inherited defect of the carcinogen-metabolism gene glutathione S-transferase M1 (GSTM1) that increases susceptibility to bladder cancer.* J. Natl. Cancer Inst. 85: 1159-1164, 1993

Cai Q, Wang Z, Zhang W, et al. *Association between glutathione S-transferases M1 & T1 gene polymorphisms & prostate cancer risk: a systematic review & meta-analysis.* Tumour Biol. 35: 247-256, 2014

Cai Q, Wu T, Zhang W, et al. *Genetic polymorphisms in glutathione S-transferases P1 (GSTP1) Ile105Val & prostate cancer risk: a systematic review & meta-analysis.* Tumour Biol. 34: 3913-3922, 2013

Castela A, Gomes P, Domingues VF, et al. *Role of oxidative stress-induced systemic & cavernosal molecular alterations in the progression of diabetic erectile dysfunction.* J Diabetes. 7: 393-401, 2015

Childs S, Haroune N, Williams L, et al. *Determination of cellular glutathione: glutathione disulfide ratio in prostate cancer cells by high performance liquid chromatography with electrochemical detection.* J Chromatogr A. 1437: 67-73, 2016

Choubey VK, Sankhwar SN, Tewari R, et al. *Null genotypes at the GSTM1 & GSTT1 genes & the risk of benign prostatic hyperplasia: a case-control study & a meta-analysis.* Prostate 73: 146-152, 2013

Ciftci H, Verit A, Savas M, et al. *Effects of N-acetylcysteine on semen parameters & oxidative/antioxidant status.* Urology 74: 73-76, 2009

Cimino S, Favilla V, Russo GI, et al. *Oxidative stress & body composition in prostate cancer & benign prostatic hyperplasia patients.* Anticancer Res. 34: 5051-5056, 2014

Clark LC, Combs GF Jr, Turnbull BW, et al. *Effects of selenium supplementation for cancer prevention in patients with carcinoma of the skin. A randomized controlled trial.* Nutritional Prevention of Cancer Study Group. JAMA 276: 1957-1963, 1996

Clark LC, Dalkin B, Krongrad A, et al. *Decreased incidence of prostate cancer with selenium supplementation: results of a double-blind cancer prevention trial.* Br. J. Urol. 81: 730-734, 1998

Combs GF Jr, Clark LC, Turnbull BW. *Reduction of cancer risk with an oral supplement of selenium.* Biomed. Environ. Sci. 10: 227-234, 1997

Combs GF Jr, Clark LC, Turnbull BW. *Reduction of cancer mortality & incidence by selenium supplementation.* Med. Klin. 92 (Suppl 3): 42-45, 1997

Cookson MS, Reuter VE, Linkov I, et al. *Glutathione S-transferase PI (GST-pi) class expression by immunohistochemistry in benign & malignant prostate tissue.* J. Urol. 157: 673-676, 1997

D'Agostini F, Bagnasco M, Giunciuglio D, et al. *Inhibition by oral n-acetylcysteine of doxorubicin-induced clastogenicity & alopecia, & prevention of primary tumors & lung metastases in mice.* International J. Oncology 13: 217-224, 1998

De Marzo AM, Coffey DS, Nelson WG. *New concepts in tissue specificity for prostate cancer & benign prostatic hyperplasia.* Urology 53 (3 Suppl 3a): 29-39, 1999

Drevet JR. *The antioxidant glutathione peroxidase family & spermatozoa: a complex story.* Mol Cell Endocrinol. 250: 70-79, 2006

Eichholzer M, Steinbrecher A, Kaaks R, et al. *Effects of selenium status, dietary glucosinolate intake & serum glutathione S-transferase α activity on the risk of benign prostatic hyperplasia.* BJU Int. 110: E879-885, 2012

Garrido N, Meseguer M, Alvarez J, et al. *Relationship among standard semen parameters, glutathione peroxidase/glutathione reductase activity, & mRNA expression & reduced glutathione content in ejaculated spermatozoa from fertile & infertile men.* Fertil Steril. 82:1059-1066, 2004

Giralt M, Cervello I, Nogues MR, et al. *Glutathione, glutathione S-transferase & reactive oxygen species of human scalp sebaceous glands in male pattern baldness.* J. Invest. Dermatol. 107: 154-158, 1996

Gopalakrishnan B, Aravinda S, Pawshe CH, et al. *Studies on glutathione S-transferees important for sperm function: evidence for catalytic activity-independent functions.* Biochem. J. 15: 231-241, 1998

Griveau JS, Le Lannou D. *Reactive oxygen species & human spermatozoa: physiology & pathology.* Int. J. Androl. 20: 61-69, 1997

Hardell L, Degerman A, Tomic R, et al. *Levels of selenium in plasma & glutathione peroxidase in erythrocytes in patients with prostate cancer or benign hyperplasia.* Eur J Cancer Prev. 4 : 91-95, 1995

Harries LW, Stubbins MJ, Forman D, et al. *Identification of genetic polymorphisms at the glutathione S-transferase Pi locus & association with susceptibility to bladder, testicular & prostate cancer.* Carcinogenesis 18: 641-644, 1997

Hou BS, Wang ZD, Shang XJ. *Glutathione & male reproduction.* Zonghua Nan Ke Xue, 14: 1023-1026, 2008

Irvine DS. *Glutathione as a treatment for male infertility.* Rev. Reprod. 1:6-12, 1996

JIMINEZ JJ, HUANG HS, YUNIS AA. *Treatment with ImuVert/n-acetylcysteine protects rats from cyclophosphamide and/or cytarabine-induced alopecia.* Cancer Investig. 10: 271-276, 1992

JONES RW, REES RW, MINHAS S, ET AL. *Oxygen free radicals & the penis.* Expert Opin Pharmacother. 3:889-897, 2002

JUNG K, SEIDEL B, RUDOLPH B, ET AL. *Antioxidant enzymes in malignant prostate cell lines & in primary cultured prostatic cells.* Free Radic. Biol. Med. 23: 127-133, 1997

KANDAR R, HAJKOVA N. *Assay of total glutathione & glutathione disulphide in seminal plasma of male partners of couples presenting for a fertility evaluation.* Andrologia. 46: 1079-1088, 2014

KERMICI M, PRUCHE F, ROGUET R, PRUNIERAS M. *Evidence for an age-correlated change in glutathione metabolism enzyme activities in human hair follicle.* Mech. Aging Dev. 53: 73-84, 1990

KHANDRIKA L, KUMAR B, KOUL S, ET AL. *Oxidative stress in prostate cancer.* Cancer Lett. 282: 125-136, 2009

KOLESNIKOVA LI, KURASHOVA NA, BAIROVA TA, ET AL. *Role of Glutathione-S-Transferase Family Genes in Male Infertility.* Bull Exp Biol Med. 163: 643-645, 2017

KOLESNIKOVA LI, VANTEEVA OA, KURASHOVA NA, ET AL. *[Glutathione-dependent enzymes & glutathione in infertility of men with different body mass].* Vestn Ross Akad Med Nauk. 1:12-6, 2015

KOLESNIKOVA LI, VANTEEVA OA, KURASHOVA NA, ET AL. *[Glutathione as an important component of thiosulfid system of infertility pathogenesis in overweight men].* Vestn Ross Akad Med Nauk. 7: 9-12, 2013

KUMAR V, YADAV CS, DATTA SK, ET AL. *Association of GSTM1 & GSTT1 polymorphism with lipid peroxidation in benign prostate hyperplasia & prostate cancer: a pilot study.* Dis Markers. 30: 163-169. 2011

LENZI A, CULASSO F, GANDINI L, ET AL. *Placebo-controlled, double blind, cross-over trial of glutathione therapy in male infertility.* Human Reproduction 8: 1657-1662, 1993

LENZI A, GANDINI L, PICARDO M. *A rationale for glutathione therapy.* Human Reproduction 13: 1419-1422, 1998

LENZI A, LOMBARDO F, GANDINI L, ET AL. *Glutathione therapy for male infertility.* Arch. Androl. 29: 65-68, 1992

LENZI A, PICARDO M, GANDINI L, ET AL. *Glutathione treatment of dyspermia: effect on the lipoperoxidation process.* Human Reproduction 9: 2044-2050, 1994

LIEBMAN B. *Clues to prostate cancer.* Nutr. Action Lett. 3: 10-12, 1996

LIU D, LIU Y, RAN L, ET AL. *GSTT1 & GSTM1 polymorphisms & prostate cancer risk in Asians: a systematic review & meta-analysis.* Tumour Biol. 34: 2539-2544, 2013

MOSKALUK CA, DURAY PH, COWAN KH, ET AL. *Immunohistochemical expression of pi-class glutathione S-transferase is down-regulated in adenocarcinoma of the prostate.* Cancer 79: 1595-1599, 1997

MURAKOSHI M, TAGAWA M, INADA R, ET AL. *Inhibition of steroid-induced prostatic hyperplasia in rats by treatment with anti-androgen (TZP-4238).* Endocr. J. 40: 479-488, 1993

NAZIROGLU M, KOKCAM I. *Antioxidants & lipid peroxidation status in the blood of patients with alopecia.* Cell Biochem Funct. 18: 169-173, 2000

OCHSENDORF FR, BUHL R, BASTLEIN A, BESCHMANN H. *Glutathione in spermatozoa & seminal plasma of infertile men.* Human Reproduction 13: 353-359, 1998

OEDA T, HENKLE R, OHMORI H, SCHILL WB. *Scavenging effect of N-acetyl-L-cysteine against reactive oxygen species in human semen: a possible therapeutic modality for male factor infertility?* Andrologia 29: 125-131, 1997

OH B, FIGTREE G, COSTA D, ET AL. *Oxidative stress in prostate cancer patients: A systematic review of case control studies.* Prostate Int. 4: 71-87, 2016

PRIE BE, IOSIF L, TIVIG I, ET AL. *Oxidative stress in androgenetic alopecia.* J Med Life. 9: 79-83, 2016

PUERTO AM, NOGUES MR, CERVELLO I, ET AL. *Glutathione S-transferase in normal human anagen hair follicles.* Rev. Esp. Fisiol. 50: 103-108, 1994

RIPPLE MO, HENRY WF, RAGO RP, WILDING G. *Prooxidant-antioxidant shift induced by androgen treatment of human prostate carcinoma cells.* J. Natl. Cancer Instit. 89: 40-48, 1997

ROUMEGUÈRE T, VAN ANTWERPEN P, FATHI H, ET AL. *Relationship between oxidative stress & erectile function.* Free Radic Res. 51: 924-931, 2017

SAFARINEJAD MR, SHAFIEI N, SAFARINEJAD S. *The association of glutathione-S-transferase gene polymorphisms (GSTM1, GSTT1, GSTP1) with idiopathic male infertility.* J Hum Genet. 55: 565-570, 2010

SAWAYA ME. *Purification of androgen receptors in human sebocytes & hair.* J. Investig.Dermaotol. 98 (6 Suppl.): 92S-96S, 1992

SHEWEITA S, SALAMA B, HASSAN M. *Erectile dysfunction drugs & oxidative stress in the liver of male rats.* Toxicol Rep. 2: 933-938, 2015

SIKKA SC. *Oxidative stress & role of antioxidants in normal & abnormal sperm function.* Front. Biosci. 1:e78-86, 1996

SIKKA SC, RAJASEKARAN M, HELLSTROM WJ. *Role of oxidative stress & antioxidants in male infertility.* J. Androl. 16: 464-481, 1995

Storey BT. *Biochemistry of the induction & prevention of lipoperoxidative damage in human spermatozoa.* Mol. Human Reproduction 3: 203-213, 1997

Tagliabue M, Pinach S, Di Bisceglie C, et al. *Glutathione levels in patients with erectile dysfunction, with or without diabetes mellitus.* Int J Androl. 28: 156-162, 2005

Taguchi Y. *Current strategies in managing prostate cancer.* Can. J. CME. :107-115, 1997

Tew KD, Clapper ML, Greenberg RE, et al. *Glutathione S-transferases in human prostate. Biochim. Biophys. Acta 926: 8-15, 1987*

Tuncayengin A, Biri H, Onaran M, et al. *Cavernosal tissue nitrite, nitrate, malondialdehyde & glutathione levels in diabetic & non-diabetic erectile dysfunction.* Int. J Androl. 26: 250-254, 2003

Upton JH, Hannen RF, Bahta AW, et al. *Oxidative stress-associated senescence in dermal papilla cells of men with androgenetic alopecia.* J Invest Dermatol. 135: 1244-1252, 2015

Ustundag-Budak Y, Sambel M, Alisik M, et al. *Thiol/disulphide homeostasis levels in erectile dysfunction patients.* Andrologia. 49: doi:10.1111/&. 12695, 2017

Van Neste L, Herman JG, Otto G, et al. *The epigenetic promise for prostate cancer diagnosis.* Prostate. 72: 1248-1261, 2012

Winter ML, Liehr JG. *Possible mechanism of induction of benign prostatic hyperplasia by estradiol & dihydrotestosterone in dogs* Toxicol. Appl. Pharmacol. 136: 211-219, 1996

Yenin JZ, Serarslan G, Yonden Z, et al. *Investigation of oxidative stress in patients with alopecia areata & its relationship with disease severity, duration, recurrence & pattern.* Clin Exp Dermatol. 40: 617-621, 2015

Yoshizawa K, et al. *Study of prediagnostic selenium level in toenails & the risk of advanced prostate cancer.* J. Natl. Cancer Inst. 90: 1219-1224, 1998

Yu B, Huang Z. *Variations in Antioxidant Genes & Male Infertility.* Biomed Res Int. doi:10.1155/2015/513196, 2015

Zachara BA, Szewczyk-Golec K, Tyloch J, et al. *Blood & tissue selenium concentrations & glutathione peroxidase activities in patients with prostate cancer & benign prostate hyperplasia.* Neoplasma. 52: 248-254, 2005

Zalata A, Hafez T, Comhaire F. *Evaluation of the role of reactive oxygen species in male infertility.* Human Reproduction 10: 1444-1451, 1995

Zhang W, Joseph E, Hitchcock C, et al. *Selenium glycinate supplementation increases blood glutathione peroxidase activities & decreases prostate-specific antigen readings in middle-aged US men.* Nutr Res. 31: 165-168, 2011

Zhou TB, Drummen GP, Jiang ZP, et al. *GSTT1 polymorphism & the risk of developing prostate cancer.* Am J Epidemiol. 180: 1-10, 2014

Zhu D, Deng Y, Pan Y, et al. *N-acetylcysteine Ameliorates the Erectile Dysfunction Caused by Chronic Intermittent Hypoxia in Rats:* Partly Involvement of Endoplasmic Reticulum Stress. Urology. 86: 844.e7-844.e14, 2015

21
Trauma, Burns & Critical Care Medicine

Trauma refers to any sort of injury, whether the emotional trauma of divorce or the physical trauma of a broken hip. In this chapter, we will talk mostly of physical trauma—although emotional trauma is known to deplete glutathione too. Motor vehicle accidents, work injuries and falls are common examples of accidental trauma. Intentional traumas include everything from gunshot wounds to surgical procedures.

Burns may be caused by heat, chemicals or radiation. Radiation burns are discussed in Chapter 2, and sunburn and UV (ultraviolet) burns in Chapter 22.

Glutathione, antioxidant protection, immune defenses, and oxidative stress all play important roles in these conditions. High or low levels of GSH determine how susceptible or tolerant an injury site is, as well as the extent of injury, recovery time and outcome.

Physical trauma

Until this century, traumatic injury was the major cause of death in human beings. In North America today, trauma has fallen to third place behind heart disease/stroke and cancer, but in some economic groups—especially poor urban male populations—trauma is still front and center.

Any critical illness depletes glutathione reserves. Writing in the journal Critical Care Medicine, Hammarqvist demonstrated that intensive care patents suffered an approximate 40% loss of glutathione compared to healthy individuals. Kretzschmar from Germany followed patients with multiple injuries all the way through intensive care—from admission to discharge or death. He found that the more severe the injuries, the higher the degree of oxidative stress and depletion of glutathione defenses. An Irish team led by Kilty suggests the measurement of glutathione S-transferases could indicate the extent of general organ damage.

At Harvard Medical School, Robinson's team showed that lab animals artificially depleted of glutathione were dramatically more prone to death and complications of blood loss (hemorrhagic shock). These results suggest that treatment of trauma should include ways to maintain glutathione levels. This would decrease the likelihood of multi-system organ failure following shock.

There's been considerable research into the role of oxidative stress and glutathione metabolism in brain and neurological tissue injuries. Head injuries often result in damage to the crucial blood-brain barrier. Subsequent circulatory problems may lead to swelling and fluid buildup in the brain. Some of the complex "secondary injuries" seen in this type of trauma depend on the action of free radicals. In emergency and critical care management, preventing these post-injury complications is an essential part of the treatment.

Glutathione metabolism counteracts the damage caused by oxyradicals. It's well known that neurological trauma increases glutathione peroxidase activity. With severe or complicated injury, these resources may become depleted. Canadians Juurlink and Paterson of the University of Saskatchewan suggest that nutritional interventions with GSH-precursors maximize antioxidant defenses, and that such strategies should be pursued aggressively.

Ellis's team at the Department of Pharmacology and Toxicology, Medical College of Virginia, tested NAC on concussion after trauma to the brain. NAC given prior to or soon after injury prevented some of the consequences of oxidative circulatory compromise. At Ohio State University, Lucas and Wheeler did the same with spinal cord injury, using the GSH-precursors gamma-glutamyl-cysteine and OTZ (see Chapter 4). The resulting elevated glutathione levels increased the survival rate of neurons in the spinal cord.

In the medical journal "Pain," Wagner and Myers of the University of California developed an interesting therapy for nerve injury and sciatic inflammation. They were able to decrease the pathological consequences of sciatic nerve injury by using the drug NAC to raise GSH levels. Subjects who were treated in advance responded best, and it was noted that the longer the delay in administering NAC after injury, the less effective the treatment was.

Surgery is intrusive and disruptive. Patients undergo a host of physiological adjustments. Although from the surgeon's point of view this is a controlled procedure with clear objectives, from the body's point of view it is still trauma. Just like recovery from accidents, the success of an operation depends on the patient's prior defenses, fitness, and immune status.

One of the more hidden reasons surgery is traumatic is because it releases billions of free radicals into the body and severely taxes the patient's antioxidant defenses. Poor surgical outcomes tend to go hand-in-hand with low antioxidant levels. As the cell's primary intracellular antioxidant, glutathione is drawn from stores in the liver and skeletal muscles and dispersed to reduce general damage. This sometimes leads to whole-body glutathione depletion. Articles from the American Journal of Physiology as well as the Annals of Surgery describe a fall in glutathione levels of 40% after abdominal surgery, increasing the patient's susceptibility to cellular oxidative injury.

An increasingly familiar surgical device—the laparoscope—is a tube with a fiber optic cable, a cam and attachments for tools. Through it the surgeon can see and work inside even small body cavities. Procedures are carried out through small surgical holes in the patient's body. This reduces cutting, recovery time and hospital stays. The traumatic effects of conventional surgery are considerably greater than those of laparoscopic surgery. A team of Hungarian surgeons noted oxidative stress and GSH levels in two groups of patients undergoing gall-bladder removal—one with laparoscopic surgery and one without. The laparoscopic group showed much lower values of oxidation and GSH depletion than the open-surgery group.

GSH not only protects from oxidative stress, it also bolsters the immune response, controls and balances the inflammatory response and helps synthesize and repair proteins involved in the healing process. This understanding has stimulated research into the use of GSH-enhancing strategies to improve and accelerate wound repair.

Plastic surgeons from the University of Michigan, Ann Arbor showed that depleted glutathione levels slow wound healing and lead to poor repair. Biochemists from the Max Plank Institute in Germany showed that as skin wounds heal, they initially increase production of glutathione peroxidase in order to fight free radical formation. As healing progresses, GSH levels fall. Pharmacologists from the Central Drug Research Institute in India demonstrated a 60 to 70% depletion of glutathione peroxidase and glutathione S-transferase levels in skin wounds after several days healing. Also confirming these mechanisms at play, Van der Laan described in the Journal of Surgical Research how NAC[1] infusion reduced tissue injury and shortened the repair period of crush injuries.

As you would expect, surgery disrupts blood flow to tissues (ischemia). What is less appreciated is that when blood flow is reestablished (reperfusion), rapid oxidation leads to a burst of free radical formation—sometimes threatening the survival of affected tissues. The Australians Knight and MacPhadden found that the glutathione precursor NAC was able to decrease the amount of reperfusion injury in skin flaps. Potential applications are being investigated in cardiac surgery to avoid reperfusion injury (see Chapter 7).

Burns

Heat or thermal burns trigger a complex series of events that only begins with the initial injury. The body responds with physiological adjustments to circulatory/fluid changes, hematological/immunological responses and an elaborate healing process. Death from heat burns is often delayed. Patients may die from circulatory shock days after the original burn due to loss of fluids. Weeks after a burn, patients may succumb to overwhelming infection (sepsis) due to the breakdown of their immune defenses.

Burn specialists know that oxidative stress in severe burn patients is dramatically marked by consistently high lipid peroxide levels, considerable free radical damage and impaired activity of glutathione and its related enzymes. These findings have prompted researchers to use antioxidants against further damage.

A German team of pediatric surgeons conducted a two-year study on children with burns and severe inflammatory diseases. They managed to correct parameters of oxidative stress in these patients using selenium substitution (see Chapter 4) to raise glutathione peroxidase and proposed this as a good supportive therapy. Other nutritionists have increased selenium delivery through TPN (Total Parenteral Nutrition or intravenous nutrition), or through tube feeding, which supplies food directly to the stomach or intestines.

One phenomenon of the early post-burn period is low hemoglobin (red blood cell) count. Scientists have questioned why. A team from Varna Medical University showed that burns depleted the glutathione and antioxidant defenses of red blood cells, and that when the oxidative byproducts had accumulated sufficiently, these cells were destroyed. The team suggested that adequate antioxidant therapy at an early stage might prevent this complication.

A Japanese team led by Kasanuma from the Environmental Health Sciences Division of Tohuku University of Medicine investigated the effects of mild heat injury on oxidative stress. Rather than burning tissue, they exposed animals to mild chronic heat (35°C, 95°F), showing that it caused oxidative damage and that GSH-related anti-oxidative systems play an important role in defending against it.

A study published in the journal "Burns" by Konukoglu described the use of NAC as a burn treatment. With it, the research team was able to decrease levels of lipid peroxidation and increase GSH levels. Using antioxidant supplementation (GSH, vitamin C, and NAC) to raise glutathione levels, several Boston studies published in the Journal of Burn Care Rehabilitation and in the journal Shock, showed a reduction in the death rate from 60% to zero in animals suffering third degree burns. This is compelling evidence that oxidation contributes to post-burn mortality.

[1] A pharmaceutical GSH precursor.

Critical Care Medicine

Because of the complexity and severity of their problems, many patients suffering from severe or life-threatening illnesses are transferred to wards with a higher level of monitoring, treatment and support. They often arrive there via the emergency department after initial stabilization, or from the surgical suites, or because their health has deteriorated. All are considered to be in "critical" condition.

The units that attend to these critically ill patients go by several names: CCU (critical care unit), ICU (intensive care unit), ITU (intensive treatment unit) and others. Some are highly specialized such as the NICU (neonatal intensive care unit) for newborns, PICU (pediatric intensive care unit) for children and the CICU (cardiac/coronary intensive care unit) for heart patients. Other specialized units are designed for burns, traumas and more.

The disorders commonly treated in critical care include cardiac instability, major trauma, respiratory distress, overwhelming infection (sepsis), multiple organ failure, severe burns and others. Patients said to be "on life support," are generally in the ICU.

One key feature relatively unaddressed in these patients is the prevalence of glutathione depletion. As you will see from the research below, this is being increasingly highlighted.

Many years of study have revealed a predictable glutathione deficiency in ICU patients. In several papers Swedish doctors from the Karolinska University have described how GSH levels change over time. Following patients with multiple organ failure, they noted within one week of standard treatment a significant increase in muscle glutathione levels as patients recovered.

This same team also investigated children in a pediatric intensive care unit. Their glutathione status correlated directly with the length of time they spent in the ICU, their dependency on mechanical breathing (life support), and multiple organ failure. GSH deficiency in pediatric ICU patients has been noted in several other childhood pathologies, including sepsis (overwhelming infection), and other critical illnesses.

Adults with ARDS (Adult Respiratory Distress Syndrome) are also known to suffer from seriously compromised antioxidant levels. Another less understood syndrome that appears in severely ill individuals is SIRS (Systemic Inflammatory Response Syndrome). South American researchers in Uruguay found that patients in the ICU with the lowest selenium and glutathione status were most likely to develop SIRS.

Several independent studies investigated whether glutathione status could predict death. Karapetsa and his team investigating sepsis patients identified persistent GSH deficiency in patients who died, and found that GSH levels recovered in survivors. Morgensen's group showed the same correlation but went further, demonstrating that this relationship was also linked to malnutrition, suggesting that nutritional status is critical to survival. Finally, a study involving over 200 patients admitted to the ICU concluded that, "glutathione redox status was an independent mortality predictor." Put simply, Rodas and his team found that a person's GSH level on admission could determine whether the patient would leave the ICU alive.

This startling information begs the question—can raising glutathione status influence the ultimate outcome of these patients? The answer appears to be—yes!

Using the glutathione precursor NAC (N-acetylcysteine), Iranian physicians significantly decreased mortality in ARDS[2] patients—especially those with underlying GSH-enzyme defects. French intensive care specialists similarly gave either GSH or NAC to septic shock patients, who improved too. A German team used a slightly different approach. In a multicenter, randomized,

[2] Acute respiratory distress syndrome.

placebo-controlled trial, they gave selenium to patients of sepsis, septic shock and ARDS. As discussed in chapter 4, the major biochemical role of selenium is its integration into the enzyme glutathione peroxidase. This was corroborated by measurable improvements in both selenium and glutathione levels. They concluded that their intervention successfully reduced mortality rates.

Conclusion

Surgery, burns, trauma and shock are all complex events, consisting of a series of biochemical, anatomical, physiological and immune responses. Oxidative stress and the release of free radicals are an inevitable part of the initial injury as well as the subsequent inflammatory reactions and the healing processes. Glutathione, an integral part of our body's mechanism to minimize damage and promote healing, acts both as an antioxidant and to support the immune system, both of which can speed up recovery.

The value of antioxidant supplementation and nutritional support has been underestimated in the past but as new approaches are developed, attitudes are changing. Strategies to maintain or increase glutathione enzyme systems have shown their worth in preliminary trials and promise significant benefit in the treatment of major trauma, surgery and burn management protocols.

Patients admitted to intensive care units often suffer from decreased glutathione status. Low GSH correlates with longer hospital stays, more complications and death. Intervention with glutathione improvement strategies improves these outcomes.

TRAUMA, BURNS & CRITICAL CARE MEDICINE

REFERENCES

Adamson B, Schwarz D, Klugston P, et al. *Delayed repair: the role of glutathione in a rat incisional wound model.* J. Surg. Res. 62: 159-164, 1996

Angstwurm MW, Engelmann L, Zimmermann T, et al. *Selenium in Intensive Care (SIC): results of prospective randomized, placebo-controlled, multiple-center study in patients with severe systemic inflammatory response syndrome, sepsis, & septic shock.* Crit Care Med. 35: 118-126, 2007

Bar-Or D, Bar-Or R, Rael LT, et al. *Oxidative stress in severe acute illness.* Redox biol. 4: 340-345, 2015

Bekyarova G, Yankova T, Marinov M. *Lipofuscin product accumulation, insufficient antioxidant defense in erythrocytes & plasma & enhanced susceptibility to oxidative haemolysis after thermal trauma.* Acta Chir. Plast. 39: 60-64, 1997

Berger MM, Soguel L, Shenkin A, et al. *Influence of early antioxidant supplements on clinical evolution & organ function in critically ill cardiac surgery, major trauma, & subarachnoid hemorrhage patients.* Crit Care. 12: R101.doi:10.1186/cc6981, 2008

Bienkowski W, Gromadzinska J, Powlowicz Z, et al. *Concentrations of selenium & lipid peroxides & glutathione peroxidase activities in plasma of thermally injured pigs.* Acta Chir. Plast. 33: 126-132, 1991

Biolo G, Massolino B, Di Girolamo FG, et al. *Intensive insulin therapy increases glutathione synthesis rate in surgical ICU patients with stress hyperglycemia.* PLoS One. 13:e0190291, 2018

Borner J, Zimmermann T, Albrecht S, et al. *Selenium administration in severe inflammatory surgical diseases & burns in childhood.* Med. Klin. 92 (Suppl 3): 17-19, 1997

Brancaccio P, Lippi G, Maffulli N. *Biochemical markers of muscular damage.* Clin Chem Lab Med. 48: 757-767, 2010

Buz A, Görgülü T, Olgun A, et al. *Efficacy of glutathione mesotherapy in burns: an experimental study.* Eur J Trauma Emerg Surg. 42: 775-783, 2016

Costa NA, Gut AL, Pimentel JA, et al. *Erythrocyte selenium concentration predicts intensive care unit & hospital mortality in patients with septic shock: a prospective observational study.* Crit Care 18: R92. doi: 10.1186/cc13860.

CSONTOS C, REZMAN B, FOLDI V, ET AL. *Effect of N-acetylcysteine treatment on the expression of leukocyte surface markers after burn injury.* Burns. 37: 453-464, 2011

CSONTOS C, REZMAN B, FOLDI V, ET AL. *Effect of N-acetylcysteine treatment on oxidative stress & inflammation after severe burn.* Burns: 38: 428-437, 2012

DYLEWSKI ML, BENDER JC, SMITH AM, ET AL. *The selenium status of pediatric patients with burn injuries.* J Trauma. 69: 584-588, 2010

ELLIS EF, DODSON LY, POLICE RJ. *Restoration of cerebrovascular responsiveness to hyperventilation by the oxygen radical scavenger n-acetylcysteine following experimental traumatic brain injury.* J. Neurosurg. 75: 774-779, 1991

EROGLU A. *The effect of intravenous alanyl-glutamine supplementation on plasma glutathione levels in intensive care unit trauma patients receiving enteral nutrition: the results of a randomized controlled trial.* Anesth Analg. 109: 502-505, 2009

FLÄRING UB, ROOYACKERS OE, WERNERMAN J, ET AL. *Glutamine attenuates post-traumatic glutathione depletion in human muscle.* Clin Sci (Lond). 104: 275-282, 2003

FLÄRING UB, ROOYACKERS OE, WERNERMAN J, ET AL. *Temporal changes in muscle glutathione in ICU patients.* Intensive Care Med. 29: 2193-2198, 2003

FLÄRING UB, ROOYACKERS OE, HEBERT C, ET AL. *Temporal changes in whole-blood & plasma glutathione in ICU patients with multiple organ failure.* Intensive Care Med. 31: 1072-1078, 2005

FLÄRING U, EKMARK L, WERNERMAN J, ET AL. *Whole blood glutathione status & ICU morbidity in critically ill children.* Acta Anaesthesiol Scand. 59: 1311-1318, 2015

FOLDI V, CSONTOS C, BOGAR L, ET AL. *Effects of fluid resuscitation methods on burn trauma-induced oxidative stress.* J Burn Care Res. 30: 957-966, 2009

FRIŠMAN E, RÁCZ O, CHMELÁROVÁ A. *Red cell antioxidant enzymes & prognostic indexes in patients with burns.* Burns. 39: 458-464, 2013

GAL I, ROTH E, LANTOS J, ET AL. *Inflammatory mediators & surgical trauma regarding laparoscopic access: free radical mediated reactions.* Acta Chir. Hung. 36: 97-99, 1997

GÄRTNER R, ALBRICH W, ANGSTWURM MW. *The effect of a selenium supplementation on the outcome of patients with severe systemic inflammation, burn & trauma.* Biofactors. 14: 199-204, 2001

GIDDAY JM, BEETSCH JW, PARK TS. *Endogenous glutathione protects cerebral endothelial cells from traumatic injury.* J. Neurotrauma. 16: 27-36, 1999

GILMONT RR, DARDANO A, YOUNG M, ET AL. *Effects of glutathione depletion on oxidant-induced endothelial cell injury.* J. Surg. Res. 80: 62-68, 1998

GOSS JR, TAFFE KM, KOCHANEK PM, ET AL. *The antioxidant enzymes glutathione peroxidase & catalase increase following traumatic brain injury in the rat.* Exp. Neurol. 146: 291-294, 1997

HAMMARQVIST F, LUO JL, COTGREAVE IA, ET AL. *Skeletal muscle glutathione is depleted in critically ill patients.* Crit. Care Med. 25: 78-84, 1997

HORTON JW. *Free radicals & lipid peroxidation mediated injury in burn trauma:* the role of antioxidant therapy. Toxicology. 189: 75-88, 2003

HUANG YX, ZHAN XH, LIU SK, ET AL. *[Effect of reduced glutathione on impairment of hepatic function after delayed resuscitation of severe burn shock].* Zhongguo Wei Zhong Bing Ji Jiu Yi Xue. 21: 92-94, 2009

HUET O, CHERREAU C, NICCO C, ET AL. *Pivotal role of glutathione depletion in plasma-induced endothelial oxidative stress during sepsis.* Crit Care Med. 36: 2328-2334, 2008

HUNT DR, LANE HW, BEESINGER D, ET AL. *Selenium depletion in burn patients. JPEN J. Parenter. Enterel.* Nutr. 8: 695-699, 1984

JUURLINK BH, PATERSON PG. *Review of oxidative stress in brain & spinal cord injury: suggestions for pharmacological & nutritional management strategies.* J. Spinal Cord Med. 21: 309-334, 1998

KARAPETSA M, PITSIKA M, GOUTZOURELAS N, ET AL. *Oxidative status in ICU patients with septic shock.* Food Chem Toxicol. 61: 106-111,2013

KASANUMA Y, WATANABE C, KIM CY, ET AL. *Effects of mild chronic heat exposure on the concentrations of thiobarbituric acid reactive substances, glutathione, & selenium, & glutathione peroxidase activity in the mouse liver.* Tohoku J. Exp. Med. 185: 79-87, 1998

KERB R, BROCKMOLLER J, SCHLAGENHAUFER R, ET AL. *Influence of GSTT1 & GSTM1 genotypes on sunburn sensitivity.* Am J Pharmacogenomics. 2: 147-154, 2002

KILTY C, DOYLE S, HASSETT B, ET AL. *Glutathione S-transferases as biomarkers of organ damage: applications of rodent & canine GST enzyme immunoassays.* Chem. Biol. Interact. 111: 123-135, 1998

KNIGHT KR, MACPHADYEN K, LEPORE DA, ET AL. *Enhancement of ischaemic rabbit skin flap survival with the antioxidant & free-radical scavenger n-acetylcysteine.* Clin. Sci. (Colch) 81: 31-36, 1991

KONUKOGLU D, CETINKALE O, BULAN R. *Effects of n-acetylcysteine on lung glutathione levels in rats after burn injury.* Burns 23: 541-544, 1997

KRETZSCHMAR M, PFEIFFER L, SCHMIDT C, ET AL. *Plasma levels of glutathione, alpha-tocopherol & lipid peroxides in polytraumatized patients; evidence for a stimulating effect of TNF alpha on glutathione synthesis.* Exp. Toxicol. Pathol. 50: 477-483, 1998

LaLonde C, Hennigan J, Nayak U, et al. *Energy charge potential & glutathione levels as predictors of outcome following burn injury complicated by endotoxemia.* Shock 9: 27-32, 1998

LaLonde C, Nayak U, Hennigan J, et al. *Excessive liver oxidant stress causes mortality in response to burn injury combined with endotoxin & is prevented with antioxidants.* Burn Care Rehabil. 18: 187-192, 1997

LaLonde C, Nayak U, Hennigan J, et al. *Antioxidants prevent the cellular deficit produced in response to burn injury.* J. Burn Care Rehabil. 17: 379-383, 1996

Lucas JH, Wheeler DG, Emery DG, et al. *The endogenous antioxidant glutathione as a factor in the survival of physically injured mammalian spinal cord neurons. J. Neuropathol.* Exp. Neurol. 57: 937-954, 1998

Luo JL, Hammarqvist F, Andersson K, et al. *Surgical trauma decreases glutathione synthetic capacity in human skeletal muscle tissue.* Am. J. Physiol. 275: E359-365, 1998

Luo JL, Hammarqvist F, Andersson K, et al. *Skeletal muscle glutathione after surgical trauma.* Ann. Surg. 223: 420-427, 1996

Lyons J, Rauh-Pfeiffer A, Ming-Yu, Y, et al. *Cysteine metabolism & whole blood glutathione synthesis in septic pediatric patients.* Crit Care Med. 29: 870-877, 2001

Manzanares W, Biestro A, Galusso F, et al. *Serum selenium & glutathione peroxidase-3 activity: biomarkers of systemic inflammation in the critically ill?* Intensive Care Med. 35: 882-889, 2009

Manzanares W, Langlois PL, Heyland DK. *Pharmaconutrition with selenium in critically ill patients: what do we know?* Nutr Clin Pract. 30: 34-43, 2015

Metnitz PG, Bartens C, Fischer M, et al. *Antioxidant status in patients with acute respiratory distress syndrome.* Intensive Care Med. 25: 180-185, 1999

Mikhal'chik EV, Piterskaya JA, Lipatova VA, et al. *Activity of antioxidant enzymes in the wound in patients with deep burns.* Bull Exp Biol Med. 147: 753-756, 2009

Mogensen KM, Lasky-Su J, Rogers AJ, et al. *Metabolites Associated With Malnutrition in the Intensive Care Unit Are Also Associated With 28-Day Mortality.* JPEN J Parenter Enteral Nutr. 41: 188-197, 2017

Moradi M, Mojtahedzadeh M, Mandegari A, et al. *The role of glutathione-S-transferase polymorphisms on clinical outcome of ALI/ARDS patient treated with N-acetylcysteine.* Respir Med. 103: 434-441, 2009

Mühl D, Woth G, Drenkovics I, et al. *Comparison of oxidative stress & leukocyte activation in patients with severe sepsis & burn injury.* Indian J Med Res. 134: 69-78, 2011

Munz B, Frank S, Hubner G, et al. *A novel type of glutathione peroxidase: expression & regulation during wound repair.* Biochem. J. 326: 579-585, 1997

Najafi A, Mojtahedzadeh M, Ahmadi KH, et al. *The immunological benefit of higher dose N-acetyl cysteine following mechanical ventilation in critically ill patients.* Daru. 22:57, 2014

Ocal K, Avian D, Cinel I, et al. *The effect of N-acetylcysteine on oxidative stress in intestine & bacterial translocation after thermal injury.* Burns 30: 778-784, 2004

Porter JM, Ivatury RR, Azimuddin K, et al. *Antioxidant therapy in the prevention of organ dysfunction syndrome & infectious complications after trauma: early results of a prospective randomized study.* Am surg. 65:478-483, 1999

Robinson MK, Rounds JD, Hong RW, et al. *Glutathione deficiency increases organ dysfunction after hemorrhagic shock.* Surgery 112: 140-147, 1992

Rodas PC, Rooyackers O, Hebert C, et al. *Glutamine & glutathione at ICU admission in relation to outcome.* Clin Sci (Lond). 122: 591-597, 2012

Sabeh F, Baxter CR, Norton SJ. *Skin burn injury & oxidative stress in liver & lung tissues of rabbit models.* Eur. J. Clin. Chem. Clin. Biochem. 33: 323-328, 1995

Sandre C, Agay D, Ducros V, et al. *Early evolution of selenium status & oxidative stress parameters in rat models of thermal injury.* J Trace Elem Med Biol. 17: 313-318, 2004

Shi EC, Fisher R, McEvoy M, et al. *Factors influencing hepatic glutathione concentrations: a study in surgical patients.* Clin. Sci. 62: 279-283, 1982

Shukla A, Rasik AM, Patnaik GK. *Depletion of reduced glutathione, ascorbic acid, vitamin E & antioxidant defense enzymes in a healing cutaneous wound.* Free Radic. Res. 26: 93-101, 1997

Sies H, Graf P. *Hepatic thiol & glutathione efflux under the influence of vasopressin, phenylephrine & adrenaline. Biochem.* J. 226: 545-549, 1985

Steiling H, Munz B, Werner S, et al. *Different types of ROS-scavenging enzymes are expressed during cutaneous wound repair.* Exp. Cell. Res. 247: 484-494, 1999

Tsai ML, Huang HP, Hsu JD, et al. *Topical N-acetylcysteine accelerates wound healing in vitro & in vivo via the PKC/Stat3 pathway.* Int J Mol Sci. 15:7563-7578, 2014

van der Laan L, Oyen WJ, Verhofstad AA, et al. *Soft tissue repair capacity after oxygen-derived free radical-induced damage in one hindlimb of the rat.* J. Surg. Res. 72: 60-69, 1997

Verona C, Hackenhaar FS, Teixeira C, et al. *Blood markers of oxidative stress predict weaning failure from mechanical ventilation.* J Cell Mol Med. 19: 1253-1261, 2015

Victor VM, Espulgues JV, Hernández-Mijares A, et al. *Oxidative stress & mitochondrial dysfunction in sepsis:* a potential therapy with mitochondria-targeted antioxidants. Infect Disord Drug Targets. 9: 376-389, 2009

Vinha PP, Martinez EZ, Vannucchi H, et al. *Effect of acute thermal injury in status of serum vitamins, inflammatory markers, & oxidative stress markers: preliminary data.* J Burn Care Res. 34 : e87-91 2013

Wagner R, Heckman HM, Myers RR. *Wallerian degeneration & hyperalgesia after peripheral nerve injury are glutathione-dependent.* Pain 77: 173-179, 1998

Wernerman J, Luo JL, Hammarqvist F. *Glutathione status in critically-ill patients: possibility of modulation by antioxidants.* Proc Nutr Soc. 58 : 677-680, 1999

Yu YM, Ryan CM, Fei ZW, et al. *Plasma L-5-oxoproline kinetics & whole blood glutathione synthesis rates in severely burned adult humans.* Am J Physiol Endocrinol Metab. 282: E247-258, 2002

22

Skin Disorders

WHAT IS THE LARGEST ORGAN in the body? Most people think it's the liver, or even the intestine. In fact, it's the skin. You might not think of it as an organ, but your skin is not just a protective barrier against the environment. It performs a large number of important functions: endocrinological, thermoregulatory, immunological, toxicological and circulatory.

The skin hosts a huge variety of diseases and disorders, and about one third of North Americans will experience some sort of skin problem. Skin disorders also affect patients differently, especially in their psychological reaction to the disease. Firstly, the problem is conspicuous and hard to forget; secondly patients are often nervous about the actual or perceived reaction of others, as well as the social or interpersonal consequences.

GSH and skin disease

Given the number of functions served by skin, it's no surprise that glutathione is involved in many of its problems. GSH is well-known to detoxify and prevent radiation damage in all tissue, and it plays just as vital a role here. Low levels of GSH have been documented in many types of skin disease, including those in Table 33.

The importance of properly-functioning GSH for the prevention of many skin diseases becomes evident when we consider genetic abnormalities in certain individuals—especially the "inborn errors of metabolism[1]" regarding GSH genes, of which there are many. Papers from all over the world studying patients of all ethnicities have established the same strong association between impaired GSH function and the development of skin disease—including skin cancer.

This chapter focuses on many of the skin diseases in Table 33. Skin cancer is discussed in a separate chapter [see Chapter 5].

[1] A large class of genetic diseases involving congenital metabolic disorders.

Acne conglobata	Acne vulgaris	Allergic dermatitis
Alopecia areata	Atopic dermatitis	Contact dermatitis
Dermatitis herpetiformis	Eczema	Ichthyosis
Lupus erythematosus	Melasma	Mycosis fungoides
Onychotillomania	Pemphigoid	Polymyositis
Pseudoporphyria	Psoriasis	Scleroderma
Seborrheic dermatitis	Sjogren's síndrome	Subacute Prurigo
Toxic epidermal necrolysis	Trichotillomania	Vasculitis
Vitiligo		

TABLE 33: *Skin diseases characterized by abnormal GSH function*

Psoriasis

Psoriasis is a common, chronic recurrent skin condition producing scaly white or red patches on the legs, knees, arms, elbows, ears, scalp or back. It may extend to just one or two patches, or cover the whole body. It can affect the joints and occasionally leads to disabling arthritis. However, extreme cases are rare and general health for most psoriatic patients is good. Lesions occur when skin cells multiply up to ten times faster than normal. This overgrowth leads to the classic, raised, silvery, flaky appearance of the condition.

No single identifiable cause of psoriasis is known. It may be triggered by different factors in different people. Fair-skinned individuals in particular may have a genetic predisposition to it. It certainly has something to do with the immune response itself. Attacks or flare-ups can be triggered by emotional or physical stress, illness, injury, infection, drug and alcohol abuse, obesity, and many different chemicals. Other chapters of this book describe the critical role of glutathione in many of these processes.

One source of relief for psoriatic patients is travel to a healing environment. The Dead Sea in Israel is popular. A medical facility—The Dead-Sea Psoriasis Treatment Center—was set up for this purpose. Researchers have tried to understand why this particular environment is beneficial. High levels of sunlight seem to affect psoriasis positively. Most interestingly, the drinking water in the area is very high in selenium. A local research team explains that the best indicator of selenium bioactivity is patients' glutathione peroxidase levels. Compared to a control group—and to their own initial GSH levels—patients spending weeks in this treatment center increased GSH peroxidase levels, often as much as 50%.

Psoriasis patients suffer from abnormal GSH enzyme activities, and researchers have linked the disease to high levels of free radicals, supporting evidence that lowered GSH activity results in greater damage.

A study using CRWPI (cysteine-rich whey protein isolate) in psoriatic patients was published in the Journal of Clinical Aesthetic Dermatology by Prussick, Prussick and Gutman (2013). Scales of PASI (Psoriasis Area and Severity Score) and sequential photographs showed the treatment to be beneficial, warranting larger clinical trials.

Case Study

ROLAND IS A 44 YEAR-OLD, energetic, sociable entrepreneur who suffered from psoriasis for ten years. Itchy, scaly eruptions often covered his entire body, and aggressive scratching led to bleeding and scabbing. His dermatologist tried many different treatments, including strong topical corticosteroids and methotrexate tablets, which he had to discontinue due to side-effects. Ultraviolet light therapy was suggested. Having the financial means, Roland preferred frequent trips to Mexico and the Caribbean rather than sitting in artificial light. Having done significant homework on his condition, he concluded that the psoriasis was caused by an immune dysfunction and started taking 40 grams/day of bioactive whey protein isolate to raise his glutathione levels. Within two weeks he was free of bleeding and scabs and described his scaling as 75% improved.

Dermatitis

Dermatitis simply means inflammation of the skin, and is a general term. Different forms of dermatitis are caused by different ailments. Toxins or irritants lead to contact dermatitis. Allergies lead to allergic or atopic dermatitis. Many intestinal or immunological diseases can trigger such forms as dermatitis herpetiformis.[2] Overproduction of oils in the skin

[2] A chronic autoimmune condition of intensely itchy watery blisters; a cutaneous manifestation of celiac disease.

can lead to seborrheic dermatitis. Dermatitis can be triggered by stress or illness. Overly hot, dry, cold or wet environments also promote dermatitis. All forms of dermatitis are characterized by red itchy skin and, in extreme cases, blistering, crusty, oozing lesions. Almost all of these conditions have been linked to abnormal glutathione activity.

In both irritant contact dermatitis and allergic contact dermatitis, glutathione levels fall both in the skin and the whole body. A group of Japanese dermatologists inhibited GSH production with the drug BSO, finding that both allergic and irritant contact dermatitis rashes became more severe. They link this both to the inhibited detoxification abilities of GSH, and to its critical role in the immune system.

Several research groups have shown that GSH precursors help the immune system respond to contact sensitivity. A Swedish team using the GSH-enhancing drugs NAC and DiNAC demonstrated significant results with contact and delayed-hypersensitivity reactions. Senaldi at the University of Geneva successfully used both topical and oral NAC to experimentally treat contact and irritant dermatitis. He suggested that a similar approach could benefit cancer patients suffering from skin inflammation secondary to TNF-alpha (tumor necrosis factor-alpha)—an inflammatory side-effect of cancer.

Contact dermatitis often arises from the use of cosmetics, including make-up, skin creams, eyeliners and similar products. One particular culprit is a group of preservatives/sanitizers used in cosmetics, known as MCI/MI (methyl-chloro-isothiazolinone/methyl-isothiolinone). A group of Swedish occupational and environmental dermatologists found that adding as little as 2% GSH to them deactivates their harmful effects.

Thimerosol is another popular preservative used in toiletries, as well as contact lens solutions. It is known to cause skin and eye reactions, probably because of its organo-mercury content. At Rome's Dermatological Institute, Santucci showed that adding L-cysteine or glutathione to solutions containing thimerosol reduced or prevented adverse reactions to this chemical.

AIDS patients are more prone to skin disease than others. Conditions include Karposi's sarcoma, seborrheic dermatitis and others. As we discussed in Chapter 12, most AIDS patients are glutathione-deficient—a factor that also contributes to these skin conditions. Passi and Morrone in Italy, as well as other teams, have shown a deficiency of glutathione peroxidase activity both in HIV-positive patients and in otherwise healthy individuals with seborrheic dermatitis.

An interesting experiment was carried out at the Welsh School of Pharmacy, where the dermatitis-inducing chemicals of plants such as poison ivy and poison oak were examined. It was found that most inflammation was due to free radicals. Using the GSH-precursor OTZ they reduced the irritation and the sensitizing effect of these noxious compounds.

Skin conditions that develop commonly in children include "atopic" dermatitis and "allergic" dermatitis. These two types share several features, including high oxidative stress, low antioxidant protection and low glutathione activity. One interesting finding, widely confirmed around the world, is the presence of key genetic abnormalities in children, that predispose them to such problems. One of the major defects found relates to glutathione transferase genes, which play a key role in inflammatory responses.

Sun and ultraviolet radiation skin damage

By far the most common cause of abnormal aging, wrinkling and cancer of the skin is exposure to sun and ultraviolet radiation. The "healthy" bronzed glow of youth may exact a price later in life. Tanning leads to skin aging, which in turn leads many people to plastic surgery, Botox injections and fillers. Most facelifts and similar treatments would be unnecessary if these patients had avoided tanning when they were younger. Many skin cancers that appear in adult life may actually have been triggered by severe sunburn years earlier as a child.

The well-known ozone layer of the upper atmosphere blunts the damaging effects of the ultraviolet A (UV-A) and ultraviolet B (UV-B) radiation found in sunlight. The ozone depletion that has so concerned us has already increased the incidence of skin cancer and we may see more dramatic increases in years to come. Physicians are seeing sunburn in more and more patients who claim to have never before been so affected by sun exposure.

Radiation releases high levels of hydroxyl-radicals in the skin. These are the most toxic of all free radicals. Such radiation comes from sunlight UV-A and UV-B, sun lamps, radiotherapy treatment and X-rays. The damaging radicals can be neutralized by glutathione but overexposure may overwhelm this protective system, causing GSH levels to fall and even more damage. For this reason, doctors have considered using antioxidant supplementation to protect the skin. Studies using various antioxidants have had mixed results, but research specifically into elevated GSH levels has been more encouraging.

Baas and his team at The Netherlands Cancer Institute used halogen lamps to sensitize their patients to light, finding that their sensitivity decreased when they were pretreated with NAC to raise glutathione levels. Another Dutch team at the Department of Medicinal Photochemistry, Leiden University tested the capacity of various oral and topical products to decrease UV skin damage. They found that NAC—whether ingested or applied directly to the skin—was a practical way to protect against UV-B radiation damage.

French researchers at Joseph Fourier University in Grenoble examined how effectively various GSH precursors limited UV-A radiation damage. They included NAC, OTZ, and selenium (most are described in detail in Chapter 4). To various degrees, all GSH-enhancing substances reduced the negative effects of UV-A radiation. The researchers concluded that elevated GSH levels protect against UV-A damage.

Similar studies at Harvard University and Hirosaki University in Japan examined just how UV-B radiation causes sunburn. Using animal subjects, they first showed that glutathione depletion resulted in significantly greater sunburn damage. Further studies with orally administered glutathione esters raised GSH levels and resulted in less damage. Other Japanese researchers subjected their animals to higher doses of UV radiation, showing that pre-treatment with glutathione esters actually decreased the number of skin tumors that developed much later on.

A German team at the University of Berlin studied the effect of UV-B damage on people with an inherited defect in the enzyme GSH S-transferase. The GSH-impaired group suffered more intense damage than the control group, so it seems that inherited GSH-transferase deficiencies determine how sensitive an individual is to sunlight.

UV-B exposure not only damages skin, at high doses it affects the immune system by suppressing the action of T-cell lymphocytes. Whatever depletes GSH levels decreases this response further, and substances that elevate glutathione levels protect it. Steenvoorden and his team at the Amsterdam Center for Drug Research used BSO to lower glutathione levels, and NAC or GSH-esters to raise them, demonstrating that elevated GSH levels protect against UV-B immunosuppression.

Case study

61 YEAR-OLD CHARLES, a Canadian boating enthusiast, dreamed of retiring to spend most of his time on the water traveling the coasts. Tall, handsome and fair-skinned, he was unfortunately prone to sunburn. Despite sunscreens and hats, being on the water often left him unprotected. His complexion grew ruddy and inflamed. His physician was worried about the possible development of pre-cancerous sun-induced lesions on his face. Charles had already started taking selenium, alpha-lipoic acid and lycopene for a potential prostate problem. After several weeks he noticed his tendency to burn was significantly decreased, despite some 'accidental' exposure. Two months later he noticed that his in-the-sun complexion wasn't so different from his winter complexion.

Glutathione and skin whitening

GSH takes part in the metabolism of melanin, the pigment that colors or darkens the skin. However, how glutathione plays this role is somewhat complicated, and its applications remain controversial.

The production of melanin—the dark pigment of skin—depends on an enzyme called "tyrosinase." Glutathione inhibits the action of tyrosinase, so that melanin production is limited. The key question is how to get GSH into that equation.

The most obvious starting point is to examine why topical GSH (applied directly to the skin) is effective. We know that GSH can be absorbed into superficial tissues, but does not penetrate into the body. Several Japanese researchers have conducted human studies using GSH creams in different forms, and have successfully whitened skin.

A more controversial question is whether oral GSH is as effective. We described in Chapter 4 its ineffectiveness as a way to raise whole body glutathione, so it would be equally unlikely to raise it in the skin. The vast majority of attempts to whiten skin using oral GSH have failed, although a small handful have found positive effects. Nevertheless, skin-whitening remains a popular marketing claim for GSH—especially among companies promoting GSH to Asian women.

Glutathione, melasma and vitiligo

The skin disorder melasma causes patients to develop gray or brown patches of skin, often on the face. It can produce a disturbing appearance but unfortunately, effective treatments remain difficult. Melasma has been correlated with increased levels of oxidative stress and decreased levels of glutathione.

Vitiligo is a common acquired[3] depigmentation disorder in which white patches of skin appear on various parts of the body. Again, oxidative stress has been shown to play a big part in the development of this skin disease. Not surprisingly, these studies also reveal that vitiligo patients suffer from low glutathione. Moreover, individuals with abnormal glutathione transferase enzymes seem more prone to developing vitiligo.

In both melanoma and vitiligo, well designed human studies using GSH-enhancing strategies have yet to be completed.

Glutathione and scleroderma

Scleroderma is a chronic autoimmune disease characterized by hardening of the connective tissues.[4] The hardening does not apply only to skin (derma). Inner tissues like blood vessels, and even the lung and kidneys can be affected in a related continuum called "systemic sclerosis."

High levels of oxidation can be found throughout the bodies of scleroderma patients. Oxidation has even been observed early in stem cell development. Such oxidative stress continues its forward momentum, resulting in increased levels of lipid peroxidation[5] and low glutathione activity. These are fixed features of scleroderma. Some researchers have suggested that certain glutathione measurements be used as a marker of the severity of the disease.

---

[3] Developed or originating after birth; not hereditary or congenital.

[4] Tissue that connects, supports, binds or separates other tissues and/or organs.

[5] A free radical breakdown product.

Glutathione and acne

Acne vulgaris is a common skin problem, especially among teenagers. It is characterized by hormonally-stimulated inflammation and overproduction of skin oils and skin cells. Many factors make acne better or worse but we cannot explore them all here. However, we will focus on the role of oxidative stress and subsequent glutathione depletion.

Acne's ongoing inflammation produces lots of free radicals, inevitably leading to loss of antioxidants—especially GSH. The oxidation of fats (lipids) in the skin (like sebum), is referred to as "lipid peroxidation," and was suggested over 50 years ago as a cause of acne.

Authors have proposed that GSH levels be correlated with the severity of the skin problem. This naturally leads researchers to question whether raising glutathione might be of potential assistance. Early studies suggest this is so. An article appearing in SkinMed[6] described how the topical GSH-enhancing drug NAC was used in a double-blind study on acne to produce statistically significant improvements.

Conclusion

Low glutathione levels characterize many skin diseases. Practical applications with GSH-raising substances have been studied in the treatment of several diseases. There has been success in some but not all cases of psoriasis. This may reflect the multiple and various causes of this disease. Many of the diseases that fall under the very general definition of dermatitis may be positively affected by raised glutathione levels. GSH is of extreme importance as a protective agent against ultraviolet radiation of the sun. Continuing research into a host of different skin diseases is ongoing, focusing on glutathione as a potential therapy.

THE SKIN

REFERENCES

ACETO A, MARTINI F, DRAGANI B, ET AL. *Purification & characterization of glutathione transferase from psoriatic skin. Biochem.* Med. Metab. Biol. 48: 212-218, 1992

ADIL M, AMIN SS, MOHTASHIM M. *N-acetylcysteine in dermatology.* Indian J Dermatol Venereol Leprol 84(6):652-659, 2018.

AFAG F, MUKTAR H. *Effects of solar radiation on cutaneous detoxification pathways.* J Photochem Photobiol B 63(1-3):61-9, 2001

AL-SHOBAILI HA. *Oxidants & anti-oxidants status in acne vulgaris patients with varying severity.* Ann Clin Lab Sci 44(2):202-7, 2014

AL-SHOBAILI HA ET AL. *Biochemical markers of oxidative & nitrosative stress in acne vulgaris: correlation with disease activity.* J Clin Lab Anal 27(1):45-52, 2013

ARICAN O, KURUTAS EB, SASMAZ S. *Oxidative stress in patients with acne vulgaris.* Mediators Inflamm (6):380-4, 2005

ARJINPATHANA N, ASAWANONDA P. *Glutathione as an oral whitening agent: a randomized, double-blind, placebo-controlled study.* J Dermatolog Treat 23(2):97-102, 2012

BAAS P, VAN MANSOM I, VAN TINTEREN H, ET AL. *Effect of n-acetylcysteine on Photoprin-induced skin photosensitivity in patients.* Lasers Surg. Med. 16: 359-367, 1995

BOWE WP, PATEL N, LOGAN AC. *Acne vulgaris: the role of oxidative stress & the potential therapeutic value of local & systemic antioxidants.* J Drugs Dermatol 11(6):742-6, 2012

CHO HR ET AL. *Glutathione S-transferase M1 (GSTM1) polymorphism is associated with atopic dermatitis susceptibility in a Korean population.* Int J Immunogenet 38(2):145-50, 2011

CHOUBEY V ET AL. *role of oxidative stress in melasma: a prospective study on serum & blood markers of oxidative stress in melasma patients.* Int J Dermatol 56(9):939-943, 2017

[6] A journal of the International Academy of Cosmetic Dermatology

CHUNG BY ET AL. *The glutathione derivative, GSH monoethyl ester, may effectively whiten skin but GSH does not.* Int J Mol Sci 17(5), 2016

CHUNG J, OH SY, SHIN YK. *Association of glutathione-S-transferase polymorphisms with atopic dermatitis risk in preschool age children.* Clin Chem Lab Med 47(12):1475-81, 2009

DWORNIAK K ET AL. *[Increased level of lipid peroxidation products & disturbances in oxidation-reduction balance in erythrocytes from patients suffering from systemic sclerosis, who are chronically treated with vitamin E].* Pol Merkur LOekarski 35(206):85-8, 2013

EMERIT I. *Free radicals & aging of the skin.* EXS 62: 328-341, 1992

EMONET N, LECCIA MT, FAVIER A, ET AL. *Thiols & selenium: protective effect on human skin fibroblasts exposed to UVA radiation. J. Photochem. Photobiol B. 40: 84-90, 1997*

FABRINI R, ET AL. *Erythrocyte glutathione transferase: a non-antibody biomarker for systemic sclerosis, which correlates with severity & activity of the disease.* Cell Death Dis 25,4:e736, 2013

FAIRRIS GM, PERKINS PJ, LLOYD B, ET AL. *The effect on atopic dermatitis of supplementation with selenium & vitamin E.* Acta. Derm. Venereol. 69: 359-362, 1989

GEORGE NM, ET AL. *Antioxidant Therapies for Ulcerative Dermatitis: A Potential Model for Skin Picking Disorder.* PLoS One 10(7):e012092, 2015

GHANIZADEH A, DERAKHSHAN N, BERK M. *N-acetylcysteine versus placebo for treating nail biting, a double blind randomized placebo controlled clinical trial. Antiinflamm Antiallergy Agents Med Chem;12:223-8. 2013*

GOODSON AG, ET AL. *Use of oral N-acetylcysteine for protection of melanocytic nevi against UV-induced oxidative stress:* towards a novel paradigm for melanoma chemoprevention. Clin Cancer Res 15(23):7434-40, 2009

GREENSTOCK CL. *Radiation & aging: free radical damage, biological response & possible antioxidant intervention. Medical Hypotheses 41: 473-482, 1993*

GRUVBERGER B, BRUZE M. *Can glutathione-containing emollients inactivate methylchloroisothiazolinone/methylisothiazolone?* Contact Dermatitis 38: 261-265, 1998

GRANDI V ET AL. *Efficacy & safety of S—acyl glutathione 2% cream vs. placebo agains UVB—induced erythema: a randomized, double—blinded clinical trial.* G Ital Dermatol Venereol, 2017

GUARNERI F, ET AL. *Polymorphism of glutathione S-transferases M1 & T1: susceptibility to solar keratoses in an Italian population.* Clin Exp Dermatol 35(7):771-5, 2010

HANADA K, GANGE RW, CONNOR MJ. *Effect of glutathione depletion on sunburn cell formation in the hairless mouse.* J. Invest. Dermatol. 96: 838-40, 1991

HANADA K, SAWAMURA D, TAMAI K, ET AL. *Photoprotective effect of esterified glutathione against ultraviolet B-induced sunburn cell formation in the hairless mouse.* J. Invest. Dermatol. 108: 727-730, 1997

HIRAI A, MINAMIYAMA Y, HAMADA T, ET AL. *Glutathione metabolism in mice is enhanced more with hapten-induced allergic contact dermatitis than with irritant contact dermatitis.J. Invest. Dermatol. 109: 314-318, 1997*

IKENO H, TOCHIO T, TANAKA H, NAKATA S. *Decrease in glutathione may be involved in pathogenesis of acne vulgaris.* J Cosmet Dermatol 10(3):240-4, 2011

JUHLIN L, EDQVIST LE, EKMAN LG, ET AL. *Blood glutathione peroxidase levels in skin diseases: effect of selenium & vitamin E treatment.Arch. Derm. Venereol. 62: 211-214, 1982*

KALKAN G ET AL. *Relationship between manganese superoxide dismutase (MnSODAla-9Val) & glutathione peroxidase (GPx1 Pro 197 Leu gene polymorphisms & alopecia areata)* Int J Clin Exp Med 8(11):21533-40, 2015

KARLKAN G ET AL. *Oxidative stress status in patients with acute urticaria.* Cutan Ocul Toxicol 33(2):109-14, 2014

KARADAG AS ET AL. *An investigation of cytochrome p450 (CYP) & glutathione S-transferase (GST) isoenzyme protein expression & related interactions with phototherapy in patients with psoriasis vulgaris.* Int J Dermatol 56(2):225-231, 2017

KARSLI N, ET AL. *Role of oxidative stress in the pathogenesis of vitiligo with special emphasis on the antioxidant action of narrowband ultraviolet B phototherapy.* J Int Med Res 42(3):799-805, 2014

KHAN R, SATYAM A, GUPTA S, SHARMA VK, SHARMA A. *Circulatory levels of antioxidants & lipid peroxidation in Indian patients with generalized & localized vitiligo.* Arch Dermatol Res 301(10):731-7, 2009

KERB R, BROCKMOLLER J, REUM T, ROOTS I. *Deficiency of glutathione S-transferases T1 & M1 as heritable factors of increased cutaneous uv sensitivity.* J. Invest. Dermatol. 108: 229-232, 1997

KIM SH ET AL. *GSTT1 & GSTM1 null mutations & adverse reactions induced by antituberculosis drugs in Koreans.* Tuberculosis (Edinb) 90(1):39-43, 2010

KIMURA J, HAYAKARI M, KUMANO T, ET AL. *Altered glutathione transferase levels in rat skin inflamed due to contact hypersensitivity: induction of the alpha-class subunit 1.* Biochem J. 335 (Pt 3): 605-610, 1998

KOBAYASHI S, TAKEHANA M, TOHYAMA C. *Glutathione isopropyl ester reduces UVB-induced skin damage in hairless mice.* Photochem. Photobiol.

63: 106-110, 1996

LJUNGHALL K, JUHLIN L, EDQVIST LE, PLANTIN LO. *Selenium, glutathione peroxidase & dermatitis herpetiformis.* Acta. Derm. Venereol. 64: 546-546. 1984

LIU L, LI C, GAO J, LI K, GAO L, GAO T. *Genetic polymorphisms of glutathione S-transferase & risk of vitiligo in the Chinese population.* J Invest Dermatol 129(11):2646-52, 2009

LU I ET AL. *Association of glutathione S-transferasee M1/T1 polymorphisms with susceptibility to vitiligo.* Gene 535(1):12-6, 2014

LUTZ W, TARKOWSKI M, NOWAKOWSKA E. *[Genetic polymorphism of glutathione s-transferase as a factor predisposing to allergic dermatitis].* Med Pr 52(1):45-51, 2001

MILLARD TP, FRYER AA, MCGREGOR JM. *A protective effect of glutathione-S-transferase GSTP1*Val(105) against polymorphic light eruption.* J Invest Dermatol 128(8):1901-5, 2008

MONTES LF, WILBORN WH, MONTES CM. *Topical acne treatment with acetylcysteine: clinical & experimental effects.* Skinmed 10(6):348-51, 2012

ORCIANI M, ET AL. *Alterations of ROS pathways in scleroderma begin at stem cell level.* J Biol Regul Homeost Agents 27(1):211-24, 2013

PASCHE-KOO F, ARECHALDE A, ARRIGHI JF, HAUSER C. *Effect of n-acetylcysteine, an inhibitor of tumor necrosis factor, on irritant contact dermatitis in the human.* Curr. Prob. Dermatol 23: 198-206, 1995

PASSI S, MORONNE A, DE LUCA C, ET AL. *Blood levels of vitamin E, polyunsaturated fatty acids of phospholipids, lipoperoxides & glutathione peroxidase in patients affected with seborrheic dermatitis.* J. Dermatol. 2: 171-178, 1991

PRUSSICK R, PRUSSICK L, GUTMAN J. *Psoriasis Improvement in Patients Using Glutathione-enhancing, Nondenatured Whey Protein Isolate: A Pilot Study.* J Clin Aesthet Dermatol 6(10):23-6, 2013

RINNERTHALER M, ET AL. *Oxidative stress in aging human skin.* Biomolecules 5(2):545-89, 2015

SANTUCCI B, CANNISTRACI C, CRISTAUDO A, ET AL. *Thimerosal positivities: the role of SH groups & divalent ions.* Contact Dermatitis 39: 123-126, 1998

SARNSTRAND B, JANSSON AH, MATUSEVICIENE G, ET AL. *N, N'-Diacetyl-L-cysteine - the disulfide dimer of n-acetylcysteine - is a potent modulator of contact sensitivity/delayed type hypersensitivity reactions in rodents.* J. Pharmacol. Exp. Ther. 288: 1174-1184, 1999

SCHMIDT RJ, KHAN L, CHUNG LY. *Are free radicals & not quinones the haptic species derived from urushiols & other contact allergenic mono- & dihydric alkylbenzines? The significance of NADH, glutathione, & redox cycling in the skin.* Arch. Dermatol. Research 282: 56-64, 1990

SCHNUCH A, WESTPHAL G, MOSSNER R, UTER W, REICH K. *Genetic factors in contact allergy—review & future goals.* Contact Dermatitis 64(1):2-23, 2011

SECKIN HY, ET AL. *Oxidative stress status in patients with melasma.* Cutan Ocul Toxicol 33(3):212-7, 2014

SFRENT-CORNATEANU R, ET AL. *Antioxidant defense capacity in scleroderma patients.* Clin Chem Lab Med, 46(6):836-41, 2008

SENALDI G, POINTAIRE P, PIGUET PF, GRAU GE. *Protective effect of n-acetylcysteine in hapten-induced irritant & contact hypersensitivity reactions.* J. Invest. Dermatol. 102: 934-937, 1994

SEUTTER E, COLSON ML, VAN DE STAAK WJ, ET AL. *Analysis in blood of dermatological patients. Glutathione & glutathione reductase 1.* Dermatologica 151: 193-198, 1975

SHANI J, LIVSHITZ T, ROBBERECH H, ET AL. *Increased erythrocyte glutathione peroxidase activity in psoriatics consuming high-selenium drinking water at the Dead-Sea Psoriasis Treatment Center.* Pharmacol. Res. Commun. 17: 479-488, 1985

SHIN JW, ET AL. *Erythrocyte malondialdehyde & glutathione levels in vitiligo patients.* Ann Dermatol 22(3):279-83, 2010

SIVARANJANI N, RAO SV, RAJEEV G. *Role of reactive oxygen species & antioxidants in atopic dermatitis.* J Clin Diagon Res 7(12):2683-5, 2013

SONTHALIA S, DAULATABAD D, SARKAR R. *Glutathione as a skin whitening agent: Facts, myths, evidence & controversies.* Indian J Dermatol Venereol Leprol 82(3):262-72, 2016

STEENVOORDEN DP, BEIJERBERGEN VAN HENEGOUWEN GM. *Cysteine derivatives protect against uv-induced reactive intermediates in human keratinocytes: the role of glutathione synthesis.* Photochem. Photobiol. 66: 665-671, 1997

STEENVOORDEN DP, BEIJERBERGEN VAN HENEGOUWEN GM. *Glutathione ethylester protects against local & systemic suppression of contact hypersensitivity induced by ultraviolet B radiation in mice.* Radiation Research 150: 292-297, 1998

STEENVOORDEN DP, HASSELBAINK DM, BEIJERBERGEN VAN HENEGOUWEN GM. *Protection against UV-induced reactive intermediates in human cells & mouse skin by glutathione precursors: a comparison of n-acetylcysteine & glutathione ethylester.* Photochem. Photobiol. 67: 651-666, 1998

TAYLOR M, BHAGWANDAS K. *Trichotillosis, skin picking & N-acetylcysteine.* J Am Acad Dermatol;72 Suppl 1:AB117. 2015

VAN DEN BROEKE LT, BEIJERBERGEN VAN HENEGOUWEN GM. *Thiols as potential uv radiation protectors: an in vitro study.* J. Photochem. Photobiol. B. 17: 279-286, 1993

VAN DEN BROEKE LT, BEIJERBERGEN VAN HENEGOUWEN GM. *The effect of n-acetylcysteine on the UVB-induced inhibition of epidermal dna synthesis in rat skin.* J. Photochem. Photobiol. B. 26: 271-276, 1994

Vadoud-Seyedi J, de Dobbeleer G, Simonart T. *Treatment of haemodialysis-associated pseudoporphyria with N-acetylcysteine: Report of two cases.* Br J Dermatol;142:580-1. 2000

Van den Broeke LT, Beijerbergen van Henegouwen GM. *Topically applied n-acetylcysteine as a protector against UVB-induced systemic immunosuppression.* J. Photochem. Photobiol. B. 27: 61-65, 1995

Walters MT, Rubin CE, Keightley SJ, Ward CD, Cawley MI. *A double-blind, cross-over, study of oral N-acetylcysteine in Sjögren's syndrome.* Scand J Rheumatol Suppl ;61:253-8. 1986

Wang IJ, Guo YL, Lin TJ, Chen PC, Wu YN. *GSTM1, GSTP1, prenatal smoke exposure, & atopic dermatitis.* Ann Allergy Asthma Immunol 105(2):124-9, 2010

Watanabe F, et al. *Skin-whitening & skin-condition-improving effects of tropical oxidized glutathione: a double-blind & placebo-controlled clinical trial in healthy women.* Clin Cosmet Investig Dermatol 7:267-74, 2014

Weschawalit S, et al. *Glutathione & its antiaging & antimelanogenic effects.* Clin Cosmet Invest Dermatol 10:147-153, 2017

Xiao BH, et al. *Glutathione Peroxidase Level in Patients with Vitiligo: A Meta-Analysis.* Biomed Res Int, 2016

Yenin Jz, et al. *Investigation of oxidative stress in patients with alopecia areata & its relationship with disease severity, duration, recurrence & pattern.* Clin Exp Dermatol 40(6):617-21, 2015

Zedan H et al. *Low glutathione peroxidase activity levels in patients with vitiligo.* J Cutan Med Surg 19(2):144-8, 2015

23
Exercise & Physical Performance

Exercise and health

STATISTICS TELL US that a sedentary lifestyle without exercise is as bad for health and longevity as smoking a pack of cigarettes a day. Countless studies show the health benefits of regular physical activity. Recent research suggests that moderate, consistent exercise may actually be more beneficial than intense workouts. The trouble is, most North Americans are not doing enough to reach this plateau. The U.S. Surgeon General reports that 75% of American adults are physically inactive, and 25% get virtually no exercise at all. Such people are at increased risk for the most common ailments and causes of death of our times. Inactivity as a lifestyle leads to heart disease, obesity, high blood pressure, diabetes, osteoporosis, stroke, depression and certain cancers.

Fortunately, in the last few decades interest in preventive health care has skyrocketed. Many people are discovering the benefits of exercise: weight control, muscle strength, bone mass and strength, increased energy, reduced stress, greater endurance, self esteem and longevity. The fitness industry is growing quickly. Enrollment in gyms and aerobic classes, and sales of fitness supplements, bicycles, skates and blades have all reached new heights. This raises new questions, especially about how much exercise is enough and whether there is such a thing as too much. How far can you push the limits of exercise? And, of course, amateur and professional athletes want to enhance their performance.

Even moderate exercise has a measurable impact on health and longevity. The Norwegian researcher Erikssen followed patients over a 22-year period and found that middle-aged men benefited from moderate fitness improvements and experienced lower risks of mortality from all causes. And it doesn't take extreme exertion to improve fitness. University of Washington doctor Lemaitre recently showed that walking for at least one hour per week reduces the risk of heart attacks as much as high-intensity physical activity.

One hour three to five times a week of light, moderate or vigorous effort is all that's needed. A light workout can provide the same benefits as a strenuous one, as long as it lasts longer. An hour of light walking, volleyball, easy gardening, stretching and baseball, thirty to sixty minutes of brisk walking, biking, raking leaves, swimming and dancing, or twenty to thirty minutes of jogging, aerobics, hockey, basketball or fast dancing provide similar health benefits.

Aging and exercise

Aging is associated with major alterations in body composition and exercise tolerance. Muscle mass, immune defense, antioxidant function and GSH levels all decrease. As our immune system ages, exercise workouts tax us more and more. Performance suffers. So does our ability to recover. Older women and men who participate in regular exercise therefore require more antioxidants in general and GSH in particular. Chapter 1 discusses the antioxidant role of GSH. Chapter 6 discusses GSH and aging.

Exercise and the immune system

Exercise appears to strengthen the immune system, but too much may have just the opposite effect. Many elite athletes come down with viral illnesses when they train intensely. A widespread virus ravaged the athletic community prior to the 1996 Atlanta Olympic Games, upsetting years of hard work. We have witnessed many such outbreaks time and again since then. However, few of us will push our immune resources to the limit. By using it in good measure, exercise can bolster our defenses against disease.

Statistical studies show that adults who exercise are less frequently ill than non-exercisers. The mechanisms of this increased resistance are very revealing. Many studies have found enhanced activity of various white blood cells—our front-line defense against infection. Fit people have a greater count of natural killer cells, macrophages and T-cell lymphocytes—crucial workers in the immune system—and more virus-fighting immune factors in their blood. Some studies have shown that the saliva of athletes contains higher levels of viral antibodies, offering greater resistance to disease. This is particularly relevant since many upper respiratory infections enter though the mouth. After several well-designed studies, Nieman's team of exercise physiologists at the Department of Health and Exercise, Appalachian State University said that people who exercise can double resistance to viral illness.

The immune system clearly responds well to moderate activity, but it has been shown that too much causes the immune system to wind down, resulting in immunosuppression. In other words, after a certain period the increase in immune factors and white cell activity initiated by exercise becomes blunted. This period depends on the intensity of activity and the condition of the athlete's defenses. Dozens of articles have documented a temporary immune deficiency after training to exhaustion. Tests conducted on marathon runners revealed that those running over 60 miles per week were twice as likely to catch a cold as those running 20. Some of these effects can be avoided by balancing and regulating nutrition and exercise levels.

Over-training syndrome

Besides the obvious possibility of physical injury, athletes who over-train run the risk of contracting various sicknesses. Their weakened immune response following exhaustive training is only one aspect of 'over-training syndrome.' Adjectives like 'burn-out,' 'staleness' and 'plateauing' are used by athletes to describe the physical sensation. British sports nutritionist Nathan Lewis has helped popularize the term "underperformance syndrome." Some respond stubbornly, by pushing even harder. This results in increasingly negative effects. Some exercise scientists have shown that decreasing the intensity of workouts may actually improve performance.

The over-trained athlete experiences a host of physiological effects that contribute to poor performance and illness. They include fluctuations in insulin secretion, alterations in glucocorticoid and hormone levels, inhibition of glucose uptake to tissues, catabolic (breakdown) effects on protein and nitrogen excretion and lactic acid over-production.

Links to immune dysfunction and intense physical training have frequently been made

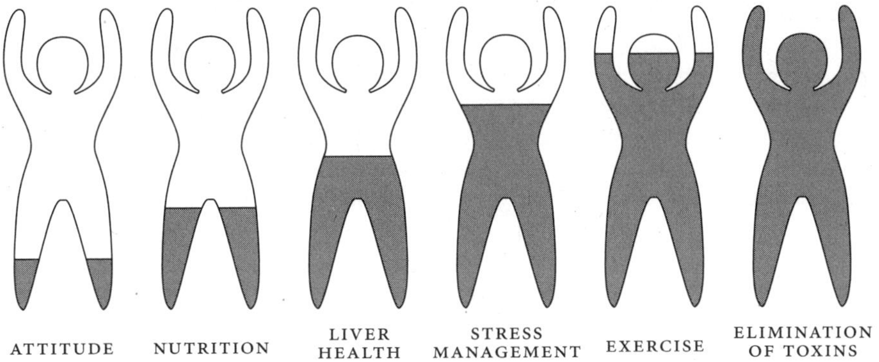

FIGURE 45: Exercise is a vital step to maximizing the immune system

by examining the role of glutathione as an intermediary. Japanese researcher Kawada and his team showed that the immune system's "natural killer cells" were better sustained in athletes taking glutathione-enhancing supplements.

Oxidative stress

While working out, athletes consume ten to fifteen times more oxygen than usual. Thus, oxidative stress is a major factor in exercise. This is because physical activity increases oxygen consumption and intensifies numerous metabolic processes. The result is the creation and circulation of liberated oxidative breakdown products, otherwise known as free radicals (see Chapter 1).

Some scientists believe that free radicals play a significant role in events leading up to muscle inflammation and damage, and the evidence is mounting. When cells need more energy, their mitochondria (power plants) work harder. When they increase energy, they also increase unhealthy by-products of lipid peroxidation. Harmful oxidation turns good fats bad, and makes bad fats like cholesterol even worse. Another consequence of increased mitochondrial activity is electron transport flux—the chain reaction of atoms snatching each other's electrons and destabilizing cellular structures (see Chapter 1). These two threats can be countered both by exogenous antioxidants like vitamins C and E—which are derived from food sources—and endogenous ones produced within the body. The most critical of these in-house antioxidants is glutathione.

The body is not entirely defenseless. Exercise also increases the level and activity of many antioxidants. A well-trained body will adapt to increased oxidative stress by developing improved physiological mechanisms, but the drive for better performance can overtake these adaptations and lead to greater muscular fatigue, injury and recovery time. And antioxidants can easily be depleted by over-training. The use of oral antioxidant supplementation is a mainstay of most athletic nutritional guidelines.

The importance of this strategy is driven home by the following study regarding glutathione levels in athletes performing "ultra endurance" events. A study showed that after a 233 km (143 mile) run, it took about one month for runners to recover their pre-race glutathione levels.

For the past decade a mixed team from the UK and USA led by Lewis have been studying oxidative stress in compromised elite athletes. They have established a direct correlation between heightened free radical activity and negative physical performance.

Another fascinating study appeared in the International Journal of Sports Medicine (2018). The question was whether lifelong exercise could improve age-related declines in antioxidant status. After all, oxidation has often been identified as a major culprit in aging. Perhaps one of the ways that exercise slows down the aging process is by improving glutathione metabolism. Four groups were included in the study: Young exercisers, young non-exercisers, old exercisers, and old non-exercisers. The four groups were then challenged with an exercise routine. Examination of glutathione and other antioxidant levels as well as subsequent breakdown products of oxidation, produced the following conclusion: regular lifelong physical activity could maintain antioxidant activity as we age, providing defense against the scourge of free radical damage.

GSH and athletic performance

Since antioxidants are especially critical to people who exercise, researchers have spent considerable time observing and testing them. This research explored two possible scenarios—to reduce the negative consequences of over-training and to improve performance. Much has been written about the role of antioxidants in sports physiology. As you might imagine, much of this research is focused on the body's most important endogenous antioxidant, glutathione. Elevated glutathione levels provide better immune defenses and reduced susceptibility to infectious disease. They also help shorten recovery time from workouts, reduce muscle fatigue and soreness, and improve performance.

Ji, Leeuwenburgh and a group of researchers at the University of Illinois carried out a series of studies on muscle injury influenced by free-radical formation. Their objective was to measure the usefulness of GSH in controlling cellular damage. It is not easy to test the body's adaptive response to exercise. Two metabolic processes in particular are somewhat unpredictable. One is the variability of GSH levels at any particular site. The other relates to the transport of GSH between tissues. Nevertheless, glutathione levels were seen to vary in proportion to the level of exertion, the individual's fitness, and his/her nutritional status.

Subjects completed a long-distance run, and Dufaux's experiments measured GSH levels before, immediately after, hours after, and days afterwards. Results showed a significant drain of glutathione. Recovery of GSH levels took from hours to days, during which subjects were susceptible to illness or injury. Similar studies were conducted on cyclists and other athletes. In all cases, GSH levels in muscle tissue were found to fall with exercise.

Researchers have shown that glutathione levels are more efficiently restored in the elite athlete than in the less well-trained. General body fitness encourages the manufacture of GSH and its more efficient release from tissues. Some scientists have gone one step further, suggesting that exercise slows the aging process by increasing one's ability to produce and distribute GSH on demand.

It is known that diabetics in particular can benefit from exercise. This is believed to result in part from the enhanced GSH metabolism of a fit body. It helps diabetics deal with the intense oxidative stress from which they characteristically suffer (see Chapter 8). Well-measured training stimulates greater GSH reserves and enhances one's ability to detoxify foreign substances. Tests show that well-exercised animals suffer less from acetaminophen toxicity than non-active ones. Some theorists even believe that the enhanced glutathione metabolism following exercise explains why the physically fit suffer less from cancer.

The glutathione-enhancing drug NAC (N-acetylcysteine) has been repeatedly demonstrated to improve strength and performance. A 2014 article in the journal "Medicine and Science in Sports and Exercise" showed significant improvement in sprint times of highly trained cyclists. Other researchers including Paschalis and his team in Greece demonstrated that improvements in physical performance are even greater in

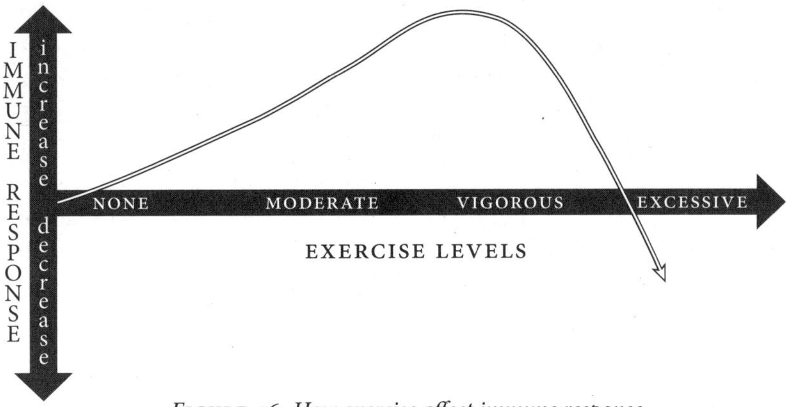

FIGURE 46: How exercise affect immune response

non-athletes when given similar GSH-enhancing supplements.

Apart from focusing on performance, NAC has also been used to suppress muscle fatigue. A large number of articles describe how NAC has decreased fatigue in athletes pre-treated with this GSH-enhancing drug. One of the major issues faced with this strategy is how to balance NAC's potential gastrointestinal side-effects with the overall improvements.

Given all this, it seems useful to take antioxidant or glutathione-enhancing supplements prior to intensive exercise. Sastre and his group at Spain's University of Valencia successfully tested this idea using vitamin C, NAC (see Chapter 4) and GSH on animal subjects. The result was reduced oxidative damage and the maintenance of reduced glutathione in blood reserves. Another group at the University of California (Berkeley) headed by Sen proved the corollary—that if greater levels improved antioxidant response, lower levels would worsen it. Using the drug BSO (which depletes glutathione), they forced GSH levels down. The ability of subjects to endure exhaustive exercise fell by 50%.

Physiologists investigating GSH's role in the immune response to exhaustive exercise have shown raised GSH levels to increase the number and activity of white blood cells. Other studies show that taking NAC before a workout diminishes oxidative stress within these white blood cells. Further studies conducted at Baylor College of Medicine in Texas—first on rodents and later on humans—showed that GSH levels raised by intravenous NAC enabled subjects to perform longer and harder in exhaustive muscle tests.

A dramatic example of increased muscle strength comes from Dr. Larry Lands of McGill University, Montreal. Thinking that oxidative stress contributes to muscular fatigue, his team gave young adults GSH precursors in the form of a cysteine-rich whey protein isolate for three months. During this time, they measured peak power and work capacity as indicators of strength and endurance and remarked that performance values could be enhanced from ten to fifteen percent.

A similar study used geriatric patients rather than fit youngsters, with similar results. A Quebec-based team of researchers led by Antony Karelis gave this same cysteine-rich whey protein to non-frail elderly subjects undergoing an exercise program for several months. Compared to a placebo group, the glutathione-enhanced group were 10% stronger. This represents a significant improvement in quality of life.

A team at the Peak Wellness Lab in Connecticut examined the effect of dietary supplementation with whey isolate protein on athletes. White blood cell levels (CD4 T-lymphocytes and neutrophils) that otherwise fall during extremely intense workouts remained elevated. Whey proteins have an extraordinarily high 'protein biological value' and are extremely effective in meeting the higher protein demands of athletes, who may require as much as two or three times as much as the average person. For this reason, whey protein is used widely in weight training to increase body mass.

Another study was carried out on AIDS and cancer patients in an attempt to counter the muscle loss (catabolism) they often suffer. This resembles the protein breakdown and muscle decline resulting from heavy exercise. A group in Germany led by Kinscherf found that NAC could slow this process. Compared to a placebo group, the NAC-supplemented group lost less body cell mass while undergoing anaerobic exertion, and interestingly carried less total body fat. The shift of body fat to body muscle is a strong focus in weight training.

Glutathione and detoxification in sports

Many athletes are exposed to substances that may adversely affect their health and performance. Some of this exposure is intentional (e.g. recreational drugs) and some of it is accidental (e.g. air pollution). A jogger running at the side of a highway may be inhaling ten times more organic and inorganic compounds than a runner in the countryside.

An excellent example of inadvertent toxic exposure can be found in enclosed skating rinks. Medical teams noticed that hockey players had an unusually high incidence of exercise-induced asthma. A team of researchers from the Human Performance Laboratory at Marywood University suspected that this was a result of repeated exposure to pollution arising from the ice-resurfacing equipment which usually ran on fuels like propane (the "Zamboni"). This machinery would regularly roll out on the ice every hour. Baumann, Rundell and their coworkers placed athletes on cysteine-rich whey isolate, and performed pulmonary function tests over time. The skaters on this bonded cysteine supplement showed significant improvement over the placebo group.

Sport enthusiasts in other high-risk environments or who work out in urban areas may consider a similar strategy to maximize the body's resistance to air pollution.

Case studies

Susan, a 35 year-old fashion merchandiser and mother of two, was a great fitness advocate. Free weights, aerobics, step and spinning classes—over fifteen years she had done them all. She was persistently dissatisfied with the "ten pounds of fat" that kept her from the muscular definition she wanted. Nutritionally conscious, she also knew that merely restricting her calories would just leave her feeling washed out. She started taking 40 grams/day of cysteine-rich whey protein isolate in combination with minimal adjustments in fat and carbohydrate intake. In three weeks she noticed better endurance during her cardiovascular workouts and was able to lift heavier weights with greater intensity. Recuperation between workouts improved, enabling her to continue without the usual soreness. Her weight remained unchanged. Despite not having made any great changes to her routine, six weeks after the dietary supplement, people at the gym commented on how "well cut" she was.

John, a national champion cyclist, understood the consequences of over-training on the immune system. He and his training partners tended to fall sick before big events if they pushed too hard. On top of that he had two children in day-care, which certainly raised his exposure to viral illnesses. Hearing that the specially prepared whey protein isolate had potential immune-boosting effects, he incorporated it into his daily diet. The frequency of viral illnesses decreased and when he did get sick, it was for only a day or two, rather than three or four. To his surprise, his performance times improved, along with his ability to recover faster from grueling competitions. After some initial hesitancy, he shared the advantages of this product with his teammates.

Conclusion

The health benefits of exercise cannot be overstated. Simply put, physically fit individuals are statistically more resistant to illness, and they live longer. They also exhibit increased antioxidative abilities. This is visibly reflected in the GSH metabolism.

However, exercise carries a risk and moderation is crucial. Over-training can lead to immune deficiency states, meaning prolonged fatigue and depletion of antioxidants, especially GSH.

The science of exercise physiology has clearly linked increased glutathione levels to improved immune function. This helps the body resist infection, decrease muscle damage, reduce recovery time, increase strength and maximize endurance. It also shifts the metabolism from fat production to muscular development.

EXERCISE & PHYSICAL PERFORMANCE

REFERENCES

Alessio HM. *Exercise-induced oxidative stress. Med. Sci. Sports Exerc. 25:218-224, 1993*

Alessio HM, Blassi ER. *Physical activity as a natural antioxidant booster & its effect on a healthy life span. Res. Q. Exerc. Sport 68:292-302, 1997*

Atalay M, Marnila P, Lilius EM, et al. *Glutathione-dependent modulation of exhausting exercise-induced changes in neutrophil function of rats. Eur. J. Appl. Physiol. 74:342-347, 1996*

Balakrishnan SD, Anuradha CV. *Exercise, depletion of antioxidants & antioxidant manipulation.* Cell Biochem Funct. 16: 269-275, 1998

Barranco-Ruiz Y, Martinez-Amat A, Casals C, et al. *A lifelong competitive training practice attenuates age-related lipid peroxidation.* J Physiol Biochem. 73:37-48, 2017

Baumann JM, Rundell KW, Evans TM, Levine AM. *Effects of cysteine donor supplementation on exercise-induced bronchconstriction.* Medicine & Science in Sports & Exercise 37:1468-1473, 2005

Bouzid MA, Filaire E, Matran R, et al. *Lifelong Voluntary Exercise Modulates Age-Related Changes in Oxidative Stress.* Int J Sports Med. 39:21-28, 2018

Bouzid MA, Hammouda O, Matran R, et al. *Influence of physical fitness on antioxidant activity & malondialdehyde level in healthy older adults.* Appl Physiol Nutr Metab. 40:582-589, 2015

Bouzid MA, Hammouda O, Matran R, et al. *Changes in oxidative stress markers & biological markers of muscle injury with aging at rest & in response to an exhaustive exercise.* PLoS One, 9:e90420, 2014

Bouzid MA, Hammouda O, Matran R, et al. *Low intensity aerobic exercise & oxidative stress markers in older adults.* J Aging Phys Act. 22:536-542, 2014

Braakhuis AJ, Hopkins WG, Lowe TE. *Effects of dietary antioxidants on training & performance in female runners.* Eur J Sport Sci. 14:160-168, 2014

Carteri RB, Schaun MI, Lopes AL, et al. *Lipid peroxidation & total glutathione after different intensities of resistance exercise in trained men.* J Sports Med Phys Fitness 55:735-741, 2015

Clarkson PM. *Antioxidants & physical performance.* Crit. Rev. Food Sci. Nutr. 35:131-141, 1995

Cobley JN, McGlory C, Morton JP, et al. *N-Acetylcysteine's attenuation of fatigue after repeated bouts of intermittent exercise: practical implications for tournament situations.* Int J Sport Nutr Exerc Metab 21:451-461, 2011

Corn SD, Barstow TJ. *Effects of oral N-acetylcysteine on fatigue, critical power, & W' in exercising humans.* Respir Physiol Neurobiol. 178:261-268, 2011

Dekany M, Nemeskeri V, Gyore I, et al. *Antioxidant status of interval-trained athletes in various sports.* Int J Sports Med. 27:112-116, 2006

Dekkers JC, Van Doornen LJ, Kemper HC. *The role of antioxidant vitamins & enzymes in the prevention of exercise-induced muscle damage.* Sports Med. 21:213-238, 1996

Douris PC, Elokda AS, H&rakis JP, et al. *Martial art training enhances the glutathione antioxidant system in middle-aged adults.* J Strength

Cond Res. 23:1518-1523, 2009

Dufaux B, Heine O, Kothe A, et al. *Blood glutathione status following distance running.* Int. J. Sports Med. 18:89-93, 1997

Eriksen G, Liestol K, Bjornholt J, et al. *Changes in physical fitness & changes in mortality.* Lancet 352: 759-762, 1998

Ferreira LF, Campbell KS, Reid MB. *N-acetylcysteine in h&grip exercise: plasma thiols & adverse reactions.* Int J Sport Nutr Exerc Metab. 21:146-154, 2011

Fielding RA, Meydani M. *Exercise, free radical generation, & aging.* Aging 9:12-18, 1997

Finaud J, Lac G, Filaire E. *Oxidative stress: relationship with exercise & training.* Sports Med. 36:327-358, 2006

Fitzgerald L. *Overtraining increases the susceptibility to infection.* Int. J. Sports Med. 12 (Suppl 1): S5-S8, 1991

Gabriel H, Kindermann W. *The acute immune response to exercise: what does it mean?Int. J. Sports Med. 18 (Suppl 1): S28-S45, 1997*

Gohil K, Viguie C, Stanley WC, et al. *Blood glutathione oxidation during human exercise.J. Appl. Physiol. 64: 115-119, 1988*

Hellsten Y, Apple FS, Sjodin B.Effect of sprint cycle training on activities of antioxidant enzymes in human skeletal muscle.J. Appl. Physiol. 81: 1484-1487, 1996

Huupponen MR, Makinen LH, Hyvonen PM, et al. *The effect of n-acetylcysteine on exercise-induced priming of human neutrophils. A chemoluminescence study.* Int. J. Sports Med. 16: 399-403, 1995

Hwang IW, Kim K, Kwon BN, et al. *Association of glutathione S-transferase M1 & T1 null/present polymorphism with physical performance in the Korean population.* Genes Genomics. 41:71-78, 2019

Hwang P, Morales Marroquin FE, Gann J, et al. *Eight weeks of resistance training in conjunction with glutathione & L-Citrulline supplementation increases lean mass & has no adverse effects on blood clinical safety markers in resistance-trained males.* J Int Soc Sports Nutr. 15:30, 2018

Jenkins RR. *Exercise, oxidative stress, & antioxidants: a review.* Int. J. Sports Nutr. 3: 356-375, 1993

Jenkins RR, Goldfarb A. *Introduction: oxidant stress, aging, & exercise.* Med. Sci. Sports Exerc. 25: 210-212,1993

Ji LL. *Oxidative stress during exercise: implication of antioxidant nutrients.* Free Radic. Biol. Med. 18: 1079-1086, 1995

Ji LL. *Antioxidant enzyme response to exercise & aging.* Med. Sci. Sports Exerc. 25: 225-231,1993

Ji LL, Fu R. *Responses of glutathione system & antioxidant enzymes to exhaustive exercise & hydroperoxide.* J. Appl. Physiol. 72: 549-554, 1992

Ji LL, Fu R, Mitchell EW. *Glutathione & antioxidant enzymes in skeletal muscle: effects of fiber type & exercise intensity.* J. Appl. Physiol. 73: 1854-1859, 1992

Karper WB, Hopewell R. *Exercise, immunity, acute respiratory infections, & homebound older adults.* Home Care Provider 3: 41-46, 1998

Kelly MK, Wicker RJ, Barstow TJ, Harms CA. *Effects of N-acetylcysteine on respiratory muscle fatigue during heavy exercise.* Respir Physiol Neurobiol. 165:67-72, 2009

Kerksick C, Willoughby D. *The antioxidant role of glutathione & N-acetyl-cysteine supplements & exercise-induced oxidative stress.* J Int Soc Sports Nutr. 2:38-44, 2005

Kinscherf R, Hack V, Fischbach T, et al. *Low plasma glutamine in combination with high glutamate levels indicate risk for loss of body cell mass in healthy individuals: the effect of N-acetyl-cysteine.* J. Mol. Med. 74:393-400. 1996

Knez WL, Jenkins DG, Coombes JS. *The effect of an increased training volume on oxidative stress.* Int J Sports Med 35:8-13, 2014

Kretzschmar M, Muller D. *Aging, training & exercise. A review of effects on plasma glutathione & lipid peroxides.* Sports Med. 15: 196-209, 1993

Laaksonen DE, Atalay M, Niskanen L, et al. *Increased resting & exercise-induced oxidative stress in young IDDM men.* Diabetes Care 19: 569-574, 1996

L&s LC, Grey VL, Smountas AA. *Effect of supplementation with a cysteine donor on muscular performance.* J. Appl. Physiol. 87:1381-135, 1999

L&s LC, Grey VL, Smountas AA. *The effect of supplementation with a cysteine donor on muscular performance.* American J. Resp. Crit. Care Med 159:A719, 1999

Lee IM. *Exercise & physical health: cancer & immune function.* Res. Q. Exerc. Sport. 66: 286-291, 1995

Leeuwenburgh C, Ji LL. *Glutathione depletion in rested & exercised mice: biochemical consequence & adaptation.* Arch. Biochem. Biophys. 316: 941-949, 1995

Lemaitre RN, Siscovick DS, Raghunathan TE, et al. *Leisure-time physical activity & the risk of primary cardiac arrest.* Arch. Intern. Med. 159: 686-690, 1999

Lemon PW. *Is increased dietary protein necessary or beneficial for individuals with a physically active lifestyle?* Nutr. Rev. 54 (Pt 2): S169-S175, 1996

Lemon PW. *Do athletes need more dietary protein & amino acids?* Int. J. Sports Nutr. 5 (Suppl): S39-S61, 1995

Leon-Lopez J, Calderon-Soto C, Perez-San-

CHEZ M, ET AL. *Oxidative stress in elite athletes training at moderate altitude & at sea level.* Eur J Sport Sci. 18:832-841, 2018

LEW H, PIKE S, QUINTANILHA A. *Changes in the glutathione status of plasma, liver, & muscle following exhaustive exercise in rats.* FEBS Lett. 185: 262-266, 1985

LEW H, QUINTANILHA A. *Effects of endurance training & exercise on tissue antioxidative capacity & acetaminophen detoxification.* Eur. J. Drug Metab. Pharmacokinet. 16: 59-61, 1991

LIFANOV AD, KHADYEVA MN, RAKHMATULLINA LSH, ET AL. *Influence of the GPX1 gene polymorphism to aerobic capacity & efficiency of glutathione supplementation in athletes.* Ross Fiziol Zh Im I M Sechenova 100:248-255, 2014

LIFE EXTENSION EDITORS. *The wonders of whey – Restoring youthful anabolic metabolism at the cellular level.* Life Ext. 5:35-38, 1999

MACKINNON LT. *Immunity in athletes.* Int. J. Sports Med. 18 (Suppl): S62-S69, 1997

MARIN E, KRETZCHMAR M, AROKOSKI J, ET AL. *Enzymes of glutathione synthesis in dog skeletal muscles & their response to training.* Acta. Physiol. Sc&. 147: 369-373, 1993

MCKENZIE MJ, GOLDFARB A, GARTEN RS, VERVAECKE L. *Oxidative stress & inflammation response following aerobic exercise: role of ethnicity.* Int J Sports Med. 35:822-827, 2014

MCKINLEY-BARNARD S, ANDRE T, MORITA M, WILLOUGHBY DS. *Combined L-citrulline & glutathione supplementation increases the concentration of markers indicative of nitric oxide synthesis.* J Int Soc Sports Nutr. 12:27, 2015

MCLEAY Y, STANNARD S, HOULTHAM S, STARCK C. *Dietary thiols in exercise: oxidative stress defence, exercise performance, & adaptation.* J Int Soc Sports Nutr. 14:12, 2017

MEDVED I, BROWN MJ, BJORKSTEN AR, MCKENNA MJ. *Effects of intravenous N-acetylcysteine infusion on time to fatigue & potassium regulation during prolonged cycling exercise.* J Appl Physiol 96:211-217, 2004

MEDVED I, BROWN MJ, BJORKSTEN AR, ET AL. *N-acetylcysteine enhances muscle cysteine & glutathione availability & attenuates fatigue during prolonged exercise in endurance-trained individuals.* J Appl Physiol. 97:1477-1485, 2004

MEDVED I, BROWN MJ, BJORKSTEN AR, ET AL. *N-acetylcysteine infusion alters blood redox status but not time to fatigue during intense exercise in humans.* J Appl Physiol 94:1572-1582, 2003

NASH MS. *Exercise & immunology.* Med. Sci. Sports Exerc. 26: 125-127, 1994

MICHAILIDIS Y, KARAGOUNIS LG, TERZIS G, ET AL. *Thiol-based antioxidant supplementation alters human skeletal muscle signaling & attenuates its inflammatory response & recovery after intense eccentric exercise.* Am J Clin Nutr. 98:233-245, 2013

MOMENI M, DE KOCK M, DEVUYST O, LIISTRO G. *Effect of N-acetyl-cysteine & hyperoxia on erythropoietin production.* Eur J Appl Physiol. 111 :2681-2686, 2011

NEHLSEN-CANNARELLA SL, NIEMAN DC, BALK-LAMBERTON AJ, ET AL. *Effects of moderate exercise training on immune response.* Med. Sci Sports Exerc. 23: 64-70, 1991

NIEMAN DC. *Exercise & resistance to infection.* Canadian J. Physiol. Pharmacol. 76: 573-580, 1998

NIEMAN DC. *Immune response to heavy exertion.* J. Appl. Physiol. 82: 1385-1394, 1997

NIEMAN DC. *Exercise & immunology: practical applications.* Int. J. Sports Med. 18 (suppl 1): S91-S100, 1997

NIEMAN DC. *Upper respiratory tract infections & exercise.* Thorax 50: 1229-1231, 1995

NIEMAN DC. *Exercise, upper respiratory tract infection, & the immune system.* Med. Sci. Sports Exerc. 26: 128-139, 1994

NIEMAN DC, HENSON DA, GUSEWITCH G, ET AL. *Physical activity & immune function in elderly women.* Med. Sci. Sports Exerc. 25: 823-831, 1993

NIEMAN DC, PEDERSEN BK. *Exercise & immune function. Recent developments.* Sports Med. 27: 73-80, 1999

NIKOLAIDIS MG, JAMURTAS AZ, PASCHALIS V, ET AL. *The effect of muscle-damaging exercise on blood & skeletal muscle oxidative stress: magnitude & time-course considerations.* Sports Med. 38:579-606, 2008

NYBERG M, MORTENSEN SP, CABO H, ET AL. *Roles of sedentary aging & lifelong physical activity in exchange of glutathione across exercising human skeletal muscle.* Free Radic Biol Med. 73:166-173, 2014

OHKUWA T, SATO Y, NAOI M. *Glutathione status & reactive oxygen generation in tissues of young & old exercised rats.* Acta. Physiol. Sc&. 159: 237-244, 1997

PACKER L. *Oxidants, antioxidants & the athlete.* J. Sports Sci. 15: 353-363, 1997

PEDERSEN BK. *Influence of physical activity on the cellular immune system: mechanisms of action.* Int. J. Sports Med. 12 (Suppl !): S23-S29, 1991

PEDERSEN BK, BRUUNSGAARD H. *How physical exercise influences the establishment of infections.* Sports Med. 19: 393-400, 1995

PEDERSEN BK, ROHDE T, ZACHO M. *Immunity in athletes.* J. Sports Med. Phys. Fitness 36: 236-245, 1996

PETERS EM. *Exercise, immunology & upper respira-*

tory tract infections. Int. J. Sports Med. 18 (suppl 1): S69-S77, 1997

Petersen AC, McKenna MJ, Medved I, et al. *Infusion with the antioxidant N-acetylcysteine attenuates early adaptive responses to exercise in human skeletal muscle.* Acta Physiol 204:382-392, 2012

Pyke S, Lew H, Quintanilha A. *Severe depletion in liver glutathione during physical exercise.* Biochem. Biophys. Res. Commun. 139: 926-931, 1986

Rai S, Chowdhury A, Reniers RLEP, et al. *A pilot study to assess the effect of acute exercise on brain glutathione.* Free Radic Res. 52:57-69, 2018

Reid MB, Stokic DS, Koch SM, et al. *N-acetylcysteine inhibits muscle fatigue in humans.J. Clin. Invest. 94: 2468-2474, 1994*

Reznick AZ, Witt EH, Silbermann M, Packer L.The threshold of age in exercise & antioxidants action.EXS 62: 423-427, 1992

Rhodes K, Braakhuis A. *Performance & Side Effects of Supplementation with N-Acetylcysteine: A Systematic Review & Meta-Analysis.* Sports Med. 47:1619-1636, 2017

Rowbottom DG, Keast D, Garcia-Webb P, Morton AR.Training adaptation & biological changes among well-trained male athletes.Med. Sci. Sports Exerc. 29: 1233-1239, 1997

Sastre J, Asensi M, Gasco E, et al. *Exhaustive physical exercise causes oxidation of glutathione status in blood: prevention by antioxidant administration. American J. Physiol. 263 (5 Pt 2): R992-R995, 1992*

Sen CK.Oxidants & antioxidants in exercise.J. Appl. Physiol. 79: 675-686, 1995

Sen CK, Atalay M, Hanninen O.Exercise-induced oxidative stress: glutathione supplementation & deficiency.J. Appl. Physiol. 77: 2177-2187, 1994

Sen CK, Marin E, Kretzchmar M, Hanninen O. *Skeletal muscle & liver glutathione homeostasis in response to training, exercise, & immobilization.* J. Appl. Physiol. 73: 1265-1272, 1992

Sen CK, Rankinen T, Vaisanen S, Rauramaa R. *Oxidative stress after human exercise: effect of n-acetylcysteine supplementation.* J. Appl. Physiol. 76: 2570-2577, 1994

Shepard RJ, Shek PN. *Impact of physical activity & sport on the immune system.* Rev. Environ. Health 11: 133-147, 1996

Shepard RJ, Shek PN. *Exercise, aging & immune function.* Int. J. Sports Med. 16: 1-6, 1995

Shiraseb F, Siassi F, Sotoudeh G, et al. *Association of blood antioxidants status with visual & auditory sustained attention.* Nutr Neurosci 18:345-354, 2015

Sinha S, Singh SN, Monga YP, Ray US. *Improvement of glutathione & total antioxidant status with yoga.* J Altern Complement Med. 13:1085-1090, 2007

Slattery KM, Dascombe B, Wallace LK, et al. *Effect of N-acetylcysteine on cycling performance after intensified training.* Med Sci Sports Exerc. 46:1114-1123, 2014

Spanidis Y, Stagos D, Orfanou M, et al. *Variations in Oxidative Stress Levels in 3 Days Follow-up in Ultramarathon Mountain Race Athletes.* J Strength Cond Res. 31:582-594, 2017

Spanidis Y, Goutzourelas N, Stagos D, et al. *Variations in oxidative stress markers in elite basketball players at the beginning & end of a season.* Exp Ther Med 11:147-153, 2016

Thompson HJ. *Effect of treadmill exercise intensity on hepatic glutathione content & its relevance to mammary tumorigenesis.* J Sports Med Fitness 32:59-63, 1992

Traustadottir T, Davies SS, Su Y, et al. *Oxidative stress in older adults: effects of physical fitness.* Age 34:969-982, 2012

Turner JE, Bosch JA, Drayson MT, Aldred S. *Assessment of oxidative stress in lymphocytes with exercise.* J Appl Physiol. 111:206-211, 2011

Yavari A, Javadi M, Mirmiran P, Bahadoran Z. *Exercise-induced oxidative stress & dietary antioxidants.* Asian J Sports Med. 6:e24898, 2015

Woods JA, Davis JM, Smith JA, Nieman DC. *Exercise & cellular innate immune function.* Med. Sci. Sports Exerc. 31: 57-66, 1999

Zarebska A, Jastrzebski Z, Ahmetov II, et al. *GSTP1 c.313A>G polymorphism in Russian & Polish athletes.* Physiol Genomics. 49:127-131, 2017

24
GSH in Life & Health Maintenance

You may say, "I'm healthy. Why worry about glutathione?" The answer is simple: "Disease prevention, quality of life, longevity, a sense of well-being." Or, to put it more bluntly, "To stay alive as long as possible and enjoy good health to the end."

One of a doctor's most challenging jobs is to convince a patient with no symptoms to take medication every day. People with high blood pressure often feel healthy and experience no symptoms, but they're highly prone to heart attacks and strokes. It's even harder to convince a diabetic teenager to avoid junk food, even though it can lead to kidney failure and blindness. I imagine financial advisors have the same difficulty convincing younger clients to tie up their hard-earned income in a retirement savings plan.

The truth is, pain and poor health are powerful motivators. Without them, logical arguments alone never provoke a truly visceral response. Preventive health maintenance requires a lifestyle commitment and special attention to personal needs. Many people find this hard.

For too long preventive medicine has taken a back seat to treatment-oriented medicine. Much of the slack has been taken up by other healthcare professionals, such as nutritionists, naturopaths and those working in complementary fields. Today, much more attention is being paid to preventive medicine, and a new school of thought is evolving.

It's a paradigm shift. Until recently, both doctors and patients regarded health as the mere absence of disease, and quality of life as secondary. Nowadays the focus is on "wellness" in its fullest sense. We owe it to ourselves and to society at large not only to stay healthy but also to maintain a sense of wellbeing—even a lust for life.

Is your health really at risk if your glutathione levels fall? If we were to impair the GSH effectiveness of young people, would this raise their incidence of disease? A group of Russian researchers found themselves ideally positioned to answer these questions. They realized that a large portion of the population was missing the gene for a GSH enzyme, glutathione-Stransferase S1 (GSTM1). They

General population	38.8
Lung cancer patients	81.0
Other cancer patients	65.0
Endometriosis patients	81.0
Alcoholic cirrhosis patients	77.0
Cystic fibrosis patients (with pulmonary manifestations)	51.0
Chronic bronchitis patients (with radiological changes)	74.0

Table 34: *Table 34: Percent missing the GSTM1 gene*

1998 (J. Gutman, first edition)	42,000
2019 (J. Gutman, curent edition)	150,000

TABLE 35: TABLE 35: Number of articles about glutathione (www.PubMed.gov)

measured first the population at large for this gene, and then a large group suffering from lung and other cancers, alcoholic cirrhosis, cystic fibrosis, chronic bronchitis, endometriosis and other diseases. It was found that a significantly higher portion of the unwell population was missing the normal gene.

Today we have the ability to "read" our DNA. Preventive medicine has entered a new era. An inexpensive genetic coding test tells us what particular problems to watch out for as we get older. A whole slew of different glutathione enzyme abnormalities have been identified, and they have strong correlations with a variety of health risks, most notable the increased likelihood of cancer or neurodegenerative disease (see chapters 5 and 28, respectively).

There's little doubt among scientists and medical professionals that good glutathione levels correspond to good health. Table 28 shows the number of articles on glutathione and aging appearing recently in major medical journals.

The references at the end of each chapter list the thousands of scientific papers consulted in the preparation of this book, providing overwhelming evidence that well-maintained glutathione levels are a precondition of general health.

This is particularly true of the aging population, as one study demonstrates with glaring simplicity. It was reported in the prestigious British medical journal The Lancet, and was entitled "Glutathione: in sickness and in health." GSH was measured in four groups of people:

1) young healthy volunteers (average 24 years); 2) a healthy elderly population with no hospital admissions, no medications and no major illnesses in the previous five years; 3) elderly patients treated at an out-patient clinic for a variety of chronic illnesses including heart disease, arthritis, diabetes and hypertension; 4) hospitalized elderly patients.

Results are shown in Figure 45. Those in the poorest health (the hospitalized elderly) have the lowest GSH levels while young volunteers—the healthiest—have high levels. Raising GSH levels keeps us well as we age.

No matter how long we live nor how much attention we pay to our health, we must eventually face our own mortality. The link between glutathione and all the major causes of death is profound, and the list of research papers supporting this evidence is still growing. The connection between GSH and many of the major causes of illness is equally

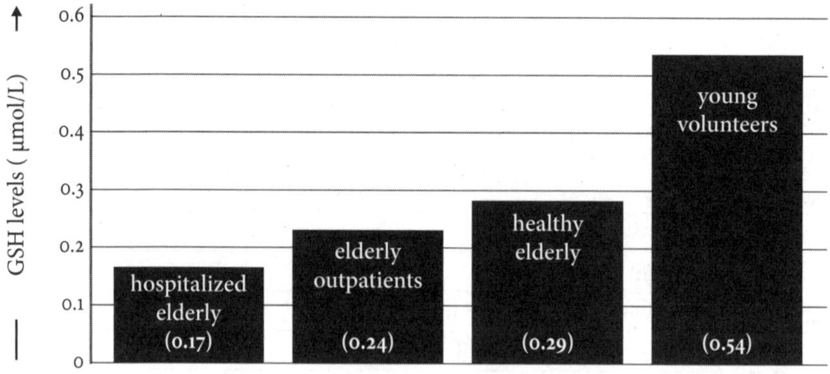

FIGURE 47: GSH levels and general health

MAJOR CAUSES OF MORBIDITY AND MORTALITY	
Heart Disease and Stroke	Chapter 7
Cancer	Chapter 5
Lung disease	Chapter 12
MAIN CAUSES OF CHRONIC ILLNESS/HOSPITAL ADMISSIONS (OTHER THAN ABOVE))	
Diabetes	Chapter 8
Arthritis	Chapter 6
Dementia, neurodegenerative diseases	Chapters 6, 26, 27, 28
AIDS	Chapter 11
MAIN CAUSES OF ACUTE HOSPITALIZATION (OTHER THAN ABOVE)	
Infectious disease	Chapters 3, 9, 12
Trauma	Chapter 21
Gastrointestinal problems	Chapter 13

TABLE 36: GSH links

unambiguous, as you can see from Table 36.

Heart disease, stroke and cancer are the leading causes of death in North America. These diseases are all to a large degree preventable, but sadly their incidence on the rise. The number of cancer cases alone is expected to increase by 30% over the next decade.

Many of the common illnesses we suffer from are avoidable. These include diabetes, bronchitis, high cholesterol levels and infectious diseases. Traditional advice for health-conscious people focuses on behavioral modification. We are told to quit smoking, drink moderately, eat well and exercise regularly. More recently we've learned the advantages of avoiding undue stress, practicing safe sex and using vitamins and other supplements.

Today, we know that glutathione maintenance is climbing up this list, propelled by the massive weight of scientific evidence. As general physicians become aware of the health potential of this marvelous molecule, they will begin to share it with their patients.

Contemplating the years of life lost to these diseases (see Figure 46) is a chilling reminder of what happens when we ignore our long-term health.

My work is killing me

This is true literally, not just figuratively. Depending on what you do, the way you die or get sick may be related to your work. A landmark study published in the journal Occupational Environmental Medicine by Canadians Carpenter and Aronson established a connection between job descriptions and the likelihood of specific causes of death. For example, barbers, hairdressers, and manicurists are seven times more likely to die of infectious disease than the average blue-collar worker. Business owners and managers are more than ten times more likely to die of kidney disease than other white-collar workers. More results of the survey are shown in Table 37 and Table 38.

The first rule of health maintenance is to identify personal and environmental risk factors. These figures can help us with part of that process. Whether you need to deal with occupational toxins or just strengthen your immune system, glutathione helps.

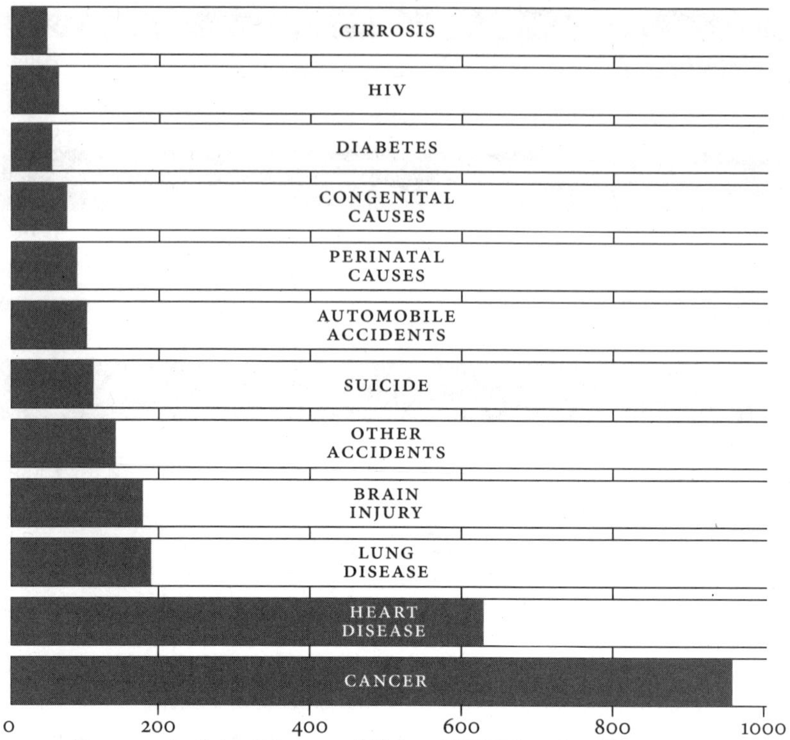

FIGURE 48: Potential years of life lost (PYLL) based on life expectancy (Source: Canadian Cancer Statistics, 1999)

Stressed out

It took the medical community a while, but it has finally acknowledged that stress is not just in the mind. It is in the body too and can be measured. We all know the effects of stress on sleep and eating habits. Now strong evidence links it to heart disease, memory problems, obesity and impaired immune defense.

Ronald Glaser of Ohio State University measured the ability of geriatric patients to respond to a flu shot. The purpose of the shot is to stimulate antibody production so that the body is prepared to confront possible infection. In particular, individuals nursing a spouse with dementia responded to the vaccine more poorly than people who were not under such stress.

Psychologist Sheldon Cohen demonstrated that individuals undergoing either work-related or interpersonal stress were more likely to catch a cold when exposed to the virus.

Others have documented that men reporting high stress levels were much more likely to suffer from a heart attack than men with little stress. As we have said before, it is not only the consequences of stress that make a demand on glutathione—the stress response itself depletes glutathione levels.

Infectious disease and the 21st century plague

"The Killer Germ," trumpets Time magazine. "War Against the Microbes," declares Business Week. The media and even TV documentaries are all doing their part to sensationalize the problem. We are facing a recurrence of infectious diseases unseen for decades, perhaps centuries.

Not long ago we thought we would once and for all annihilate such scourges as polio, scarlet fever, cholera and smallpox. But the same pharmaceutical technology that almost made these microbes extinct seems also to be partly responsible for the emergence of newer and more resistant ones. Overuse of antibiotics, both in the human population and in livestock, has given these pathogens an opportunity to develop antibiotic resistance. This leaves us without effective weapons against them, making their elimination increasingly difficult—perhaps impossible.

Outbreaks of antibiotic-resistant infections are on the rise. Whole wings of hospitals have been shut down to contain such problems as MRSA (Methicillin Resistant Staphlococcus Aureus). Other examples are outbreaks of toxic E. Coli that have sickened and killed thousands worldwide, rampaging Strep A, and deadly flus that strike every several years.

Flesh-eating disease, mad cow disease and super-bugs, Ziki, AIDS, Ebola, dengue fever, chikungunya fever, Lyme disease and others conjure up nightmare scenes that have fed the imagination of Hollywood script-writers. These may sound like exotic and remote diseases, but they are only a plane-ride away from New York, London, Mexico City or Montreal. The next new plague is always, "just around the corner."

Why do some people fall prey to infection while others resist? How is it that two people with the same bug recuperate at very different rates? These are complex questions with equally complex answers, but it always comes down to the state of the immune system. Rather than spending all our money and time on the development of newer and more powerful antibiotics and antiviral agents, we should apply some of it to enhancing the defensive capabilities of the immune system.

Since viruses and bacteria are always mutating, they eventually become resistant to drugs. As we've discovered to our cost, this is inevitable. To develop offensive weapons without paying attention to our defense

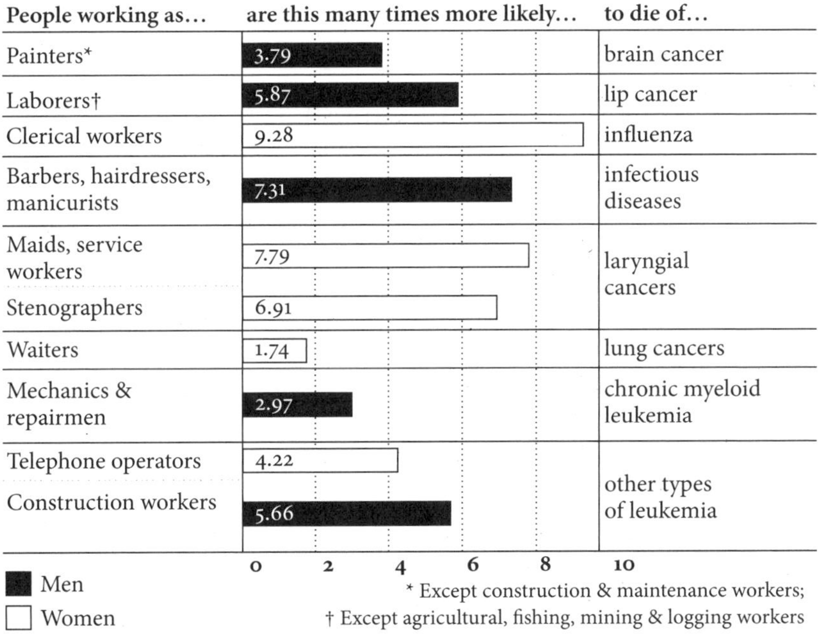

Table 37: Occupational hazards for blue-collar workers [Adapted from Aronson KJ, Howe GR, Carpenter M, Fair ME: Occupational Environmental Medicine (UK), 1999]

People working as…	are this many times more likely…	to die of…
Inspectors & foremen	3.94	ischemic heart disease
Civil engineers	3.94	prostate cancer
Funeral directors and embalmers	6.00	other cancer
Foremen, textile occupations	5.79	all cancers
Owners & managers	10.45	nephritis
Foremen	5.10	chronic myeloid leukemia
Purchasing agents & buyers	5.90	lung cancers

■ Men
□ Women

0 2 4 6 8 10

TABLE 38: Occupational hazards for white-collar workers [ADAPTED FROM ARONSON KJ, HOWE GR, CARPENTER M, FAIR ME: OCCUPATIONAL ENVIRONMENTAL MEDICINE (UK), 1999]

system is an unsound strategy. By enhancing the immune system of the population at large, we make it difficult for microbes to get a foothold. And even when we're infected, we would fight the bug more efficiently. Elevated glutathione levels enhance the immune system. Healthcare professionals, teachers, retail salespersons, restaurant workers and others who work with the public, those who spend time in crowded places such as movie theatres, restaurants, gyms and airports and those prone to any illness for any reason can increase their resistance by raising their glutathione levels.

Complementary or alternative medicine

Alternative medicine is not an alternative "to" medicine but an "addition." Conventional medicine does not adequately address such issues as wellness, balance, nutrition and spiritual health. The fusion of these two fields is long overdue. In fact, after years of fruitless bickering, the two approaches are being integrated into what is called "complementary medicine" or "integrative medicine." Instead of choosing between them, we are learning how they best work together.

However, the causes of conflict are not imaginary. Any integration of alternative and conventional medicine into a coherent system requires compromise. Alternative therapies are not perceived as credible, and cannot gain acceptance without scientific scrutiny and validation. For their part, conventional doctors must reconsider the mind-body connection—most importantly, how their personal relationship with patients impacts healing.

As is often the case, such broad changes in our society are being driven by market forces. Nationwide polls across North America reveal increasing use of alternative medicine as conventional medicine becomes too expensive, not accessible or not enough.

Traditional doctors and health professionals are often surprised by the demographic profile of people using alternative medicine. The conventional view that alternative medicine is driven by the poor and uneducated is mistaken. On the contrary, most users are city-dwellers and high earners. Also, those who use alternative medicine most often tend to be the more educated ones.

This growing demand for complementary practices has stimulated growth in many sectors of society, not just the economy. More medical schools in North America are adding courses on alternative medicine to their curricula, and this number continues to rise.

U.S. health insurers are beginning to offer coverage for alternative treatments. Independent manufacturers of vitamins, supplements and herbal products are being bought up by brand-name drug companies.

Since the turn of the millennium, the market for supplements, "medical foods," "pharmafoods" or "nutriceuticals" has increased by $2.5 billion dollars per year, and is still growing. This is not simply a cash-grab by a few well-positioned companies, but a well-funded source of ideas and scientific discovery. It will change how long and how well we live.

Conclusion

Both doctors and patients need to develop an open-minded, cautious approach to all possible diagnostic and therapeutic tools. Whether conventional or complementary, the emphasis should be on what works. That is the approach we have taken in this book. We have looked at both conventional and complementary ways of elevating glutathione levels. All information is based on hard scientific research and the reader is encouraged to pursue the references listed at the end of each chapter. The volume, variety and reliability of research data is staggering, and places glutathione squarely at the forefront of this natural approach to health.

Whether you want to simply treat an existing disease or are attempting to avoid future health problems, raised glutathione levels address the vast majority of the most common and most serious afflictions of modern society. The role of GSH as our body's most important antioxidant, its ability to rid the body of toxins, pollutants and carcinogens, and its critical role in the immune function will establish this molecule as a primary focus of disease prevention and anti-aging.

GSH IN LIFE & HEALTH MAINTENANCE

REFERENCES

Angell M, Kassirer JP. *Alternative medicine – the risks of untested & unregulated remedies.* New England J. Med. 17: 339: 839-841, 1998

Aronson KJ, Howe GR, Carpenter M, Fair ME. *Surveillance of potential associations between occupations & causes of death in Canada, 1965-91.* Occup. Environ. Med. 56:265-269, 1999

Astin JA. *Why patients use alternative medicine: results of a national study.* JAMA 279: 1548-1553, 1998

Ballatori N, Krance SM, Notenboom S, et al. *Glutathione dysregulation & the etiology & progression of human diseases.* Biol chem. 390: 191-214, 2009

Baranov VS, Ivaschenko T, Bakay B, et al. *Proportion of the GSTM1 0/0 genotype in some Slavic populations & its correlation with cystic fibrosis & some multifactorial diseases.* Human Genetics 97: 516-520, 1996

Barnett PA, Spence JD, Manuck SB, et al. *Psychological stress & the progression of carotid artery disease.* J. Hypertens. 15: 49-55, 1997

Berman BM, Singh BK, Lao L, et al. *Physicians' attitudes toward complementary or alternative medicine: A regional survey.* J. Am. Board Fam. Pract. 8:361-365, 1995

Blumberg DL, Grant WD, Hendricks SR, et al. *The physician & unconventional medicine.* Altern. Therapies 1: 31-35, 1995

Cacioppo JT, Berntson GG, Malarkey WB, et al. *Autonomic, neuroendocrine, & immune responses to psychological stress: the reactivity hypothesis.* Ann. N. Y. Acad. Sci. 840: 664-673, 1998

Cohen S, Frank E, Doyle WJ, et al. *Types of stressors that increase susceptibility to the common cold in healthy adults.* Health Psychol. 17: 214-223

Cooper KL, Harris PE, Relton C, et al. *Prevalence of visits to five types of complementary & alternative medicine practitioners by the general population:* a systematic review. Complement Ther Clin Pract. 19: 214-220, 2013

Cooper RA, Stoflet SJ. *Trends in the education & practice of alternative medicine clinicians.* Health

Aff. 15: 226-238, 1996

Cottrell K. *Herbal products begin to attract the attention of brand-name drug companies.* Can. Med. Assoc. J. 155: 216-219, 1996

CTV/Angus Reid Group *Use of alternative medicines & practices.* Angus Reid Group (Winnipeg), 1997

Currais A, Maher P. *Functional consequences of age-dependent changes in glutathione status in the brain.* Antioxid Redox Signal. 19: 813-822, 2013

de Almeida Andrade F, Schlechta Portella CF. *Research methods in complementary & alternative medicine: an integrative review.* J Integr Med. 16: 6-13, 2018

De Matteis S, Heederik D, Burdorf A, et al. *Current & new challenges in occupational lung disease.* Eur Respir Rev. DOI: 10.1183/16000617.0080-2017

Droge W, Hack V, Breitkreutz R, et al. *Role of cysteine & glutathione in signal transduction, immunopathology & cachexia.* Biofactors 8: 97-102, 1998

Eisenberg DM, Kessler RC, Foster C, et al. *Unconventional medicine in the United States: Prevalence, cost, & patterns of use.* New England J. Med. 328: 246-252, 1994

Ernst E, Resch KL, White AR. *Complementary medicine: What physicians think of it: a meta-analysis.* Arch. Inter. Med. 155: 2405-2408, 1995

Everson SA, Lynch JW, Chesney MA, et al. *Interaction of workplace demands & cardiovascular reactivity in progression of carotid atherosclerosis: population based study.* BMJ 314: 553-558, 1997

Fischer HF, Junne F, Witt C, et al. *Key issues in clinical & epidemiological research in complementary & alternative medicine—a systematic literature review.* Forsch Komplementmed 2: 51-60, 2012

Franco R, Cidlowski JA. *Apoptosis & glutathione : beyond an antioxidant.* Cell Death Differ. 16: 1303-1314, 2009

Franco R, Schoneveld OJ, Pappa A, et al. *The central role of glutathione in the pathophysiology of human diseases.* Arch Physiol Biochem. 113: 234-258, 2007

Franzel B, Schwiegershausen M, Heusser P, et al. *How to locate & appraise qualitative research in complementary & alternative medicine.* BMC Complement Altern Med 13:125, 2013

Fraternale A, Paoletti MF, et al. *GSH & analogs in antiviral therapy.* Mol Aspects Med. 30: 99-110, 2009

Glaser R, Kiecolt-Glaser JK. *Stress-associated immune modulation: relevance to viral infections & chronic fatigue syndrome.* Am. J. Med. 105: 35S-42S, 1998

Glaser R, Kiecolt-Glaser JK, Malarkey WB, et al. *The influence of psychological stress on the immune response to vaccines.* Ann. N. Y. Acad. Sci. 840: 649-655, 1998

Glaser R, Rabin B, Chesney M, et al. *Stress-induced immune modulation: implications for infectious diseases?* JAMA 281: 2268-2270, 1999

Go YM, Jones DP. *Redox theory of aging: implications for health & disease.* Clin Sci (Lond). 131: 1669-1688, 2017

Harris PE, Cooper KL, Relton C, et al. *Prevalence of complementary & alternative medicine (CAM) use by the general population: a systematic review & update.* Int J Clin Pract. 66:924-939, 2012

Harris P, Rees R. *The prevalence of complementary & alternative medicine use among the general population: a systematic review of the literature.* Complement Ther Med. 8: 88-96, 2000

Homma T, Fujii J. *Application of Glutathione as Anti-Oxidative & Anti-Aging Drugs.* Curr Drug Metab. 16: 560-571, 2015

Janssen-Heininger YM, Nolin JD, Hoffman SM, et al. *Emerging mechanisms of glutathione-dependent chemistry in biology & disease.* 114:1962-1968, 2013

Jonas WB, Eisenberg D, *The evolution of complementary & alternative medicine (CAM) in the USA over the last 20 years.* Forsch Komplementmed. 20: 65-72, 2013

Kanherkar RR, Stair SE, Bhatia-Dey N, et al. *Epigenetic Mechanisms of Integrative Medicine.* Evid Based Complement Alternat Med. 2017:4365429.

Katz DL, William AL, Girard C, et al. *The evidence base for complementary & alternative medicine: methods of Evidence Mapping with application to CAM.* Altern Ther Health Med. 9: 22-30, 2003

Khachatourians GG. *Agricultural use of antibiotics & the evolution & transfer of antibiotic-resistant bacteria.* CMAJ 159: 1129-1136, 1998

Kiecolt-Glaser JK, Glaser R. *Psychoneuroimmunology & immunotoxicology: implications for carcinogenesis.* Psychosom. 61: 271-272, 1999

Kivimäki M, Kawachi I. *Work Stress as a Risk Factor for Cardiovascular Disease.* Curr Cardiol Rep. 17: 630, 2015

Kolesnichenko LS, Kulinskii VI, Ias'ko MV, et al. *The effect of emotional-painful stress, hypoxia, & adaptation to it on the activity of enzymes for metabolizing glutathione & concentration of glutathione in rat organs.* Vopr. Med. Khim. 40: 10-12, 1994

Kolesnichenko LS, Mantorova NS, Shapiro LA, et al. *Effect of emotional stress on the activity of enzymes of glutathione metabolism.* Vopr. Med.

Khim. 33: 85-88, 1987

Kral BG, Becker LC, Blumenthal RS, et al. *Exaggerated reactivity to mental stress is associated with exercise-induced myocardial ischemia in an asymptomatic high-risk population.* Circulation 96: 4246-4253, 1997

Leigh JP. *Economic burden of occupational injury & illness in the United States.* Milbank Q. 89: 728-772, 2011

Litchy AP. *Naturopathic physicians: holistic primary care & integrative medicine specialists.* J Diet Suppl. 8: 369-377, 2011

Lubos E, Loscalzo J, Handy DE. *Glutathione peroxidase-1 in health & disease: from molecular mechanisms to therapeutic opportunities.* Antioxid Redox Signal. 15: 1957-1997, 2011

Lynch JW, Everson SA, Kaplan GA, et al. *Does low socioeconomic status potentiate the effects of heightened cardiovascular responses to stress on the progression of carotid atherosclerosis?* Am. J. Public Health 8: 389-394

Maher P. *The effects of stress & aging on glutathione metabolism.* Ageing Res Rev. 4: 288-314, 2005

Maizes V, Rakel D, Niemiec C. *Integrative medicine & patient-centered care.* Explore (NY) 5: 277-289, 2009

Mansfield KL, Jizhou L, Phipps LP, et al. *Emerging Tick-Borne Viruses in the Twenty-First Century.* Front Cell Infect Microbiol. 7: 298, 2017

Mari M, Morales A, Colell A, et al. *Mitochondrial glutathione, a key survival antioxidant.* Antioxid Redox Signal. 11: 2685-2700, 2009

Marwick C. *Growing use of medicinal botanicals forces assessment by drug regulators.* JAMA 273: 607-609, 1995

McCarty MF, DiNicolantonio JJ. *An increased need for dietary cysteine in support of glutathione synthesis may underlie the increased risk for mortality associated with low protein intake in the elderly.* Age (Dordr). 37: 96, 2015

McEwen BS, Sapolsky RM. *Stress & cognitive function.* Curr. Opin. Neurobiol. 5: 205-216, 1995

McIntosh LJ, Hong KE, Sapolsky RM. *Glucocorticoids may alter antioxidant enzyme capacity in the brain: baseline studies.* Brain Res. 791: 209-214, 1998

McIntosh LJ, Sapolsky RM. *Glucocorticoids may enhance oxygen radical-mediated neurotoxicity.* Neurotoxicology 17: 873-882, 1996

Morris D, Khurasany M, Nguyen T, et al. *Glutathione & infection.* Biochem Biophys Acta. 1830: 3329-3349, 2013

National Institute of Health. *Alternative medicine – Expanding medical horizons: A report to the NIH on alternative medical systems & practices in the United States.* NIH publication 94-066. Washington DC. Government Printing Office, 1994

Nuttal SL, Martin U, Sinclair AJ, Kendall MJ. *Glutathione: in sickness & in health.* Lancet 35: 645-646, 1998

Oparil S, Oberman A. *Nontraditional cardiovascular risk factors.* Am. J. Med. Sci. 317: 193-207, 1999

Peeke PM, Chrousos GP. *Hypercortisolism & obesity.* Ann. N. Y. Acad. Sci. 771: 665-676, 1995

Rebrin I, Sohal RS. *Pro-oxidant shift in glutathione redox state during aging.* Adv Drug Deliv Rev. 60: 1545-1552, 2008

Reid M, Jahoor F. *Glutathione in disease.* Curr Opin Clin Nutr Metab Care. 4: 65-71, 2001

Rosenthal T, Alter A. *Occupational stress & hypertension.* J Am Soc Hypertens. 6: 2-22, 2012

Rozanski A, Blumenthal JA, Kaplan J. *Impact of psychological factors on the pathogenesis of cardiovascular disease & implications for therapy.* Circulation 99: 2192-2217, 1999

Rushton L. *The Global Burden of Occupational Disease.* Curr Environ Health Rep. 4: 340-348, 2017

Sapolsky RM. *Why stress is bad for your brain.* Science 273: 749-750, 1996

Sapolsky RM. *Stress, Glucocorticoids, & Damage to the Nervous System: The Current State of Confusion.* Stress 1: 1-19, 1996

Sharpley CF. *Psychosocial stress-induced heart rate reactivity & atherogenesis: cause or correlation?* J. Behav. Med. 21: 411-432, 1998

Singh RJ. *Glutathione: a marker & antioxidant for aging.* J Lab Clin Med. 140: 380-381, 2002

Smith A. *The scale of perceived occupational stress.* Occup Med (Lond). 50: 294-298, 2000

Spence JD. *Neurocardiology. Stress & atherosclerosis.* Baillieres Clin. Neurol. 6: 275-282, 1997

Stayner LT, Collins JJ, Guo YL, et al. *Challenges & Opportunities for Occupational Epidemiology in the Twenty-first Century.* Curr Environ Health Rep. 4: 319-324, 2017

Steptoe A, Deaton A, Stone AA. *Subjective wellbeing, health, & ageing.* Lancet. 385: 640- 648, 2015

Sweileh WM. *Global research trends of World Health Organization's top eight emerging pathogens.* Global Health 13:9, 2017

Takala J, Hämäläinen P, Saarela KL, et al. *Global estimates of the burden of injury & illness at work in 2012.* J Occup Environ Hyg. 11: 326-337, 2014

Templeman K, Robinson A. *Integrative medicine models in contemporary primary health care.* Complement Ther Med. 19: 84-92, 2011

Tew KD, Townsend DM. *Glutathione-s-transfer-*

ases as determinants of cell survival & death. Antioxid Redox Signal. 17: 1728-1737, 2012

Toleikis PM, Godin DV. *Alteration of antioxidant status in diabetic rats by chronic exposure to psychological stressors.* Pharmacol. Biochem. Behav. 52: 355-366, 1995

Townsend DM, Tew KD, Tapiero H. *The importance of glutathione in human disease.* Biomed Pharmacother. 57: 145-155, 2003

Treister-Goltzman Y, Peleg R. *Trends in publications on complementary & alternative medicine in the medical literature.* J Complement Integr Med. 12: 111-115, 2015

Veziari Y, Leach MJ, Kumar S. *Barriers to the conduct & application of research in complementary & alternative medicine: a systematic review.* BMC Complement Altern Med. 17:166, 2017

Vouga M, Greub G. *Emerging bacterial pathogens: the past & beyond.* Clin Microbiol Infect. 22: 12-21, 2016

Wilson MD, Conroy LM, Dorevitch S. *Occupational stress & subclinical atherosclerosis: a systematic review.* Int J Occup Environ Health. 20: 271-280, 2014

Woolhouse ME. *Population biology of emerging & re-emerging pathogens.* Trends Microbiol. 10: S3-S7, 2002

Wu G, Fang YZ, Yang S, et al. *Glutathione metabolism & its implications for health.* J Nutr. 134: 489-492, 2004

Wu H, Wang J, Cacioppo JT, et al. *Chronic stress associated with spousal care giving of patients with Alzheimer's dementia is associated with down-regulation of B-lymphocyte GH mRNA.* J Gerontol A Biol Sci Med Sci. 54: M212-215, 1999

PART THREE

GLUTATHIONE IN THE BRAIN & NERVOUS SYSTEM

[CHAPTERS 25 TO 34]

The third part of this book describes the glutathione metabolism in the brain and nervous system, and demonstrates how glutathione can help prevent or treat a variety of disorders there.

25

Parkinson's Disease

Also known as shaking palsy, Parkinson's disease is one of North America's most common debilitating illnesses. It is often thought of as a disease of old age—one person in a hundred will develop it by retirement age, but half of those may have it by age 40.

Parkinson's disease progresses as nerve cells degenerate in the part of the mid-brain controling movement.[1] In normal health, messages from the motor cortex to the reticular formation initiate free movement, and neurotransmitters released from the basal ganglia in response to the same messages slow down and dampen movement, providing the suppleness and dexterity we take for granted (see Figure 47). These two neurotransmitters are dopamine, which stimulates the damping effect, and acetylcholine, which inhibits it.

Symptoms and causes

Its exact cause is usually unknown, but Parkinson's disease is characterized by cell damage in an area of the brain called the "basal ganglia." Dopamine production slows and characteristic symptoms appear, beginning with weakness or stiffness accompanied by a light tremor of the hands or head. Over time the tremors worsen, muscles stiffen and there is visible deterioration in balance and coordination. In advanced stages, symptoms include generalized rigidity, drooling, loss of appetite, stooped posture, a shuffling walk and a fixed facial expression. Eventually, communication skills may be impaired. Dementia is common, as are depression and other emotional problems.

Genetic factors too play a role. Other contributing causes include certain medications, pesticides, carbon monoxide, cyanide, manganese, street heroin, specific viruses

[1] The substantia nigra layer of the basal ganglia

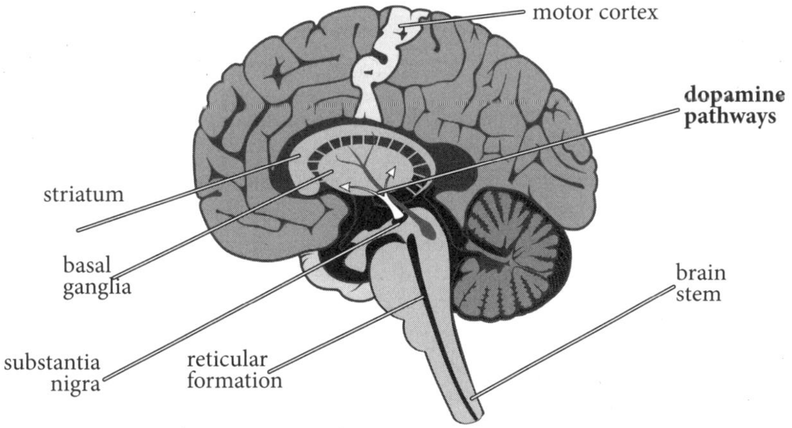

FIGURE 49: Parts of the brain affected by Parkinson's, showing dopamine pathways

and repetitive head trauma, as suffered by boxer Mohammed Ali (dementia pugilistica). Researchers at the National Institute of Health in Bethesda recently identified a gene programmed for the production of a protein called alpha synuclein—hopefully a clue to further discoveries about Parkinson's disease, and innovative ways to treat it.

Treatment

There is so far no definitive cure for Parkinson's disease but it is treatable—most effectively at the outset. Therefore, the earlier the diagnosis the better. So far, treatments include medication that attempts to replace or supplement the body's production of dopamine, restoring neurochemical balance. Neurosurgical techniques and fetal tissue implants have had some success. Some scientists are implanting electrodes in the brain, trying to stimulate specific neural pathways. Drugs such as selegiline[2] may help. A team headed by researchers Jenner and Olanow from the Neurodegenerative Disease Research Centre in London have shown that selegiline may increase GSH activity. Recently, newer drugs like pramipexole and ropenerole have emerged as more effective treatments. Even more exciting is the advent of stem cell technology, which has shown great promise.

Parkinson's disease and glutathione

Research has revealed two important findings. First, biochemical analysis of affected brain tissue shows damage consistent with extensive oxidative stress and the circulation of free radicals that follows it. Second, GSH levels in these tissues are particularly low. What's striking about Parkinson's is that there's about a 40% decrease in glutathione during the early stages of the disease. Adams and his researchers at the University of Southern California were able to show that in advanced Parkinson's Disease, glutathione levels fall to a mere 2% of normal. Whether the drop in GSH is a cause or a symptom of this damage remains unclear. But there is good news—elevated GSH levels slow brain tissue damage. Some symptoms may even be reversed.

Since free radical damage is an invariable part of Parkinson's Disease, researchers have experimented with a number of high-dose antioxidants, including both well-known ones and glutathione therapy. Not only is GSH an exceptional antioxidant, the substantia nigra of Parkinson's patients is especially deficient in it, so its need is great. Gabby's research team in Israel showed that elevated GSH levels more effectively reduce dopaminergic toxicity than the antioxidant vitamins C and E. Paradoxically, while brain cells need dopamine to function, dopamine at certain times actually becomes toxic to the same tissues. This may be why drugs which raise L-dopa levels, like Sinemet, work only for a few years before the benefits wear off and the patient deteriorates.

Jenner and his team at the Parkinson's Disease Experimental Research Laboratories in London have extensively examined GSH in the progression of this disease. They found that GSH levels fall steadilly at the very onset of Parkinson's Disease and believe elevated GSH levels can help prevent neural damage.

Offen's team at the Beilinson Medical Center in Israel considered the neurons actually involved in dopamine metabolism, and the cell-death that accompanies Parkinson's characteristic loss of dopamine. To slow down this decline they used antioxidants, finding that the thiol (sulfur-containing) antioxidants GSH, NAC and dithioleitol worked well. In the cautious language of medical science, Offen described them as "markedly protective" of brain cells. This corroborated the findings of Gabby's work (above), further

[2] An enzyme blocker that slows the breakdown of dopamine and other neurotransmitters.

supporting the theory that GSH may prevent or delay dopamine-induced cell death.

Studying individuals that lack specific genetic coding for normal glutathione function provides indirect evidence of the critical importance of GSH in protecting against this disease. This includes abnormalities in the glutathione enzymes GSH-S-transferase, GSTT1, GSTM1 and other inborn errors of the glutathione metabolism. The advancing sophistication of genetic testing will soon identify people at risk and suggest preventive measures.

Sechi's team in Italy studied a group of untreated Parkinson's patients in the early stages of the disease, giving them intravenous GSH therapy twice a day for a month. All patients improved significantly, with more than 40% decrease in their disability. The improvement faded away two to four months after the last GSH treatment.

Other authors have drawn attention to GSH-enhancing drugs in the treatment of this disease. There is much evidence to support the usefulness of elevated glutathione levels. Today, fortunately, there are ways to raise GSH levels without the use of pharmaceutical drugs—see Chapter 4.

Since the last edition of this book, there have been extensive human trials into raising glutathione levels in Parkinson's disease. It is not yet considered a "standard of care" by the medical community, but these studies continue to accumulate and cannot be ignored, compelling neuroscientists to keep exploring GSH-based therapies.

Given the mounting evidence linking GSH deficiency to Parkinsonian patients, Martinez-Banaclocha (2012) wrote the aptly titled "N-acetyl-cysteine in the treatment of Parkinson's disease—*What are we waiting for*?" Her call resulted in a flurry of studies using that approach. With MR (magnetic resonance) imaging, Holmay's team clearly showed how this GSH precursor could raise GSH in the brain. Katz (2015) used high levels of oral NAC to increase GSH levels in the fluid surrounding the spine and brain—cerebrospinal fluid (CSF). This was verified by Reyes et al (2016). Unfortunately, NAC did not result in the robust clinical improvement that was anticipated.

A Thai team using cysteine-rich whey protein isolate (CRWPI) was the first to establish that this natural protein could raise GSH levels in Parkinson's disease as well as raising BCAAs[3] (branch chain amino acids). This opened up the possibility of larger trials, a welcome addition to potential treatment using natural supplementation.

Case studies

Wally, a seventy-four year-old baseball fan, was diagnosed with Parkinson's disease in May 1997. The disease progressed rapidly and his doctors placed him on Sinemet (carbidopa/levodopa[4]). By November he was experiencing severe headaches—presumably from the medication—and he discontinued it. Up to this point he had lived a very active life, but now he deteriorated to the point where he could not get out of bed or even rise from a chair without help. He says movement felt like "walking in cement." He was constantly fatigued and soon needed a wheelchair to go outdoors. The doctors used other medications, including Eldepryl (selegiline hydrochloride) and Requip (ropinirole hydrochloride). They helped slightly. In March 1998 he started taking a CRWPI[5]—a type of natural protein which raises GSH levels. After five days his headaches were gone. Within two weeks his fatigue had lessened. Two months later Wally was walking well again and was eventually able to visit the new Anaheim Angels baseball stadium, Edison Field, and to jog around the block. This was his only therapeutic intervention, and seven months later his active lifestyle continued.

---

[3] Branched-chain amino acids: of the nine essential amino acids, leucine, isoleucine and valine are BCAAs.

[4] A dopamine precursor.

[5] Cysteine-Rich Whey Protein Isolate

62 YEAR-OLD CAROL maintained an active legal practice until 1990. After being diagnosed with Parkinson's disease in 1986, she continued working for a while, but eventually had to quit. The stress aggravated her symptoms, and the symptoms in turn increased her stress. She was treated with a number of different medications but her health continued to deteriorate until she needed help at home to carry out day-to-day tasks. She quit driving and stopped the daily walks she loved. Then, within days of starting to take a bioactive whey protein isolate she felt her strength return. Weeks later she was once more exploring her neighborhood, and after nine months driving again.

Conclusion

Parkinson's disease is characterized by the loss of the brain cells that regulate dopamine. Significant evidence points to the joint role of very high oxidative stress and very low GSH levels as critical contributing causes. Studies have demonstrated that protecting these cells from damage and death by raising GSH levels can succeed both in the laboratory and in patients, and is a welcome addition to conventional medical treatments.

PARKINSON'S DISEASE

REFERENCES

ADAMS JD JR, KLAIDMAN LK, ODUNZE IN, SHEN HC, MILLER CA. *Alzheimer's & Parkinson's disease. Brain levels of glutathione, glutathione disulfide, & vitamin E.* Molecular Chemical Neuropathology 14(3):213-226, 1991

ADAMS JD JR, ODUNZE IN. *Oxygen free radicals & Parkinson's disease. Free Radical Biol Med 10(2):161-169, 1991*

ALLEN GF, ULLAH Y, HARGREAVES IP, LAND JM, HEALES SJ. *Dopamine but not l-dopa stimulates neural glutathione metabolism. Potential implications for Parkinson's & other dopamine deficiency states.* Neurochem Int 62(5):684-94, 2013

ARAKAWA M, ITO Y. *N-acetylcysteine & neurodegenerative diseases: basic & clinical pharmacology.* Cerebellum. 2007;6(4):308-14. doi: 10.1080/14734220601142878. Epub 2007 Jan 19

CACCIATORE I, BALDASSARRE L, FORNASARI E, MOLLICA A, PINNEN F. *Recent advances in treatment of neurodegenerative diseases based on GSH delivery.* Oxid Med Cell Longev 2012:240146, 2012

CACCIATORE I. ET AL. *A glutathione derivative with chelating & in vitro neuroprotective activities: synthesis, physicochemical properties, & biological evaluation.* ChemMedChem 8(11):1818-29, 2013

CHINTA SJ, ANDERSEN JK. *Redox imbalance in Parkinson's disease.* Biochim Biophys Acta 1780(11):1362-7, 2008

CORNETTA T. ET AL. *Epidemiological, clinical, & molecular study of a cohort of Italian Parkinson disease patients: association with glutathione-S-transferase & DNA repair gene polymorphisms.* Cell Mol Neurobiol 33(5):673-80, 2013

DI MONTE DA, CHAN P, SANDY MS. *Glutathione in Parkinson's disease: a link between oxidative stress & mitochondrial damage?* Annals of Neurology 32(suppl): S111-115, 1992

DIAS V, JUNN E, MOURADIAN MM. *The role of oxidative stress in Parkinson's disease.* J Parkinsons Dis 3(4):461-91, 2013

EBADI M, SRINIVASAN SK, BAXI MD. *Oxidative stress & antioxidant therapy in Parkinson's disease.* Progress in Neurobiology 48(1):1-19, 1996

GABBY M, TAUBER M, PORAT S, SIMANTOV R. *Selective role of glutathione in protecting human neuronal cells from dopamine-induced apoptosis.* Neuropharmacology 35(5):57 – 578, 1996

GARCIA-GARCIA A, ZAVALA-FLORES L, RODRIGUEZ-ROCHA H, FRANCO R. *Thiol-redox signaling, dopaminergic cell death, & Parkinson's disease Antioxid Redox Signal. 2012 Dec 15;17(12):1764-84*

GOKCE COKAL B. ET AL. *Serum glutathione peroxidase, xanthine oxidase, & superoxide dismutase activities & malondialdehyde levels in patients with Parkinson's disease.* Neurol Sci 38(3):425-431, 2017

GU F, CHAUHAN V, CHAUHAN A. *Glutathione redox imbalance in brain disorders.* Curr Opin Clin Nutr Metab Care 18(1):89-95, 2015.

HOLMAY MJ, TERPSTRA M, COLES LD, MISHRA U, AHLSKOG M, OZ G, CLOYD JC, TUITE PF. *N-Acetylcysteine boosts brain & blood glutathione in Gaucher & Parkinson diseases.* Clin Neuropharmacol 36(4):103-6, 2013

JENNER P. *Oxidative damage in neurodegenerative disease.* The Lancet 344:796-798, 1994

JENNER P. *Oxidative stress in Parkinson's disease & other neurodegenerative disorders.* Pathologie

Biologie 44(1):57-64, 1996

JENNER P, OLANOW CW. *Oxidative stress & the pathogenesis of Parkinson's disease.Neurology 47(6 suppl 3):S161-170, 1996*

JOHNSON WM, WILSON-DELFOSSE AL, MIEYAL JJ.DYSREGULATION OF GLUTATHIONE HOMEOSTASIS IN NEURODEGENERATIVE DISEASES. *Nutrients 4(10):1399-440, 2012*

KATZ M, WON SJ, PARK Y, ORR A, JONES DP, SWANSON RA, GLASS GA. *Cerebrospinal fluid concentrations of N-acetylcysteine after oral administration in Parkinson's disease.* Parkinsonism Relat Disord 21(5):500-3, 2015

KUMAR A, DHULL DK, GUPTA V, CHANNANA P, SINGH A, BHARDWAJ, RUHAL P, MITTAL R. *Role of Glutathione-S-transferases in neurological problems.* Expert Opin Ther Pat 27(3):299-309, 2017

KUMAR H, LIM HW, MORE SV, KIM BW, KOPPULA S, KIM IS, CHOI DK. *The role of free radicals in the aging brain & Parkinson's Disease: convergence & parallelism.* Int J Mol Sci 13(8):10478-504, 2012

LIMÓN-PACHECO JH, GONSEBATT ME. *The glutathione system & its regulation by neurohormone melatonin in the central nervous system.* Cent Nerv Syst Agents Med Chem 10(4):287-97, 2010

LIU H, PENG J, GAO J, ZHENG F, TIE C. *Glutathione S-transferase T1 & M1 null genotypes & Parkinson's disease risk: evidence from an updated meta-analysis.* Neurol Sci 36(9):1559-65, 2015

MARTIN HL, TEISMANN P. *Glutathione—a review on its role & significance in Parkinson's Disease.* FASEB J 23(10):3263-72, 2009

MARTINEZ-BANACLOCHA M. *Cysteine Network (CYSTEINET) Dysregulation in Parkinson's Disease: Role of N-acetylcysteine.* Curr Drug Metab. 2016;17(4):368-85.

MARTINEZ-BANACLOCHA MA. *N-acetyl-cysteine in the treatment of Parkinson's disease. What are we waiting for?* Med-Hypotheses 79(1):8-12, 2012

MAZZETTI AP, FIORILE MC, PRIMAVERA A, LO BELLO M. *Glutathione transferases & neurodegenerative diseases.* Neurochem Int 82:10-8, 2015

MCBEAN GJ, ASLAN M, GRIFFITHS HR, TORRAO RC. *Thiol redox homeostasis in neurodegenerative disease.* Redox Biol 5:186-94, 2015

MORRIS G, ANDERSON G, DEAN O, BERK M, GALECKI P, MARTIN-SUBERO M, MAES M. *The glutathione system: a new drug target in neuroimmune disorders.* Mol Neurobiol 50(3):1059-84, 2014

OWEN AD, SCHAPIRA AHV, JENNER P, MARSDEN CD. *Oxidative stress & Parkinson's disease.* Annals of the New York Academy of Science 786:217-223, 1996

OFFEN D, ZIV I, STERNIN H, MELAMED E, HOCHMAN A. *Prevention of dopamine-induced cell death by thiol antioxidants: possible implications for treatment of Parkinson's disease.* Experimental Biology 141(1):32-39, 1996

PERRY TL, GODIN DV, HANSEN S. *Parkinson's disease: a disorder due to nigral glutathione deficiency?* Neuroscience Letter 33(3):305-310, 1982

REIDERER P, SOFIC E, RAUSCH WD, SCHMIDT B ET AL. *Transition metals, ferritin, glutathione, ascorbic acid in Parkinsonian Brains.* Journal of Neurochemistry 52: 515-520, 1989

REYES RC ET AL. *Neuronal GSH Content & Antioxidant Capacity can be Normalized In Situ by N-acetyl Cysteine Concentrations Attained in Human Cerebrospinal Fluid.* Neurotherapeutics 13(1):217-25, 2016

REYNOLDS A, LAURIE C, MOSLEY RL, GENDELMAN HE. *Oxidative stress & the pathogenesis of neurodegenerative disorders.* Int Rev Neurobiol 82:297-325, 2007

SECHI G, DELEDDA MG, BUA G, SATTA WM, DEIANA GA, PES GM, ROSATI G. *Reduced intravenous GSH in the treatment of early Parkinson's disease.* Progress in Neuro-Psychopharmacology & Biological Psychiatry 20(7):1159-70, 1996

SEGURA-AGUILAR J, PARIS I, MUÑOZ P, FERRARI E, ZECCA L, ZUCCA FA. *Protective/toxic roles of dopamine in Parkinson's disease.* J Neurochem 129(6):898-915, 2014

SIAN J, DEXTER DT, LEES AJ, DANIEL S, JENNER P, MARSDEN CD. *Glutathione-related enzymes in brain in Parkinson's disease.* Annals of Neurology 36(3):356-361, 1994

SIAN J, DEXTER DT, LEES AJ, DANIEL S, AGID Y, JAVOY-AGID F, JENNER P, MARSDEN CD. *Alterations in GSH levels in Parkinson's disease & other neurodegenerative disorders affecting basal ganglia.* Annals of Neurology 36(3): 348-355, 1994

SIMONIAN NA, COYLE JT. *Oxidative stress in neurodegenerative diseases.* Annual Review of Pharmacology & Toxicology 36:83-106, 1996

SMEYNE M, SMEYNE RJ. *GSH metabolism & Parkinson's disease.* Free Radic Biol Med. 62:13-25, 2013

SPENCER JPE, JENNER P, HALLIWELL B. *Superoxide-dependent depletion of reduced glutathione by L-Dopa & dopamine. Relevance to Parkinson's disease.* Neuroreport 6(11):1480-84, 1995

TOSUKHOWONG P. ET AL. *Biochemical & clinical effects of Whey protein supplementation in Parkinson's disease: A pilot study.* J Neurol Sci 367:162-70, 2016

WANG D, ZHAI JX, ZHANG LM, LIU DW. *Null genotype of GSTT1 contributes to increased Parkinson's disease risk in Caucasians: evidence from a meta-analysis.* Mol Biol Rep 41(11):7423-30, 2014

YUAN Y. ET AL. *Plasma antioxidant status & motor features in de novo Chinese Parkinson's disease patients.* Int J Neurosci 126(7):641-6, 2016

ZHANG F, DRYHURST G. *Effects of L-cysteine on the oxidation chemistry of dopamine: new reaction pathways of potential relevance to idiopathic Parkinson's disease.* Journal of Medical Chemistry 37(8):1084-98, 1994

26

Alzheimer's Disease

ALZHEIMER'S DISEASE (AD) is the most common form of dementia in North America and currently afflicts more than five million people. It's predicted that that figure will rise to 16 million American cases by year 2050. Studies estimate that five to ten percent of adults over the age of 65, and one in three over age 80, will be affected. Given that more people are living longer, this represents an enormous, growing burden. Alzheimer's disease follows heart disease, cancer and stroke as the fourth most common cause of death.

Alzheimer's is a degenerative disease of the nervous system resulting in progressive deterioration of memory, comprehension, intellectual function and behavior. It may have a subtle onset with a slow progression for up to twenty years, or the patient may deteriorate rapidly with a devastating decline in mental capacity over a short period of time. The average duration is about seven years.

Not to be confused with the simple forgetfulness of normal aging, Alzheimer's is a devastating brain disease that leads to profound memory loss, dramatic mood changes, emotional outbursts, childlike behavior, inability to retain new information and general disorientation—particularly at night. Health and general skill sets decline until one is unable to care for oneself and dies.

Causes

Alzheimer's disease is characterized by a degeneration of brain nerve cells and a shrinkage of brain mass. Although its exact cause has yet to be determined, certain changes in the brain can be clearly identified. Firstly, there is a decline in levels of neurotransmitters which relay information from neuron to neuron, such as acetylcholine (ACh) and

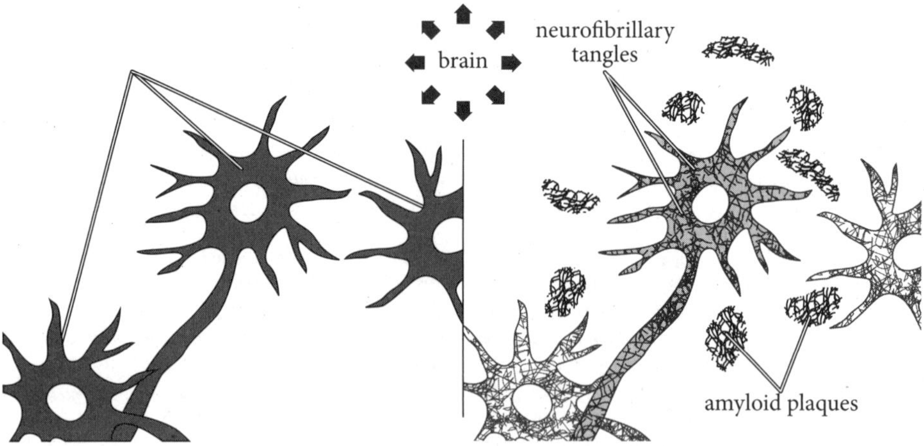

FIGURE 50: Normal (l) vs. Brain with Alzheimer's Disease (r) showing amyloid plaques and neurofibrillary tangles

gamma-aminobutyric acid (GABA). Two other striking features are neurofibrillary tangles and the formation of neural plaque or 'amyloid' (see Figure 48). Amyloid is the remnant of damaged brain tissue—sticky clumps of abnormal protein that interrupt normal cell-to-cell signaling. To make things worse, amyloid triggers an immune system response and increases inflammation, leading to the eventual destruction of surrounding tissue. The result is the 'shrinking brain' seen in CT-scans of advanced Alzheimer's patients (see Figure 49).

Several theories attempt to explain these changes. Alzheimer's was once called 'senile dementia' and thought to be just an extreme form of the normal aging process. We know now that it is an abnormal condition that can be delayed by a number of factors.

Recent research identified a blood protein called Apolipoprotein E (ApoE) which appears to be altered in Alzheimer's patients, causing nerve cell damage. Further studies have shown how this protein interacts with heavy metals like aluminum and mercury and other elements such as iron, zinc and calcium, leading to plaque formation. A strong argument has been made that damage in these tissues is promoted by oxidative stress and free radical formation.

GSH and Alzheimer's disease

How and where does GSH fit into this picture? GSH can play a critical role in the elimination and detoxification of the heavy metals involved in the progress of Alzheimer's Disease. Appropriate quantities of iron, copper, zinc, aluminum and other elements are critically important to human physiology. Problems occur when they accumulate excessively, or end up in the wrong tissue. Jomova and his team wrote a review on metals and Alzheimer's Disease insisting that the research community must focus on the protective role of antioxidants like glutathione in their search for new treatments.

Some studies have shown that when aluminum is 'pulled' from cells by chelators (small molecules that bind very tightly to metal ions and escort them out of the body), the symptoms of Alzheimer's can be reduced or delayed. As we outlined in Chapter 2, one of our primary defenses against these toxins is a satisfactory GSH enzyme system. And, as researchers determine exactly how free radicals contribute to brain cell destruction, the role of GSH as the primary intracellular antioxidant will come to the fore.

Much research has focused on the role of antioxidants in alleviating Alzheimer's symptoms and its progression, especially vitamin E, because of its availability and low price. But as we saw in Chapter 1, these antioxidants interact in complex ways. Many of them depend on adequate GSH levels to function properly. A large number of post-mortem studies have compared normal brain tissue with diseased brain tissue. They reveal significant changes in GSH and GSH peroxidase levels, as well as elevated levels of the powerful oxidant lipid peroxide, against which GSH is a primary defense.

Fibroblast cells grown in Alzheimer-damaged brain tissue are more prone to damage by free radicals than normal cells. This increased vulnerability likely occurs in the cells' mitochondria (energy generators). Adams and his research team found GSH levels diminished in the hippocampus (the brain region active in short-term memory). Jenner and his co-workers found similar declines in the cerebral cortex (the brain region of higher intellectual function).

As early as 2006 Lott et al. linked glutathione deficiency to the formation of Beta amyloid plaque. Other researchers (Gamba et al, Sinha et al.) have followed up with studies using the GSH precursor NAC in both vitro (test-tube) and in-vivo (live animal) experiments. Both produced encouraging results.

Saharan and Mandal reviewed the role of GSH in Alzheimer's disease from both

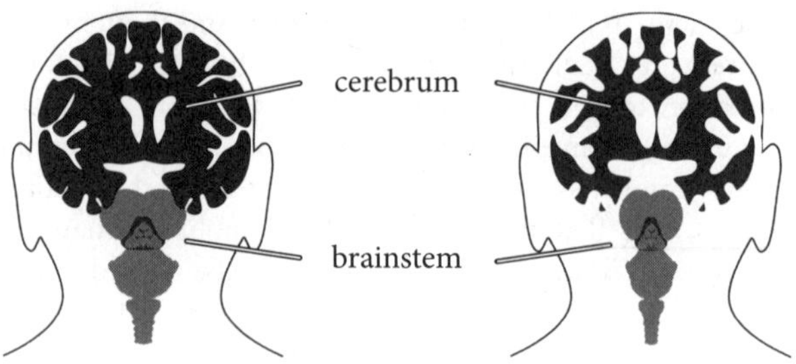

FIGURE 51: Normal brain (left) and Alzheimer's brain (right)

pathological and diagnostic perspectives, concluding that not only is GSH deficiency part of the problem, but GSH levels could mark the onset and progression of the disease.

Alzheimer's disease is a multifactorial problem, but certain features of it claim our attention. Although it's unclear whether oxidative damage is the cause or just an effect of Alzheimer's, there's no doubt that diminished oxidative stress can slow down or diminish the damage caused by this disease. In addition, the part apparently played by heavy metals and other toxins must be addressed. In either case, elevated GSH levels can play a critical role in the fight against these dangers.

Case study

Despite excellent care at home, Max eventually had to be institutionalized for his Alzheimer's disease. His 78-year-old wife's arthritis and heart disease left her unable to give him the high-maintenance care he needed. Previously a gregarious salesman who loved to tell a joke, in his present condition he was unaware of even who was in the room. His history of smoking one to two packs a day left him with chronic bronchitis, requiring frequent inhalation therapy. To treat his ever-thickening secretions, the respiratory therapist started using Mucomyst (n-acetylcysteine –a GSH-promoting drug). After several weeks on the Mucomyst, Max began to smile when his wife entered his room and was visibly pleased by her visits.

Conclusion

In Alzheimer's Disease, certain proteins seem to react with heavy metals and other toxins, leading to plaque formation. Oxidative stress and free radical formation definitely play a role in promoting this damage. When heavy metals are removed by chelators, the symptoms of Alzheimer's can be reduced or delayed.

It is unclear whether oxidative damage is the cause or just an effect of Alzheimer's. Nevertheless, antioxidants have been shown useful in intervention. All antioxidant function is maximized by maintaining adequate GSH levels. By diminishing oxidative stress disease, the progression of this disease can be retarded or diminished.

ALZHEIMER'S DISEASE

REFERENCES

AASETH J. ET AL. *Treatment strategies in Alzheimers's disease: a review with focus on selenium supplementation. Biometals.* 29(5):827-39, 2016

ADAMS JD JR, KLAIDMAN LK, ODUNZE IN, SHEN HC, MILLER CA. *Alzheimer's & Parkinson's disease. Brain levels of glutathione, glutathione disulfide, & vitamin E.* Molecular Chemical Neuropathology 14:213-226, 1991

ARIMON M. ET AL. *Oxidative stress & lipid peroxidation are upstream of amyloid pathology.* Neurobiol Dis. 84:109-19, 2015

BALAZS L, LEON M. *Evidence of an oxidative challenge in the Alzheimer's brain.* Neurochemical Research 19:1131-1137, 1994

BENZI G, MORETTI A. *Are reactive oxygen species involved in Alzheimer's disease?* Neurobiol Aging 16:661-674, 1995

CEBALLOS-PICOT I, MERAD-BOUDIA M, NICOLE A, THEVENIN M, HELLIER G, LEGRAIN S, BERR C. *Peripheral antioxidant enzyme activities & selenium in elderly subjects & in dementia of Alzheimer's type: place of the extracellular glutathione peroxidase.* Free Radical Biology & Medicine 20:579-587, 1996

CONNOR RJ, MENZIES SL, ST. MARTIN SM, MUFSON EJ. *A histochemical study of iron, transferrin, & ferritin in Alzheimer's diseased brains.* Journal of Neuroscience Research 31: 75-83, 1992

COSTA M. ET AL. *N-acetylcysteine protects memory decline induced by streptozotocin in mice.* Chem Biol Interact, 253:10-7, 2016

DA COSTA M. ET AL. *N-acetylcysteine treatment attenuates the cognitive impairment & synaptic plasticity loss induced by streptozotocin.* Chem Biol Interact. 272:37-46, 2017

GAMBA P. ET AL. *Up-regulation of β-amyloidogenesis in neuro-like human cells by both 24- & 27-hydroxycholesterol: protective effect of N-acetyl-cysteine.* Aging Cell 13(3):561-572, 2014

GOSH D, LEVAULT KR, BREWER GJ. *Dual-energy precursor & nuclear erythroid-related factor 2 activator treatment additively improve redox glutathione levels & neuron survival in aging & Alzheimer mouse neurons upstream of reactive oxygen species.* Neurobiol Aging 35(1):179-90, 2014

HAMEL E. *Cerebral circulation: function & dysfunction in Alzheimer's disease.* J Cardiovasc Pharmacol. 65(4):317-24, 2015

ISLAM MT. *Oxidative stress & mitochondrial dysfunction-linked neurodegenerative disorders.* Neurol Res. 39(1):73-82, 2017

JENNER P. *Oxidative damage in neurodegenerative disease.* Lancet 344:796-798, 1994

JOMOVA K, VONDRAKOVA D, LAWSON M, VALKO M. *Metals, oxidative stress & neurodegenerative disorders.* Mol Cell Biochem. 345(1-2):91-104, 2010

LIU H. ET AL. *Glutathione metabolism during aging & in Alzheimer disease.* Ann N Y Acad Sci 1019:346-9, 2004

LOHR JB, BROWNING JA. *Free radical involvement in neuropsychiatric illnesses.* Psychopharmacological Bulletin 31:159-165, 1995

LOTT IT, HEAD E, DORAN E, BUSCIGLIO J. *Beta-amyloid, oxidative stress & down syndrome.* Curr Alzheimer Res 3(5): 521-8, 2006

LOVELL MA, EHMANN WD, BUTLER SM, MARKESBERY WR. *Elevated thiobarbituric acid-reactive substances & antioxidant enzyme activity in the brain in Alzheimer's disease.* Neurol 45:1594-1601, 1995

MARI M. ET AL. *Mitochondrial glutathione: features, regulation & role in disease.* Biochim Biophys Acta 1830(5):3317-28, 2013

PETER C. ET AL. *Therapeutic approaches to modulating glutathione levels as a pharmacological strategy in Alzheimer's disease.* Curr Alzheimer Res 12(4):298-313, 2015

POCERNICH CB, BUTTERFIELD DA. *Elevation of glutathione as a therapeutic strategy in Alzheimer disease.* Biochim Biophys Acta 1822(5):625-30, 2012

SAHARAN S, MANDAL PK. *The emerging role of glutathione in Alzheimer's disease.* J Alzheimers Dis 40(3):519-29, 2014

SINHA M, BIR A, BANERJEE A, BHOWMICK P, CHARKRABARTI S. *Multiple mechanisms of age-dependent accumulation of amyloid beta protein in rat brain: Prevention by dietary supplementation with N-acetylcysteine, α-lipoic acid & α-tocopherol.* Neurochem Int. 95:92-9, 2016

SKVARC DR ET AL. *The effect of N-acetylcysteine (NAC) on human cognition, a systematic review.* Neurosci Biobehav Rev. 78:44-56, 2017

TREPANIER G, FURLING D, PUYMIRAT J, MIRAULT ME. *Immunocytochemical localization of seleno-glutathione peroxidase in the adult mouse brain.* Neuroscience 75:231-243, 1996

27

Cognitive Impairment

When it comes to aging, two things in particular scare my patients. First and foremost is fear of being unable to care for themselves. Even scarier is the thought of losing their intellect. A poll taken some years ago revealed that Americans are twice as fearful of losing their mental capacity as their physical ones. Additional polls show that a good 60% of adults worry about memory loss.

The term "memory loss" is only part of what people dread. In medicine we use a more precise term: 'cognitive impairment.' This is defined by the Centers of Disease Control and Prevention (CDC) as follows:

"Cognitive impairment is when a person has trouble remembering, learning new things, concentrating, or making decisions that affect their everyday life. Cognitive impairment ranges from mild to severe. With mild impairment, people may begin to notice changes in cognitive functions, but still be able to do their everyday activities. Severe levels of impairment (dementia) can lead to losing the ability to understand the meaning or importance of something and the ability to talk or write, resulting in the inability to live independently."

No matter how you define cognitive impairment, the number of people suffering from it is large and growing larger. A recent surge in numbers has actually been due to our improved ability to make the diagnosis of early impairment, giving rise to the new diagnosis of MCI (Mild Cognitive Impairment), a field of newly surging interest. The Mayo Clinic (the number-one ranked US hospital) defines MCI as follows:

"Mild Cognitive Impairment (MCI) is an intermediate stage between the expected cognitive decline of normal aging and the more-serious decline of dementia. It can involve problems with memory, language, thinking and judgment that are greater than normal age-related changes."

Think of cognitive impairment as a spectrum of metal decline. At point zero is the optimally-functioning brain of a twenty-year old; at the other end is an immobile person in a vegetative state.

Cognitive impairment places an immense fiscal, medical and emotional burden on families and on communities. A study commissioned by the Alzheimer's Society revealed that people with cognitive impairment are admitted to hospital three times more often than other patients. Alzheimer's Disease and similar dementias are consid-

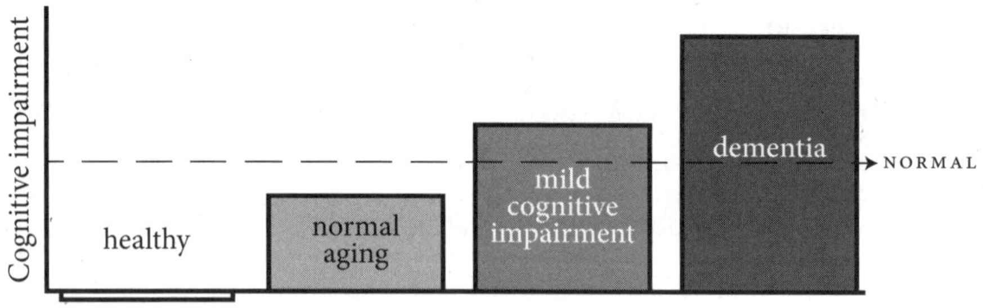

FIGURE 52: *The spectrum of metal decline*

Poor memory, especially short-term memory
Frequently asking the same question
Repeating the same story
Not recognizing familiar people
Not recognizing familiar places
Difficulty planning or carrying out tasks
Poor judgment and reaction
Changes in behavior

TABLE 39: Common signs of cognitive impairment

ered the third most expensive ailments in the USA, adding up to billions of dollars annually—and this is just the fiscal burden. It doesn't include the unpaid care of not-for-profit groups, friends and family who tend to their loved ones on a daily basis and endure tremendous financial and emotional stress.

When the topic of cognitive impairment comes up, most people think immediately of Alzheimer's, but there are other sorts of dementia. Many of the neurodegenerative diseases mentioned in this book may be the underlying cause, and while age is the primary risk factor, there are many other diseases that might lead to cognitive decline: some psychiatric conditions, stroke, head trauma, drug abuse, sleep disturbance, obesity, diabetes and even physical inactivity.

The glutathione connection

Many conditions contribute to dementia. Aging, neurodegenerative disease and circulatory disorders are most typical but there are dozens of others. One thing they all have in common is glutathione: there is less of it in impaired brains.

As we've seen in this book, GSH is the most active and abundant antioxidant in the body. It's also been called the master antioxidant which, though not a quantifiable scientific term, points to its pivotal role in cellular health as a recycler of other antioxidants. Lowered GSH is both a cause and result of aging. GSH levels drop with age. Increasing oxidative stress (hence lowering GSH) accelerates aging. In either case, any opportunity to replenish it should be seized.

Researchers from California's Salk Institute have stated, "Brain glutathione (GSH) decreases with age in humans, and a loss of GSH can impact cognitive function." In an appropriately-titled article "Functional Consequences of Age-dependent Changes in Glutathione Status in the Brain," they came to this profound conclusion:

"We argue here that many of the changes in brain function associated with age are linked through GSH metabolism."

Do low glutathione levels predicate aging, or is it that aging depletes glutathione levels? It's a chicken-and-egg question. While people with genetic GSH abnormalities are more likely to suffer neurodegenerative and cognitive defects, research also clearly shows that increased oxidative stress damages the brain and leads to neurodegeneration.

Either way, glutathione loss is a slippery slope. The less you have, the greater the free radical damage and the more quickly remaining glutathione is consumed. This quickly gets out of hand, so the most urgent need is to slow down or stop the downward spiral. As you'll see from the studies below, improving glutathione status in the brain may be extremely beneficial.

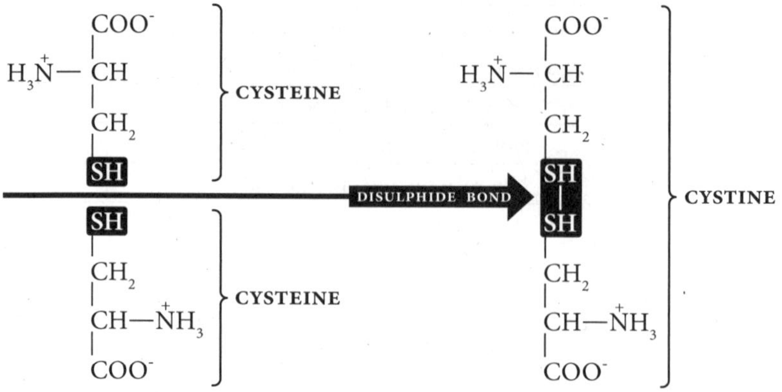

FIGURE 53: Cystine is made up of two cysteine molecules linked by an easily disrupted disulfide bond. CYSTEINE and CYSTINE can cross the BBB (Blood-Brain-Barrier). Glutathione cannot.

Raising glutathione in the brain

The brain is separated from the rest of the body by the blood-brain-barrier (BBB), which allows certain molecules through while barring others—among others, the glutathione molecule. Although some researchers believe it can sometimes make it through, it's never in large quantities. Furthermore, eating glutathione does not effectively raise glutathione levels. Glutathione is quickly broken down by the digestive enzyme GGT (gamma-glutamyl-transferase), which is especially high in the human gut.

What's curious is that autopsies, animal studies and neuroimaging studies have all shown that glutathione levels in the brain are much higher than in blood and other tissues. So, 1) Why does the brain need so much glutathione? 2) If the blood-brain barrier doesn't let it in, how does it get there?

This is what we know:

1. The brain consumes far more energy and oxygen than any other organ. Although it consists of only 2% of the body's mass, it consumes 20% of the oxygen. As we know, burning more oxygen results in more oxidative stress and releases more free radicals. Antioxidants come to the rescue—or try to—but are soon exhausted. Glutathione—the 'master antioxidant'—is literally your first-line defense. Healthy brains depend on high levels of glutathione to "put out the fires."
2. As for how glutathione gets into the brain, the obvious answer is that if it can't pass through the blood-brain barrier it must be manufactured within the brain. Glutathione's scarcest building blocks are two smaller molecules called cysteine and cystine (notice the different spelling). These are able to pass through the blood-brain barrier and into the brain. Using them as raw materials, each brain cell manufactures its own supply of glutathione on demand.

When doctors need to therapeutically increase GSH levels anywhere in the body, they most often use the drug N-acetylcysteine (NAC). It's proven and highly effective for short-term use. However its side-effects accumulate eventually to toxic levels, making it unsuitable for continuous use. A natural alternative is specially-formulated whey protein, a food product rich in both cysteine and cystine, and free of side-effects.

Another way glutathione can be raised in brain neurons concerns the cellular biology of the brain. This is a bit more complicated.

Scientists have known for decades that neurons are only one of several types of brain cell. Until recently, it was believed

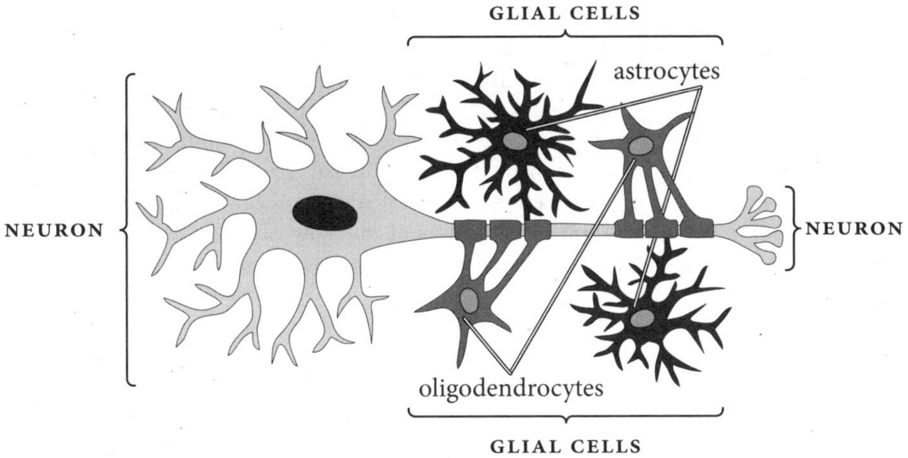

FIGURE 54: Neurons are not the only sort of brain cell

that neurons alone were responsible for the transmission and reception of signals, neurotransmitter metabolism, storage of information and other brain functions. Neurons account for only 15% of brain mass. The 85% of non-neurons—called 'glia'—were believed to not contribute to any cognitive function. They were just a sort of glue (glia' in Latin) holding the neurons together.

Today, that belief is obsolete. We've learned that glia cells play an extraordinary role in healing and other functions. In his book 'The Other Brain,' Douglas Fields PhD provides a tantalizing look at new discoveries that are revolutionizing brain science. He describes glia as, 'the brain's immune system,' and he's not the only one.

Where does glutathione come into it? Certain types of glia are responsible for transporting both cysteine and cystine into the brain, where they're released into the tiny intracellular gaps between glia and neurons. Neurons pick it up from there and are then able to manufacture glutathione.

Populations with GSH abnormalities and cognitive decline

There's no question that glutathione abnormalities contribute to a number of different neurodegenerative diseases. We've discussed this in our chapters on Alzheimer's, Parkinson's and Huntington's Diseases as well as ALS and Down Syndrome. All these disorders exhibit varying degrees of mental decline.

However, they're not the only causes. Aging and stress play a role too. Brazilian researchers examined aging people and noticed that those with greater oxidative stress had a weakened cognitive function, a reduced quality of life and a shorter lifespan.

The Journal of Alzheimer's Disease published an article correlating GSH levels with 'mini-mental-status' scores, concluding that glutathione levels may accurately predict the course of mental decline.

Even more surprising, this link between glutathione levels and mental capacity has been remarked on in other fields of medicine:

General anesthetics can cause cognitive deficits, and research has focused on boosting glutathione levels during the operative period. People with sleep apnea tend to suffer cognitive difficulties. (See Chapter 27). Researchers at the Brain & Mind Research Institute in the University of Sydney, Australia have linked the impaired glutathione function of these patients to mental decline.

Cognitive difficulties are also commonly found in different psychiatric problems. Major depression, bipolar disease, and psychosis all demonstrate a tendency towards glutathione abnormalities and cognitive decline. Active research is looking at intervention using glutathione precursors.

The relationship between oxidative stress and impaired thinking can be confirmed even in healthy individuals. A cross-sectional study of 400 women between 20 and 40 years of age showed that increasing antioxidant status and glutathione levels improved their scores on visual and auditory attention tests.

As if obesity did not already carry enough risks, it appears that low glutathione is yet another one, and it's been specifically associated with impaired brain function. A 2016 publication in the journal Experimental and Clinical Endocrinology and Diabetes revealed significant cognitive impairment plus glutathione abnormalities in the unhealthy obese—those with a combination of high blood pressure, diabetes and high cholesterol (metabolic syndrome).

MCI, Alzheimer's Disease and cognition

Mild Cognitive Impairment (MCI) is a risk factor for the development of Alzheimer's Disease. Not all MCI patients progress to full-blown dementia, but it becomes increasingly likely as the person ages. Many doctors consider MCI and Alzheimer's to be progressive stages of the same disease.

Bearing in mind that both MCI and Alzheimer's patients have similarly low antioxidant levels, intervention with antioxidants could become a critically important way to lessen the likelihood of it turning into Alzheimer's Disease. We've known since the early 2000s that in early Alzheimer's disease, critical biomolecules are damaged by oxidative stress. This damage is apparent even before symptoms are—suggesting a preventive approach through glutathione augmentation.

Studies in Italy and elsewhere have confirmed that accurately measured glutathione levels predict the progress and severity of MCI/Alzheimer's disease. This is what we call a 'biomarker' that can be used to measure the status of a disease. It suggests how aggressively doctors should intervene by supplementing antioxidants and glutathione.

Measuring this biomarker has become even easier through new brain scanning technologies such as Magnetic Resonance Spectroscopy (MRS) that can directly measure glutathione levels in the brain. As we mentioned regarding the studies above, glutathione levels correlate to severity of the disease, so this should make it easier to diagnose and treat.

Appearing in Neuroscience and Biobehavioral Reviews in 2017, an international team of neuroscientists reviewed the use of NAC in cognitive decline. Alzheimer's Disease was the most commonly treated condition. They concluded that "The available data suggested statistically significant cognitive improvements following NAC treatment." While raised glutathione levels may have positive cognitive effects, larger studies will be needed before this can be considered a standard of care.

Conclusions

Increased oxidative stress and antioxidant depletion are apparent during cognitive decline, and have been correlated with glutathione abnormalities. Improved access to glutathione measurement tests now provides a potential marker of the diagnosis, severity and progress of cognitive dysfunctions, especially mild cognitive impairment (MCI) and Alzheimer's disease. We expect to see more research into the use of elevated brain glutathione to combat cognitive impairment.

COGNITIVE IMPAIRMENT

REFERENCES

Alzheimer's Association. *Characteristics, Costs & Health Service Use for Medicare Beneficiaries with a Dementia Diagnosis: Report 1: Medicare Current Beneficiary Survey.* Chicago: Alzheimer's Association; 2009.

Alzheimer's Association. *Alzheimer's Disease Facts & Figures.* Chicago: 2010

Alzheimer's Association. *Medicare & Medicaid costs for people with Alzheimer's disease.* Chicago: Alzheimer's Association; 2001

Arce-Varas N, Abate G, Prandelli C et al. *Comparison of Extracellular & Intracellular Blood Compartments Highlights Redox Alterations in Alzheimer's & Mild Cognitive Impairment Patients.* Curr Alzheimer Res. 14(1):112-122, 2017

Aydemir Ö et al. *Oxidative stress markers, cognitive functions, & psychosocial functioning in bipolar disorder: an empirical cross-sectional study.* Rev Bras Psiquiatr 36(4):293-7, 2014

Baierle M, Nascimiento SN, Moro AM et al. *Relationship between inflammation & oxidative stress & cognitive decline in the institutionalized elderly.* Oxid Med Cell Longev 2015: 804198, 2015

Baldeiras I, Santana I, Proença MT et al. *Oxidative damage & progression to Alzheimer's disease in patients with mild cognitive impairment.* J Alzheimers Dis 21(4):1165-77, 2010

Bermejo P, Martin-Aragn S, Benedi J et al. *Peripheral levels of glutathione & protein oxidation as markers in the development of Alzheimer's disease from Mild Cognitive Impairment.* Free Radic Res 42(2):162-70, 2008

Cristalli DO, Arnal N, Marra FA, de Alaniz MJ, Marra CA. *Peripheral markers in neurodegenerative patients & their first-degree relatives.* J Neurol Sci 314(1-2):48-56, 2012

Cruz R, Almaguer Melian W, Bergado Rosado JA. *Glutathione in cognitive function & neurodegeneration.* Rev Neurol 1-15; 36(9):877-86, 2003

Currais A, Maher P. *Functional consequences of age-dependent changes in glutathione status in the brain.* Antioxid Redox Signal 19(8):813-22, 2013

Cutler NE, Whitelaw NW, Beattie BL. *American Perceptions of Aging in 21st C.* Washington (DC): National Council on Aging; 2002

Dean OM, Bush AL et al. *Effects of N-acetyl cysteine on cognitive function in bipolar disorder.* Psychiatry Clin Neurosci 66(6):514-7, 2012

Deepmala, Slaterry J et al. *Clinical trials of NAC in psychiatry & neurology: A systematic review.* Neurosci Biobehav Rev 55:294-321, 2015

Duffy SL et al. *Glutathione relates to neuropsychological functioning in mild cognitive impairment.* Alzheimers Dement 10(1):67-75, 2014

Dringen R. *Metabolism & functions of glutathione in brain.* Prog Neurobiol 62(6):649-71, 2000

Farah R, Gilbey P et al. *Antioxidant Enzyme Activity & Cognition in Obese Individuals with or without Metabolic Risk Factors.* Exp Clin Endocrinol Diabetes 124(9):568-571, 2016

Galecki P et al. *Thiol protein groups correlate with cognitive impairment in patients with recurrent depressive disorder.* Neuro Endocrinol Lett 34(8):780-6, 2013

Gironi M et al. *Oxidative imbalance in different neurodegenerative diseases with memory impairment.* Neurodegener Dis 8(3):129-37, 2011

Gu F, Chauhan V, Chauhan A. *Glutathione redox imbalance in brain disorders.* Curr Opin Clin Nutr Metab Care 18(1):89-95, 2015

Hara Y, McKeehan N, Dacks PA, Fillit HM. *Evaluation of the Neuroprotective Potential of N-Acetylcysteine for Prevention & Treatment of Cognitive Aging & Dementia.* J Prev Alzheimers Dis 4(3):201-206, 2017

Johnson WM, Wilson-Delfosse AL, Mieyal JJ. *Dysregulation of GSH homeostasis in neurodegenerative diseases.* Nutrients 4(10):1399-440, 2012

López N, Tormo C, De Blas I, Llinares I, Alom J. *Oxidative stress in Alzheimer's disease & mild cognitive impairment with high sensitivity & specificity.* J Alzheimers Dis 33(3):823-9, 2013

Lovell MA, Markesbery WR. *Oxidative Damage in mild cognitive impairment & early Alzheimers's disease.* J Neurosci Res 85(14):3036-40, 2007

Mandal PK, Saharan S, Tripathi M, Murari G. *Brain glutathione levels—a novel biomarker for mild cognitive impairment & Alzheimer's disease.* Biol Psychiatry 78(10):702-10, 2015

Mangialasche F et al. *Biomarkers of oxidative & nitrosative damage in Alzheimer's & mild cognitive impairment.* Ageing Res Rev 8(4):285-305, 2009

Martinez-Cengotitabengoa M et al. *Cognitive impairment is related to oxidative stress & chemokine levels in first psychotic episodes.* Schizophr Res 137(1-3):66-72, 2012

Martinez-Cengotitabengoa M et al. *Basal low antioxidant capacity correlates with cognitive deficits in early onset psychosis.* A 2 year follow-up study. Schizophr Res 156(1):23-9, 2014

Mecocci P. *Oxidative stress in mild cognitive impairment & Alzheimer disease: a continuum.* J Alzheimers Dis 6(2):159-63, 2004

Padurariu M et al. *Changes of some oxidative stress markers in the serum of patients with mild cognitive impairment & Alzheimer's disease.* Neuroschi Lett 469(1):6-10, 2010

Rae CD, Williams SR. *Glutathione in the human brain: Review of its roles & measurement by magnetic resonance spectroscopy.* Anal Biochem 529:127-143, 2017

Rapado-Castro M et al. *Cognitive effects of adjunctive N-acetyl cysteine in psychosis.* Psychol Med 47(5):866-876, 2017

Revel F, Gilbert T et al. *Influence of oxidative stress biomarkers on cognitive decline.* J Alzheimers Dis 45(2):553-60, 2015

Research!America. *American Speaks: Poll Data Summary. Volume 7. Alexandria:Research, 2006*

Rinaldi P et al. *Plasma antioxidants are similarly depleted in mild cognitive impairment & in Alzheimer's disease.* Neurobiol Aging 24(7):915-9, 2003

Sales LV, Bruin VM et al. *Cognition & biomarkers of oxidative stress in obstructive sleep apnea.* Clinics (Sao Paulo) 68(4):449-55, 2013

Schrag M et al. *Oxidative stress in blood in Alzheimer's disease & mild cognitive impairment: a meta-analysis.* Neurobiol Dis 59:100-10, 2013

Shiraseb F et al. *Association of blood antioxidants status with visual & auditory sustained attention.Nutr Neurosci 18(8):345-54, 2015*

Skvarc DR et al. *The Post-Anaesthesia NAC Cognitive Evaluation (PANACEA) trial: study protocol for a randomised controlled trial.* Trials 17:395, 2016

Skvarac DR et al. *The effect of N-acetylcysteine (NAC) on human cognition – A systematic review. Neurosci Biobehav Rev 78:44-56, 2017*

Song F, Poljak A, Smythe GA, Sachdev P. *Plasma biomarkers for mild cognitive impairment & Alzheimer's.* Brain Res Rev 61(2):69-80, 2009

Song W et al. *Cysteine-rich whey protein isolate (Immunocal) ameliorates deficits in the* GFAP.HMOX1 *mouse model of schizophrenia.* Free Radic Biol Med 110:162-175, 2017

Torres LL et al. *Peripheral oxidative stress biomarkers in mild cognitive impairment & Alzheimer's disease.* J Alzheimers Dis 26(1):59-68, 2011

Umur EE et al. *Increased iron & oxidative stress are separately related to cognitive decline in elderly.* Geriatr Gerontol Int 11(4):504-9, 2011

Zhou H, Yuan Y, Qi Z, Tong Q, Zhang K. *[Study on changes of plasma levels of oxidative stress biomarkers & its relation with cognition function in patients with parkinson's disease].* Zhonghua Yi Xue Za Zhi 95(41):3357-60

28

Other Neurodegenerative Problems

NEURODEGENERATION refers to the breakdown of nerves (neurons) over time. Depending on severity, the result is some level of deterioration in movement, thought, sensation and/or balance. It can lead to heart and breathing problems. Neurodegeneration is life-altering and can be life-threatening.

There are many types of neurodegenerative diseases. Some we inflict upon ourselves through alcoholism, drug abuse, or accidental exposure to toxins, including pesticides, herbicides, heavy metals and more. Others have a genetic or epigenetic[1] basis. Many are not completely understood. The most common neurodegenerative diseases include Alzheimer's Disease (Chapter 26), Parkinson's Disease (Chapter 25), and Multiple Sclerosis (Chapter 30). Several more will be covered in this chapter, including ALS (amyotrophic lateral sclerosis), Huntington's Disease, and Friedreich's ataxia. I have also included Down Syndrome. Despite being a multi-system disorder, in certain ways it strongly parallels other neurodegenerative diseases.

What has become strikingly evident over the last quarter-century is one feature common to all neurodegenerative diseases—oxidative stress. Along with free radical damage, this always taxes the glutathione system and leads to GSH depletion. Renowned brain researcher Dan Linseman says, "The brain is especially vulnerable to oxidative damage because of its high lipid (fat) content and high rate of oxygen consumption." Each particular neurodegenerative disease begins with the oxidation of specific neurons.

ALS (amyotrophic lateral sclerosis)

ALS is also known as "Lou Gehrig's Disease", after the famous American baseball player who quit playing when he was diagnosed with this disease. Before that, he'd been known as "The Iron Horse" because of his tremendous durability. His retirement at age 36 shocked the baseball community. Announcing it, he described himself as, "The luckiest man on the face of the earth." He died two years later. Another famous individual afflicted by ALS was the cosmologist Stephen Hawking, who survived remarkably to the age of 75, while making extraordinary contributions to our knowledge of the universe.

Lou Gehrig's Disease is one of several "motor neuron" diseases, so-called because they mostly affect the nerve cells controlling movement. Patients can develop ALS in middle age, but most are diagnosed around age 60. The average life span after diagnosis is three to five years. Typically, patients suffer painless muscle weakness over time, followed by paralysis of the swallowing mechanism or the muscles involved in breathing.

ALS appears in several forms—some with a genetic basis and some termed "sporadic." Sporadic ALS may be triggered by exposure to environmental toxins, or follow military

[1] Changes in gene expression that do not involve alterations in the DNA sequence; as opposed to genetic changes, which do.

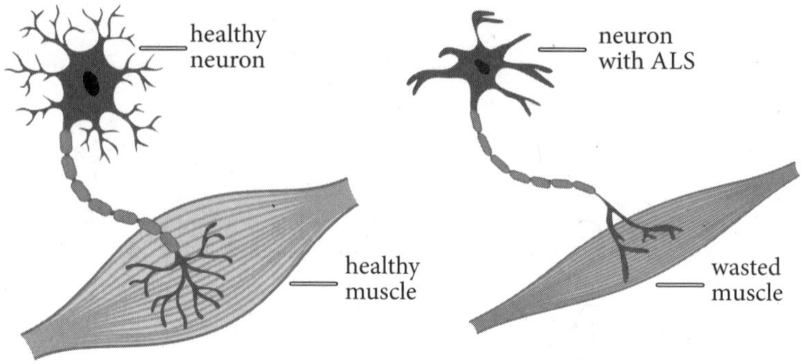

FIGURE 55: Motor neuron disease mostly affects the nerve cells controlling skeletal muscles, and hence bodily motion

service, chronic head trauma, excessive physical exertion or sports injuries. Regardless of the cause, it is always marked by increased oxidative stress and lowered glutathione activity. In "Frontiers of Molecular Neuroscience," authors Valle and Carri review closely-related evidence of a more general cysteine disturbance coming into play.

In Chapter 1, we described how cysteine is the hardest-to-find amino acid limiting glutathione synthesis. Denver scientist Dan Linseman and his team tested a mouse version of ALS, and had promising results to share. Onset of the disease was delayed after feeding the mice a cysteine-rich whey protein isolate, and there was less muscle degeneration than usual.

Translating laboratory research into human studies is a bit more challenging. As far back as 1998, the Italians Chio, Cucatto, Terreni and Schiffer attempted to treat ALS patients with glutathione. Their failure to show improvement was almost certainly due to the way the GSH was administered—by intramuscular injection (600 mg/day of glutathione), which is not an effective way to raise systemic GSH levels.

More recently, research by a number of different scientists using NAC (the glutathione precursor N-acetylcysteine) has shown more promising results, though results are inconsistent. Work is needed before this becomes a viable solution.

Huntington's Disease

In the past, this was called "Huntington's Chorea." Chorea is Latin for "dance," referring to the rapid muscle twitching and movements that affects hands and feet. Although these movements are the most visible feature, Huntington's also results in deterioration of cognition (thinking) and emotional instability. Unlike Alzheimer's or Parkinson's Diseases, which generally start late in life, Huntington's usually appears in the third or fourth decade. A juvenile form has been identified, but it's much less common than the adult form. Life expectancy is about fifteen to twenty years after diagnosis.

Both Adult and Juvenile Huntington's Disease follow a genetic pattern called "autosomal dominant." This implies that the gene from only one parent is enough to transmit this disease. If there is any history of this disease in your family, genetic testing is recommended.

Huntington's has been shown to degrade specific proteins in the brain. It starts in the striatum—a region critical to movement control—and eventually affects the rest of the brain. If you suspect the role of oxidative stress, you'd be right. Quite predictably, glutathione levels are low as well.

Examination of oxidative stress and glutathione levels across various age groups reveals that younger (asymptomatic) patients had the same biochemical abnormalities as older (symptomatic) patients. This would imply that the damage occurs relatively slowly but progresses steadily.

Glutathione-elevating drugs like NAC (N-acetylcysteine) have shown promise in animal models of Huntington's disease, including symptoms of depression. However, good human studies are still needed.

Friedreich's Ataxia

Ataxia from the Greek "a-taxis" means "without order" or "lack of coordination." The loss of voluntary muscle control leads to problems walking, picking things up, speaking and even swallowing. There are several types of ataxia, but the most common inherited form is Friedreich's Ataxia, named after the German physician who first described it in the 1890s.

In Friedreich's Ataxia, the nerve degeneration takes place mostly in the spinal cord, which at least spares the patient from cognitive or mental decline. The condition usually affects people under 20 years of age. The first general signs are stumbling and frequent falling. After about ten to twenty years the person becomes wheelchair bound and totally dependent on others.

Friedreich's Ataxia shares the same fate as all nerve cells in the neurodegenerative diseases discussed in this chapter—increased free radical damage and oxidative stress accompanied by abnormal glutathione activity.

Importantly, these abnormalities are most prevalent in the mitochondria[2] of cells. The mitochondria are tiny structures within cells that supply cellular energy. Many authors describe the mitochondria as the "batteries" of the cell. For this reason, Friedreich's and other neurodegenerative diseases are said to be "mitochondrial diseases."

A unique feature of Friedreich's Ataxia is lack of the protein "Frataxin." This deficiency is always accompanied by increased oxidative damage. In laboratory experiments, raised glutathione levels has proven helpful against Friedreich's Ataxia, but few trials on human beings have been completed. Hopefully, as more anecdotal evidence about increased glutathione accumulates, researchers will investigate more closely, with properly controlled studies.

Down syndrome

Down syndrome is also known as trisomy 21, and was once called mongoloidism, inappropriately comparing its distinctive facial characteristics with the mongoloid peoples of Asia. Ironically, some parts of the Far East refer to it as 'caucausianism.'

This congenital[3] disorder occurs during fetal development, when chromosomes divide mistakenly to produce a third 21st chromosome when there should only be two. It is not an inherited trait and it occurs more often in older pregnancies. It is relatively common, occurring once in about every 700 births.

Down syndrome leads to several easily recognizable traits, including moderate to severe mental retardation, typically flattened facial features, slanted eyes, low-set ears and a large tongue. Less obvious is a tendency toward congenital heart defects, poor vision, leukemia and susceptibility to infectious disease. In a suitable environmental setting, Down syndrome patients may lead happy and productive—though shorter—lives.

Oxidative stress and free radical formation have been studied in Down syndrome. There is still debate, but some factors are clear. The gene for an enzyme involved in oxidation/antioxidation reactions called 'superoxide

---

[2] Energy-producing organelles that float free inside cells; muscle cells need more energy and may have thousands, while some cells have none.

[3] A defect present from birth.

dismutase' (SOD) is located on chromosome 21. It may be that decreased SOD activity overproduces hydrogen peroxide in Down syndrome—a source of potent free radicals. Researchers have noted that this places heightened demands on the antioxidant defenses, including glutathione.

Down syndrome patients who make it to older ages seem more prone to the development of Alzheimer's Disease (see Chapter 26). Scientists, including those working at the University of California (San Diego) think this is due to changes in free radical metabolism that increase destruction of nerve cells. Simple experiments to measure the blood serum levels of glutathione in Down patients reveal significant alterations in GSH activity.

In more complex studies, GSH activity in Down patients without Alzheimer's disease were compared to those who had both, revealing that glutathione defenses (already abnormal) are impaired even further in the Down/Alzheimer's group. The same University of California team went so far as to suggest that these findings provide a possible route to early treatment.

In attempts to further identify issues linking Alzheimer's Disease with Down Syndrome, a research study published in the Journal of Alzheimer's Disease in 2012 tracked levels of oxidative stress (including GSH and SOD levels) during memory decline. Results were clear—antioxidant levels predicted memory

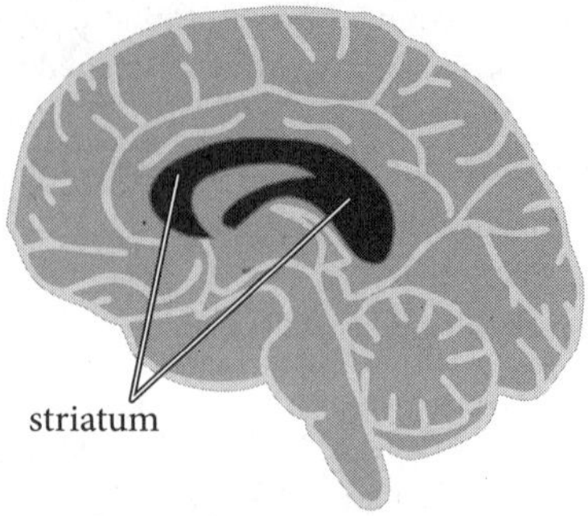

FIGURE 56: The striatum is just above the brain stem, under the cerebral cortex

decline that worsened over time. The group also suggested that research should focus on antioxidant supplementation in similar neurodegenerative disorders.

An interesting animal experiment from 1997, published in the journal Brain Research, showed that in brain cells affected by Down syndrome, those with the lowest GSH were most likely to die. By chemically lowering GSH still further, cell death rates increased. This leaves no doubt that low GSH levels accelerate neurodegeneration and brain cell death, and that elevated levels can slow it down.

In 2014 and 2015 a Brazilian research team began putting this knowledge to practical use, using antioxidants in different Down Syndrome populations. They showed that antioxidant supplementation consistently reduced oxidative damage in both children and teenagers with Down Syndrome.

Conclusion

From the point of view of biochemistry, all neurodegenerative diseases discussed in this book—ALS, Friedreich's Ataxia, Huntington's Chorea and Down Syndrome in this chapter as well as Alzheimer's (Chapter 26) and Parkinson's (Chapter 25) diseases—share one thing in common. That is, high oxidative stress and low glutathione. Attempts to raise glutathione levels have been more complex than the underlying biochemistry suggests, and results vary with each disease. Nevertheless, future research will begin to address these life-altering afflictions with antioxidant therapy.

OTHER NEURODEGENERATIVE PROBLEMS

REFERENCES

ABETI R, PARKINSON MD, HARGREAVES IP, ET AL. *Mitochondrial energy imbalance & lipid peroxidation cause cell death in Friedreich's ataxia.* Cell Death Dis 7:e2237, 2016

ANTILA E, WESTERMARK T. *On the etiopathogenesis & therapy of Down syndrome.* Int. J. Dev. Biol. 33: 183-188, 1989

BAEZ S, SEGURA-AGUILAR J, WIDERSTEN M, ET AL. *Glutathione transferases catalyze the detoxification of oxidized metabolites (o-quinones) of catecholamines & may serve as an antioxidant system preventing degenerative cellular processes.* Biochem J. 324(Pt. 1): 25-28, 1997

BAVARSAD SHAHRIPOUR R, HARRIGAN MR, ALEXANDROV AV. *N-acetylcysteine (NAC) in neurological disorders: mechanisms of action & therapeutic opportunities.* Brain Behav 4(2):108-22, 2014

BANDMANN O, VAUGHEN J, HOLMANS P, ET AL. *Association of slow acetylator genotype for N-acetyltransferase 2 with familiar Parkinson's disease.* Lancet 350: 1136-1139, 1997

BLASCO H, GARCON G, PATIEN F, ET AL. *Panel of Oxidative Stress & Inflammatory Biomarkers in ALS: A Pilot Study.* Can J Neurol Sci 44(1):90-95, 2017

BONNEFONT-ROUSSELOT D, LACOMBLEZ L, JAUDON M, ET AL. *Blood oxidative stress in amyotrophic lateral sclerosis.* J Neurol Sci 178(1):57-62, 2000

BRADLEY JL, HOMAYOUN S, HART PE, SCHAPIRA AH, COOPER JM. *Role of oxidative damage in Friedreich's ataxia.* Neurochem Res 29(3):561-7, 2004

BULTEAU AL, PLANAMENTE S, ET AL. *Changes in mitochondrial glutathione levels & protein thiol oxidation in Δyfh1 yeast cells & the lymphoblasts of patients with Friedreich's ataxia.* Biochim Biophys Acta 1822(2):212-25, 2012

BRUGGE KL, NICHOLS S, DELIS D, ET AL. *The role of alterations in free radical metabolism in mediating cognitive impairments in Down syndrome.* EXS 62: 190-198, 1992

CALABRESE V, LODI R, TONON C, ET AL. *Oxidative stress, mitocondrial dysfunction & celular stress response in Friedreich's ataxia.* J Neurol Sci 233(1-2):145-62, 2005

CARLETTI B, PIERMARINI E, TOZZI G, ET AL. *Frataxin silencing inactivates mitochondrial Complex I in NSC34 motoneuronal cells & alters glutathione homeostasis.* Int J Mol Sci 15(4):5789-806, 2014

CHEN CM, WU YR, CHENG ML ET AL. *Increased oxidative damage & mitochondrial abnormalities in the peripheral blood of Huntington's disease patients.* Biochem Biophys Res Commun 359(2):335-40, 2007

CHIO A, CUCATTO A, TERRENI AA, SCHIFFER D. *Reduced glutathione in amyotrophic lateral sclerosis: an open, crossover, randomized trial.* Ital J Neurol Sci 19(6):363-6, 1998

CLAUSEN J, JENSON GE, NIELSEN SA. SELENIUM IN CHRONIC NEUROLOGICAL DISEASES. MULTIPLE SCLEROSIS & BATTEN'S DISEASE. *Biol. Trace Elem. Res. 15: 179-203, 1988*

D'AMICO E, FACTOR-LITVAK P, SANTELLA RM, MITSUMOTO H. *Clinical perspective on oxidative stress in sporadic amyotrophic lateral sclerosis.* Free Radic Biol Med 65:509-27, 2013

DAVEY GP, PEUCHEN S, CLARK JB. *Energy thresholds in brain mitochondria. Potential involvement in neurodegeneration.* J. Biol. Chem. 273: 12753-12757, 1998

DEEPMALA, SLATTERY J, KUMAR N, ET AL. *Clinical trials of N-acetylcysteine in psychiatry & neurology: A systematic review.* Neurosci Biobehav Rev 55:294-321, 2015

EVANS PH. *Free radicals in brain metabolism & pathology.* Br. Med. Bull. 49: 577-587, 1993

GARLET TR, PARISOTTO EB, ET AL. *Systemic oxidative stress in children & teenagers with Down syndrome.* Life Sci 93(16):558-63, 2013

HE J, LI T, CHEN J, LIU Y, XIONG F, YANG J, SONG C. *Plasma antioxidant enzymes & lipoperoxidation status in children with Down syndrome.* Clin Biochem 49(1-2):61-5, 2016

HELVESTON W, HURD R, UTHMAN B, WILDER BJ. *Abnormalities of glutathione peroxidase & glutathione reductase in four patients with Friedreich's disease.* Mov Disord 11(1):106-7, 1996

ISLAM MT. *Oxidative stress & mitochondrial dysfunction-linked neurodegenerative disorders.* Neurol Res 39(1):73-82, 2017

JAIN A, MARTENSSON J, STOLE E, ET AL. *Glutathione deficiency leads to mitochondrial damage in brain.* Proc. Natl. Acad. Sci. USA 88: 1913-1917, 1991

JAUSLIN ML, WIRTH T, MEIER T, SCHOUMACHER F. *A cellular model for Friedreich Ataxia reveals small-molecule glutathione peroxidase mimetics as novel treatment strategy.* Hum Mol Genet 11(24):3055-63, 2002

JENNER P. *Oxidative stress in Parkinson's disease & other neurodegenerative disorders.* Pathol. Biol. (Paris) 44: 57-64, 1996

JENSEN GE, CLAUSEN J. *Leukocyte glutathione peroxidase activity & selenium level in Batten's disease.* Scand. J. Clin. Lab. Invest. 43: 187-196, 1983

JOHNSON WM, WILSON-DELFOSSE AL, MIEVAL JJ. *Dysregulation of glutathione homeostasis in neurodegenerative diseases.* Nutrients 4(10):1399-440, 2012

KISH SJ, MORITO CL, HORNYKIEWICZ O. *Brain glutathione peroxidase in neurodegenerative disorders.* Neurochem Pathol 4(1):23-8, 1986

KLEPAC N, RELJA M, ET AL. *Oxidative stress parameters in plasma of Huntington's disease patients, asymptomatic Huntington's disease gene carriers & healthy subjects: a cross-sectional study.* J Neurol 254(12):1676-83, 2007

LOTT IT, HEAD E, DORAN E, BUSCIGLIO J. *Beta-amyloid, oxidative stress & down syndrome.* Curr Alzheimer Res 3(5):521-8, 2006

MAERTENS P, DYKEN P, GRAF W, ET AL. *Free radicals, anticonvulsants, & the neuronal ceroid-lipofuscinoses.* American J. Med. Genet. 57: 225-228, 1995

MASON RP, CASU M, BUTLER N, ET AL. *Glutathione peroxidase activity is neuroprotective in models of Huntington's disease.* Nat Genet 45(10):1249-54, 2013

MAY PC, GRAY PN. *The mechanism of glutamate-induced degeneration of cultured Huntington's disease & control fibroblasts.* J. Neurol. Sci. 70: 101-112, 1985

MUCHOVA J, GARAIOVA I, SUSTROVA M, ET AL. *The redox state of glutathione in erythrocytes of individuals with Down syndrome.* Bratisl Lek Listy, 109(2):70-4, 2007

MUYDERMAN H, CHEN T. *Mitochondrial dysfunction in amyotrophic lateral sclerosis – a valid pharmacological target?* Br J Pharmacol 171(8):2191-205

PARISOTTO EB, GARLET TR, CAVALLI VL, ET AL. *Antioxidant intervention attenuates oxidative stress in children & teenagers with Down syndrome.* Res Dev Disabil 35(6):1228-36, 2014

PARISOTTO EB, GIARETTA AG, ZAMONER A, ET AL *Persistence of the benefit of an antioxidant therapy in children & teenagers with Down syndrome.* Res Dev Disabil 45-46:14-20, 2015

PASTORE A, TOZZI G, GAETA LM, ET AL. *Actin glutathionylation increases in fibroblasts of patients with Friedreich's ataxia: a potential role in the pathogenesis of the disease.* J Biol Chem 278(43):42588-95, 2003

PEREZ-SEVERIANO F, MONTES S, ET AL. *Study of oxidative damage & antioxidant systems in two Huntington's disease rodent models.* Methods Mol Biol 1010:177-200, 2013

PEÑA-SÁNCHEZ M, RIVERÓN-FORMENT G, ZALDIVAR-VAILLANT T, ET AL. *Association of status redox with demographic, clinical & imaging parameters in patients with Huntington´s disease.* Blin Biochem 48(18):1258-63, 2015

PIERMONTE F, PASTORE A, TOZZI G, ET AL. *Glutathione in blood of patients with Friedreich's ataxia.* Eur J Clin Invest 31(11):1007-11, 2001

PERCY ME, DALTON AJ, MARKOVIC VD, ET AL. *Red cell superoxide dismutase, glutathione peroxidase & catalase in Down syndrome patients with & without manifestations of Alzheimer's disease.* American J. Med. Genet. 35: 459-467, 1990

REITER RJ. *Oxidative processes & antioxidative defense mechanisms in the aging brain.* FASEB 9: 526-533, 1995

RODRIGUEZ-SUREDA V, VILCHES A, ET AL. *Intracellular oxidant activity, antioxidant enzyme defense system, & cell senescence in fibroblasts with trisomy 21.* Oxid Med Cell Longev 2015:509241, 2015

ROSS EK, WINTER AN, WILKINS HM ET AL. *A Cystine-Rich Whey Supplement (Immunocal ®) Delays Disease Onset & Prevents Spinal Cord Glutathione Depletion in the hSOD1(G93A) Mouse Model of Amyotrophic Lateral Sclerosis.* Antioxidants (Basel) 3(4):843-65, 2014

SHOICHET SA, BAUMER AT, ET AL. *Frataxin promotes antioxidant defense in a thiol-dependent manner resulting in diminished malignant transformation in vitro.* Hum Mol Genet 11(7):815-21, 2002

SOROLLA MA, RODRIGUEZ-COLMAN MJ, ET AL. *Protein oxidation in Huntington disease.* Biofactors 38(3):173-85, 2012

SPARACO M, GAETA LM, SANTORELLI FM, ET AL. *Friedreich's ataxia: oxidative stress & cytoskeletal abnormalities.* J Neurol Sci 287(1-2):111-8, 2009

STACK EC, MATSON WR, FERRANTE RJ. *Evidence of oxidant damage in Huntington's disease: translational strategies using antioxidants.* Ann N Y Acad Sci 1147:79-72, 2008

STABEL-BUROW J, KLEU A, SCHUCHMANN S, HEINEMANN U. *Glutathione levels & nerve cell loss in hippocampal cultures from trisomy 16 mouse – a model of Down syndrome.* Brain Res. 765: 313-318, 1997

SULTHANA SM, KUMAR SN ET AL. *Levels of non enzymatic antioxidants in Down syndrome.* Indian J Pediatr 79(11):1473-6, 2012

TABRIZI SJ, CLEETER MW, XUEREB J, ET AL. *Biochemical abnormalities & excitotoxicity in Huntington's disease brain.* Ann. Neurol. 45: 25-32, 1999

TOZZI G, NUCCETELLI M, LO BELLO M, ET AL. *Antioxidant enzymes in blood of patients with Friedreich's ataxia.* Arch Dis Child 86(5):376-9, 2002

VALLE C, CARRI MT. *Cysteine Modifications in the Pathogenesis of ALS.* Front Mol Neurosci 10:5, 2017

WESTERMARCK T, SANDHOLM M. *Decreased erythrocyte glutathione peroxidase activity in neuronal lipofuscinosis (NCL) – corrected with selenium supple-*

mentation. Acta Pharmacol. Toxicol. (Copenh.) 40: 70-74, 1977

Wright DJ, Renoir T, Smith ZM et al. *N-Acetylcysteine improves mitochondrial function & ameliorates behavioral deficits in the R6/1 mouse model of Huntington's.* Transl Psychiatr 5:e492, 2015

Wright DJ, Gray LJ, et al. *N-acetylcysteine modulates glutamatergic dysfunction & depressive behavior in Huntington's disease.* Hum Mol Genet 25(14):2923-2933, 2016

Teksen F, Sayli BS, Aydin A, et al. *Antioxidative metabolism in Down syndrome. Biol. Trace Elem. Res. 63: 123-127, 1998*

Zanella A, Izzo C, Meola G, et al. *Metabolic impairment & membrane abnormality in red cells from Huntington's disease.* J. Neurol. Sci. 47: 93-103, 1980

Zis P, Dickinson M, Shende S. Walker Z, Strydom A. *Oxidative stress & memory decline in adults with Down syndrome: longitudinal study.* J Alzheimers Dis 31(2):277-83, 2012

29

Autism and Glutathione

Autism is an abnormal development of the nervous system in children. Its incidence has grown in recent decades, and whether this disorder is truly on the rise or is simply diagnosed more often is open to debate. In either case, most estimates put the incidence of Autism at 1 or 2 cases for every 200 children. These numbers are still rising.

Known more properly as autistic spectrum disorder (ASD), autism is usually diagnosed before the age of three. One early sign is a child's resistance to cuddling and affection. This is followed by a pattern of difficulty forming interpersonal relationships. Over time, autistic children withdraw into their own world, expressing minimal interest in family, friends and much of the surrounding environment. Language, communication skills, eye contact, physical contact and relationships do not develop normally.

Aside from social difficulties, autistic children often exhibit repetitive body movements such as rocking, hand flapping or finger flipping. Repeating words or phrases (echolalia) is a common symptom. Insistence on familiar patterns and adherence to rigid routines are often apparent. Autistic individuals are sometimes preoccupied by lights or moving objects. Distressingly, some are prone to self-mutilation or injury.

Causes of Autism

The cause of autism remains unknown. Theories abound, and most researchers agree that several mechanisms are at play. Some forms of autism have been shown to run in families and may have a genetic component. Examining the personal genome (DNA coding) of autistic individuals reveals defects in certain glutathione enzymes (GSTs). There is also evidence that environmental factors may provoke this syndrome. In fact, it seems most likely that several forms of autism exist, and conventional wisdom suggests that a genetic predisposition towards this syndrome may remain dormant or be triggered by specific environmental factors.

Renowned neuro-pharmacologist Dr. Richard Deth hypothesizes that autism is a 'redox/methylation' disorder. Methylation is a subtle change in DNA that alters its code. This is referred to as an 'epigenetic' trigger, leading to abnormalities in the way the genetic code plays out, in this case expressing autistic symptoms rather than normal behavior. Methylation is exquisitely sensitive to 'redox' (the antioxidant/oxidant balance), so it makes sense that the master antioxidant glutathione would be implicated.

While it's likely that several different forms of autism exist, it's also clear that older theories linking autism to parental neglect or behavior are considered false.

Reliable testing for autism remains elusive and in all likelihood will never be established. It's becoming increasingly clear that autism is the interrelated end-point of several pathways. Dozens of 'biomarkers' and 'autism genes' have so far been identified, and research continues, but there is no one single cause that appears in every case. Autism is called a 'complex disorder' not because it's 'complicated' but to indicate that it results from several interacting causes.

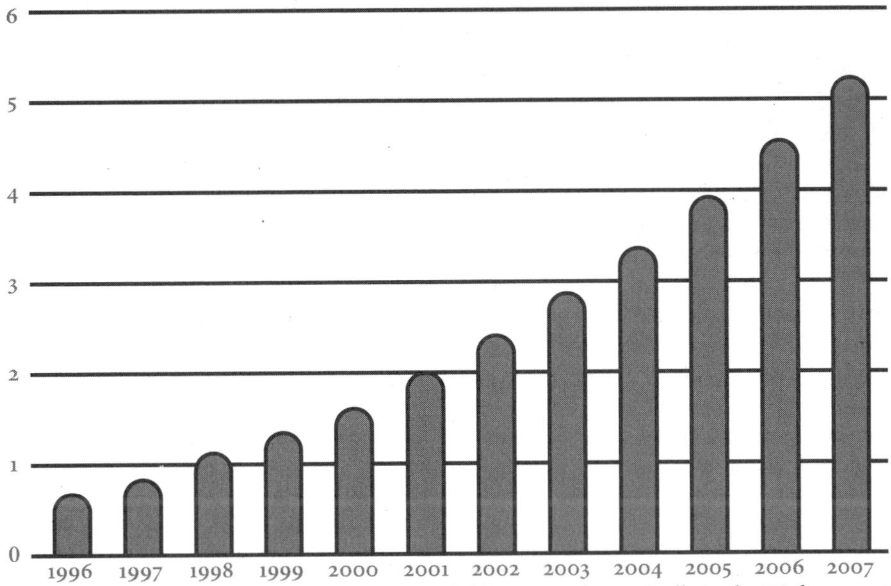

FIGURE 57: Reports of autism cases per 1,000 children grew dramatically in the US from 1996 to 2007. It is unknown how much, if any, growth came from changes in rates of autism [Eubulides]

Autism has been linked to a number of different diseases, including congenital rubella (German measles), fragile X syndrome, abnormal purine metabolism, William's syndrome, tuberous sclerosis, Down syndrome and others. Theories on the cause of autism abound. They include autoimmunity, chronic inflammatory state, exposure to teratogens during first trimester pregnancy, viral infection, phospholipid abnormalities, oxytocin administration during delivery, and exposure to toxins, notably mercury.

Scientists continue to identify factors that might be modified either to treat or prevent autism. Environmental toxins that are theoretically within our control seem to be contributing factors in the development of this disorder, giving great impetus to the search for specific triggers that can subsequently be avoided or controlled.

The Mercury-Thimerosal Link

Mercury is a heavy metal and also a potent neurotoxin that is poisonous or destructive to nerve tissue. Much of the mercury and heavy metals we're exposed to comes from eating fish, but other sources include mercury amalgams (dental fillings), industrial pollution and some preservatives. The effects of mercury and heavy metal poisoning have been well documented, and their detoxification depends on glutathione.

Exposure to mercury in adults leads to predictable changes in nervous and mental functions. The effects of mercury in newborn and young children are less clear. Studies carried out at the National Center for Health Statistics, Centers for Disease Control and Prevention have indicated that approximately 8% of American women of childbearing age show concentrations higher than the US EPA's (Environmental Protection Agency) recommended dose of mercury. Several public advocacy agencies have challenged the Food and Drug Administration by pushing for stricter guidelines on safe levels of fish consumption in women and children.

Thimerosal is a preservative used in pharmacological applications, including contact lens cleaning solutions and vaccines.

It consists of about 50% ethyl mercury. From 1988 to 2002, American children were routinely exposed to this compound during their first six months of life—and sometimes even before. Pregnant women with Rh-negative blood indirectly exposed their fetuses to thimerosal when they received a RhoGAM, an injectable drug given to prevent problems in case the baby's blood type was Rh-positive. The influenza vaccine (flu-shot) is another source of potential mercury exposure. Routine immunizations including the MMV vaccine (measles, mumps and varicella) and others all formerly contained thimerosal. Most state governments have already removed thimerosal from many immunizations. Other states seem poised to ban this preservative outright.

The question of whether thimerosal causes autism is still undecided. Proponents of this theory point to epidemiological studies (population statistics) showing that as the use of immunizations increased in the United States, so did the rate of autism. As we said at the outset of this chapter, this does not necessarily mean there are more occurrences of autism, merely that more cases have been diagnosed. While the debate continues and no clear answer is apparent, the conservative approach would be to avoid substances with potentially harmful results. This does not necessarily mean avoiding immunizations, just limiting the use of products with mercury-based preservatives.

IMPORTANT NOTE: Mercury has been commonly identified as a prominent suspect, but it's not the only one. Many other toxins have been studied as potential causes of autism. These include pesticides, PCBs (polychlorinated biphenyls), phthalates, solvents, other heavy metals and many air pollutants.

Glutathione and autism

The earliest-found article on glutathione and autism dates back several decades to France, where a Parisian team sought to identify various scenarios in which autism might occur. They were apparently the first to notice that glutathione activity was below average in autism patients. Other than some other obscure reports (also of French origin), this association between glutathione and autism was ignored for several years, even in major studies on autism.

Fortunately, the work was picked up again in Turkey at the turn of the millennium by two separate groups of researchers: one team of child psychiatrists and one of biochemists. Both demonstrated that diminished glutathione activity is common to autistic children, and statistically significant. They proposed that neurological damage was caused by oxidative stress.

In the interim, North American scientists were at work studying the 'etiology' of autism (looking for a single cause). It now became clear that this was unlikely.

Back in 2003 Eigsti and Shapiro from Columbia University (NY) reviewed the body of scientific work on genetic, biochemical and anatomical differences found in autism. They stated that, "Autism is a heterogeneous disorder and is likely to have multiple possible etiologies." Rather than a simple determinant, they found various intersecting causes and conditions that differed from one case to another. They noticed various anatomical differences that they said were, "reflective of an early developmental change in the growth or pruning of neural tissue."

Seeking common pathways, Eigsti and Shapiro experimented with dietary ways to alleviate symptoms. One gluten-free and casein-free regimen led to some promising outcomes. A review in the Journal of Nutrional Biochemistry by Trivedi and his team highlighted that both gluten and caseine may release peptides (small proteins) with opioid activity, having consequences for both the gastrointestinal tract and the brain. Some teams focused more on environmental toxins, while others investigated potential allergens and their elimination.

By the early 2000s, a research team led by Jill James from the University of Arkansas had

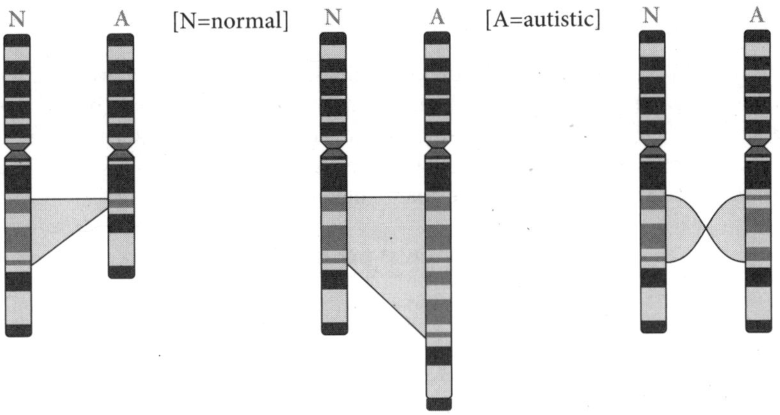

Figure 58: Types of redox-caused chromosome abnormalities in autism

[Acknowledgment: Richard Wheeler, https://en.wikipedia.org/wiki/User:Zephyris]

started assembling disparate pieces of this puzzle. Noting that previous studies indicated a higher than average load of oxidative stress in autistic children, and that environmental toxins such as mercury were also implicated, it appeared that glutathione played a greater role than previously imagined.

The key finding was that many autistic children were unable to protect themselves from heavy metals—including known neurotoxins. The team from Arkansas demonstrated a significant deficiency in GSH activity in up to 80% of cases examined. They also noted that several genes coding for normal glutathione metabolism were faulty in autistic children. James' team followed up with a more intrusive study in 2012, testing post-mortem human brains. When compared to non-autistic brains of a similar age, they revealed obvious glutathione abnormalities.

Janet Kern and her associates at University of Texas Southwestern Medical Center used a dietary supplement to raise GSH. A small pilot study with specially-prepared bioactive whey protein was carried out on autistic children to make sure they could tolerate it, since many autistic children are sensitive to a variety of different foods. The children had no digestive issues with the bioactive isolate.

Kern and associates also observed an improvement in the children's behavior, though this was not the primary objective of the study and there were too few subjects to be statistically significant. However, a multidisciplinary research study at Florida's Nova Southeastern University, under Principal Investigator Dr. Ana Maria Castejon, is currently investigating the role of glutathione in autism, and has already revealed promising results. Her final publication is pending.

Various diet-based studies have given widely differing results according to how glutathione is delivered. Oral glutathione (eating it) is not effective. Successful treatments relied on injecting or ingesting glutathione precursors, thus enabling individual cells to manufacture glutathione for themselves. Injecting the pharmaceutical drug NAC (N-acetyl-cysteine) successfully raised glutathione, but a high proportion of autistic children experienced side effects. The Nrf2 activator sulphoraphane is also known to stimulate glutathione synthesis. A study adding sulphoraphane to the diet of autistic males (13 to 27 years) showed improvement in behavioral scales which subsequently dropped back to baseline after the treatment.

Although it is too early to expect raising GSH to be a universally accepted treatment, many clinicians are anticipating that further research will bear considerable fruit. On an anecdotal level, there are abundant testimonials attesting to dramatic improvements in autism by increasing glutathione levels.

Conclusion

Autism is a multi-factorial disease involving a combination of genetic, epigenetic and environmental triggers. No single cause for autism is likely to be found, but one notable problem identified is a deficiency in normal glutathione activity. Early trials suggest that raising glutathione offers a potential advantage in the fight against autism, and research efforts to establish this strategy are being actively investigated.

AUTISM

REFERENCES

Adams JB, Baral M, Geis E, et al. *The severity of autism is associated with toxic metal body burden & red blood cell glutathione levels.* J. Toxicol Aug 26, 2009.

Alabdali A, Al-Ayadhi L, El-Ansary A. *A key role for an impaired detoxification mechanism in the etiology & severity of autism spectrum disorders.* Behav Brain Funct. Apr 28;10:14, 2014

Arnt TL, Stodgell CJ, Rodier PM. *The teratology of autism.* Int. J. Dev. Neuroscience 23(2-3): 189-199, 2005

Ashwood P, Van de Water J. *Is autism an autoimmune disease?* Autoimmune Review 3(7-8): 557-562, 2004

Baron-Cohen S. *Autism: Research into causes & intervention.* Pediatric Rehabil. 7(2):73-78, 2004

Bespaltova IN, Buxbaum JD. *Disease susceptibility genes for autism.* Ann. Med. 35(4):274-281, 2003

Blaxill MF, Redwood L, Bernard S. *Thimerosal & autism? A plausible hypothesis that should not be dismissed.* Med Hypothesis 62(5):788-794, 2004

Bowers K, Li Q, Bressler J, Avramopoulos D, Newschafer C, Fallin MD. *Glutathione pathway gene variation & risk of autism spectrum disorders.* J Neurodev Disord. 3(2):132-143, 2011.

Chauhan A, Audhya T, Chauhan V. *Brain region-specific glutathione redox imbalance in autism.* Neurochem Res. 37(8): 1681-1689. 2012.

Chez MG, Chin K, Hung PC. *Immunizations, immunology, & autism.* Semin. Pediatr. Neurol. 11(3):214-217, 2004

Deth R. *Autism: a redox/methylation disorder.* Glob Adv Health Med. 2(6):68-73, 2013.

Durieux AMS, Horder J, Mendez MA, et al. *Cortical & subcortical glutathione levels in adults with autism spectrum disprder.* Autism Res. 9(4):429-435. 2016.

Endres D, Tebartz van Elst L, Meyer SA, et al. *Glutathione metabolism in the prefrontal brain of adults with high-functioning autism spectrum disorder: an MRS study.* Mol Autism. Mar 7;8:10. 2017.

Eigsti IM, Shapiro T. *A systems neuroscience approach to autism: biological, cognitive, & clinical perspectives.* Ment. Retard. Dev. Disabil. Res. Rev. 9(3):205-215, 2003

Esparham AE, Smith T, Belmont JM, et al. *Nutritional & metabolic biomarkers in autism spectrum disorders: An exploratory study.* Integr Med. 14(2):40-53.

Frustaci A, Neri M, Cesario A, et al. *Oxidative stress-related biomarkers in autism: systematic review & meta-analyses.* Free Rad Biol Med. 52(10):2128-2141. 2012.

Frye RE, Delatorre R, Taylor H, et al. *Redox metabolism abnormalities in autistic children associated with mitochondrial disease. Transl Psychiatry Jue 18, 2013.*

Frye RE, James SJ. *Metabolic pathology of autism in relation to redox metabolism.* Biomark Med. 8(3):321-330. 2014.

Geier DA, Geier MR. *Neurodevelopmental disorders following thimerosal-containing childhood immunizations: a follow-up analysis.* Int. J. Toxicol. 23(6):369-376, 2004

Geier DA, Geier MR. *A two-phased population epidemiological study of the safety of thimerosal-containing vaccines: a follow-up analysis.* Med. Sci. Monit. 11(4):CR160-170, 2005

Geier MR, Geier DA. *The potential importance of steroids in the treatment of autistic spectrum disorders & other disorders involving mercury toxicity.* Med. Hypothesis 64(5):946-954, 2005

Geier DA, Kern JK, Homme KG, Geier MR. *The risk of neurodevelopmental disorders following Thimerosal-containing Hib vaccine in comparison to Thimerosal-free Hib vaccine administered form 1995 to 19999 in the United States.* Iny J Hyg Environ Health. 22(4):677-683, 2018,

Ghanizadeh A, Akhondzadeh S, Hormozi M, et al. *Glutathione-related factors & oxidative stress in autism, a review.* Curr Med Chem. 19(23):4000-4005. 2012.

Goldson E. *Autism spectrum disorders: an overview.* Adv. Pediatr. 51:63-109, 2004

Golse B, Debray-Ritzen P, Durosay P, Puget K, Michelson AM. *Alterations in two enzymes: superoxide dismutase & glutathione peroxidase in developmental infantile psychosis (infantile autism).* Rev. Neurol. (Paris) 134(11):699-705, 1978

Gu F, Chauhan V, Chauhan A. *Impaired synthesis & antioxidant defense of glutathione in the cerebellum of autistic subjects: alterations in the activities & protein expression of glutathione-related enzymes.* Free Rad Biol Med. 65:488-496. 2013.

Gu F, Chauhan V, Chauhan A. *Glutathione redox imbalance in brain disorders.Curr Opin Clin Nutr Metab Care. 28(1):89-95. 2015.*

Hendren RL, James SJ, Widjaja F, et al. *Randomized, placebo-controlled trial of methyl B12 for children with autism.* J Child Adolesc Psychopharmacol. Nov;26(9):774-783. Epub 2016 Feb 18 2016.

Hessel L. *Mercury in vaccines. Bull.* Acad. Natl. Med. 187(8):1501-1510. 2003

Hidgson NW, Waly MI, Al-Farsi YM et al. *Decreased glutathione & elevated hair mercury levels are associated with nutritional deficiency-based autism in Oman.* Exp Biol Med. 239(6):697-706, 2014.

James SJ, Melnyk S, Fuchs G, et al. *Efficacy of methylcobalamin & folinic acid treatment on glutathione redox status in children with autism.* Am J Clin Nutr. 89(1):425-430, 2009.

James SJ, Cutler P, Melnyk S, Jernigan S, Janak L, Gaylor DW, Neubrander JA. *Metabolic biomarkers of increased oxidative stress & impaired methylation capacity in children with autism.* American J. Clin. Nutrition 80(6):1611-1617, 2004

Jick H, Kaye JA. *Epidemiology & possible causes of autism.* Pharmacotherapy 23(12):1524-1530, 2003

Kern JK, Geier DA, Adama JB, Garver CR, Audhya T, Geier MR. *A clinical trial of glutathione supplementation in autism spectrum disorders.* Med Sci Monit. 17(12):CR677-682, 2011.

Kern JK, Grannemann BD, Gutman J, Trivedi MH. *Oral tolerability of whey protein isolate in autism as a potential means of glutathione augmentation: a pilot study.* JANA 2008, in press

Kern JK, Jones AM. *Evidence of toxicity, oxidative stress, & neuronal insult in autism.* J Tox Envir Health 9(6):485-499, 2006

Kidd PM. *Autism, an extreme challenge to integrative medicine. Part 1: The knowledge base.* Altern. Med. Rev. 7(4):292-316, 2002

Libbey JE, Sweeten TL, McMahon WM, Fujinami RS. *Autistic disorder & viral infections.* Neurovirol. 11(1):1-10, 2005

Main PA, Angley MT, O'Doherty CE, Thomas P, Fenech M. *The potential role of the antioxidant & detoxification properties of glutathione in autism spectrum disorders: a systematic review & meta-analysis.* Nutr Metab (Lond). 24:9;35, 2012.

Meguid NA, Dardir AA, Abdel-Raouf ER, Hashish A. *Evaluation of oxidative stress in autism: defective antioxidant enzymes & increased lipid peroxidation.* Biol Trace Elem Res. 143(1):58-65, 2011.

Milward C, Ferriter M, Calver S, Connell-Jones G. *Gluten- & Caseine-free diets for autistic spectrum disorder.* Cochrane Database Syst. Rev. (2):CD003498, 2004

Minarini A, Ferrari S, Galletti M, et al. *N-acetylcysteine in the treatment of psychiatric disorders: current status & future prospects.* Expert Opin Drug Metab Toxicol. 13(3):279-292, 2017.

Nadeem A, Ahmad SF, Attia SM, et al. *Dysregulated enzymatic antioxidant network in peripheral neutrophils & monocytes in children with autism.* Prog Neuropsychopharmacol Biol Psychiatry 88:352-359, 2019.

Parker SK, Schwartz B, Todd J, Pickering LK. *Thimerosal-containing vaccines & autistic spectrum disorder;: a critical review of published original data.* Pediatrics 114(3):793-804, 2004

Pelios LV, Lund SK. *A selective overview of issues on classification, causation, & early intensive behavioral intervention for autism.* Behav. Mod. 25(5):678-697, 2001

Ragbar MH, Samms-Vaughan M, Ma J, et al. *Interaction between GSTT1 & GSTP1 allele variants as a risk modulating-factor for autism spectrum disorders.* Res Autism Spectr Disörd 1:12:1-9, 2015.

Rose S, Bennuri SC, Wynne R, Malnyk S, James SJ, Frye RE. *Mitochondrial & redox abnormalities in autism lymphoblastoid cells: a sibling control study.* FASEB J. 31(3):904-909, 2017.

Rose S, Melnyk S, Pavliv O, et al. *Evidence of oxidative damage & inflammation associated with low glutathione redox status in the autism brain.* Transl Psychiatry. Jul 10, 2012.

Rossignol DA, Genuis SJ, Frye RE. *Environ mental toxicants & autism spectrum disorders: a systematic review.* Transl Psychiatry. Feb 11:4, 2014.

Rutter M. *Aetiology of autism: findings & questions.* J Intellect. Disabil. Research 49(Pt 4):231-238, 2005

Rutter M. *Incidence of autism spectrum disorders: change over time & their meaning.* Acta Paediatr. 94(1):2-15, 2005

Schiavone S, Trabace L. *Pharmacological targeting of redox regulation systems as new therapeutic approach for psychiatric disorders: A literature overview.* Pharmacol Res . 107:195-204, 2016.

Schober et al. *Blood mercury levels in US children & women of childbearing age, 1999-2000.* JAMA 289(13):1667-1674, 2003

Serajee FJ, Nabi R, Zhong H, Huq M. *Polymorphisms in xenobiotic metabolism genes & autism.* J. Child. Neurol. 19(6):413-417, 2004

Singh K, Connors SL, Macklin EA, et al. *Sulforaphane treatment of autism spectrum disorder (ASD).* Proc Natl ACad Sci USA. 111(43):15550-15555, 2014.

Sogut et al. *Changes in nitric oxide levels & antioxidant enzyme activities may have a role in the pathophysiological mechanisms involved in autism.* Clin. Chim. Acta. 33(1-2):111-117, 2003

Tidmarsh L, Volkmar FR. *Diagnosis & epidemiology of autism spectrum disorders.* Canadian J. Psychiatry 48(8):517-525, 2003

Trivedi MS, Shah JS, Al-Mughairy S, Hodgson NW, Simms B, Trooskens GA, Van Criekinge W, Deth RC. *Food-derived opioid peptides inhibit cysteine uptake with redox & epigenetic consequences.* J Nutr Biochem 25(10):1011-1018, 2014.

Tuchman R. *Autism.* Neurol, Clin. 21(4):915-932, 2003

Vargason T, Howsmon DP, Melnyk S, James SJ, Hahn J. *Mathematical modeling of the methionine cycle & transsulfutation pathway in individuals with autism spectrum disorder.* J Theor Biol 416:28-37, 2016.

Veenstra-Vanderweele J, Christian SL, Cook EH Jr. *Autism as a paradigmatic complex genetic disorder.* Annu. Rev. Genomics Hum. Genet. 5:379-405, 2004

Wahl RU. *Could oxytocin administration during labor contribute to autism & related behavioral disorders? – A look at the literature.* Med. Hypothesis 63(3):456-460, 2004

Wassink TH et al. *The search for autism disease genes.* Ment. Retard. Dev. Disabil. Res. Rev. 10(4):272-283, 2004

Welsh JP, Ahn ES, Placantonakis DG. *Is autism due to brain desynchronization?* Int. J. Dev. Neurosci. 23(2-3):253-263, 2005

Wink LK, Adams R, Wang Z, et al. *A randomized placebo-controlled pilot study of N-acetylcysteine in youth with autism spectrum disorder.* Apr 21;7:26, 2016.

Wiznitzer M. *Autism & tuberous sclerosis.* J. Child. Neurol. 19(9):675-679, 2004

Yorbik O, Sayal A, Akay C, Akbiyik DI, Sohmen T. *Investigation of antioxidant enzymes in children with autistic disorder.* Prostaglandins Leukot. Essent. Fatty Acids 67(5):341-343, 2002

Zoruglu SS et al. *Increased oxidative stress & altered activities of erythrocytes free radical scavenging enzymes in autism. Eur. Arch. Psychiatry Clin. Neurosci. 254(3):143-147, 2004*

30

Multiple Sclerosis

Multiple sclerosis (MS) has been referred to as "the great crippler of young adults." It usually strikes victims in the prime of their life and is one of the most dreaded degenerative diseases of the nervous system. The symptoms of MS are quite variable, ranging from one or two attacks of weakness in a limb or blurred vision to a relentless, progressive deterioration of speech, movement and other basic functions.

MS affects various parts of the nervous system by damaging myelin, the fatty sheath that insulates nerve fibers, just as a plastic sheath insulates electrical wire. This demyelination leaves scars or plaques that short-circuit the electrical signals passing through the nerve fibers. The scarring process is called sclerosis. Figure 57 shows the degeneration of the myelin sheath and the weakening of the nerve signal.

Depending on which nerves are affected, patients may suffer localized weakness or stiffness, visual difficulties, diminished bladder or bowel control and other neurological dysfunctions. Attacks may be mild, lasting only days and followed by remission.

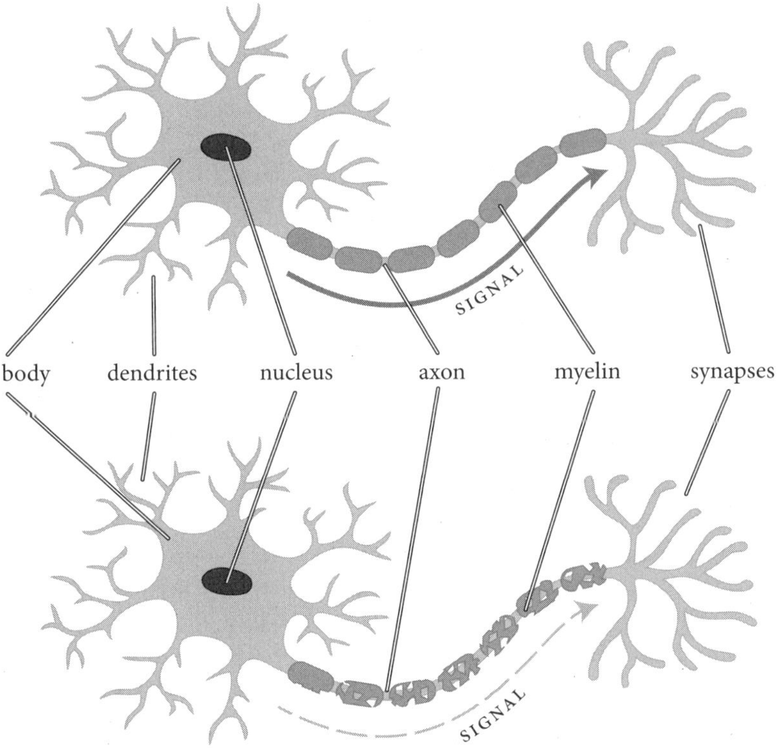

Figure 59: Normal nerve cell (top) and cell with myelin damage (bottom)

However, after some years this eventually turns into a constant decline. Some experience this rapid progression from the outset and are quickly disabled.

The causes of MS are still unclear. However, many possible causes have been suggested. Some point to environmental and/or genetic factors, while other researchers believe that certain viruses may be involved. A widely held view holds that MS is an autoimmune disease in which the immune system mistakenly attacks healthy tissue. Still others are investigating dietary factors or exposure to toxins such as lead, mercury, pesticides and carbon monoxide. Yet another theory considers the role of allergies.

Conventional medicine treats the symptoms of MS, but cannot cure it. However, some newer drugs show promise in diminishing the rate of relapse. Diets of all sorts have been widely tested without consistent results. Everything about this disease is difficult to study because symptoms vary so widely, patients often recover spontaneously and one can never be sure whether or not a treatment has been helpful or not.

Multiple sclerosis belongs to a group of nervous system diseases called neurodegenerative disorders that also includes Alzheimer's, Parkinson's and ALS (amyotrophic lateral sclerosis, or Lou Gehrig's disease). Their specific causes are unknown, but a number of studies suggest that an important role is played by the formation of oxygen-derived free radicals and/or inadequate antioxidant defenses.

Oxidation and multiple sclerosis

The myelin sheaths destroyed by MS are made of lipids, fatty substances highly sensitive to damage by lipid peroxidation—a particularly aggressive type of oxidation. Our key metabolic defenses are GSH and SOD (super-oxide dismutase). It has been shown that elevating these natural defense systems reduces the damage of oxidative stress.

Measuring the breakdown products of oxidation has revealed significantly higher levels in MS patients. Toshniwal and Zarling at Chicago's Loyola University went further, showing that the measure of oxidative stress corresponded to the severity of the MS attack.

Some authors, including LeVine from the University of Kansas, suggest that the pathology leading to demyelination begins when the immune system cooperates with a free radical generating system in the myelin sheaths. This explanation combines two potential causes of MS—autoimmune disorder and oxidative stress. LeVine describes a demyelination episode as follows: macrophages (immune cells meant to protect) seek out myelin and release powerful chemicals (lipases, proteinases, H_2O_2 and others) producing tremendous levels of oxidative stress.

Such a hypothesis suggests that the way to help MS patients is by either blunting the immune response or minimizing oxidative stress. Immunosuppressive drugs that blunt the immune response have had only limited success, which has driven researchers to seek improved antioxidant protection. For this, glutathione modulation seems very promising.

Glutathione and multiple sclerosis

Many studies have compared groups of MS patients to healthy individuals. Among other things, they measured levels of reactive metabolites that result from oxidation, and protective enzymes—especially GSH.

The fact that individuals with genetically impaired glutathione enzymes are more prone to MS points indirectly to glutathione's protective role against nerve damage. An Italian group headed by Calabrese drew samples of cerebrospinal fluid (CSF) through spinal taps from MS patients. CSF analysis is a good indicator of brain metabolism. They found consistently low GSH-peroxidase levels in the cerebro-spinal fluid of MS patients and concluded that the fundamental MS anti-oxidation activity is abnormal, and that oxidative stress plays a causative role.

Another study looking at CSF was performed in Sweden by Ronquist and Frithz, who tested spinal taps from a large number of patients, including those with stroke, seizures, brain tumors and MS. The cerebrospinal fluid of MS patients was found to be almost entirely lacking in GSH.

Further evidence of the involvement of free radical elevation and GSH depletion in MS was found by Helen Langemann in Switzerland, who measured GSH levels within MS plaques themselves. Without exception, they were depleted.

Several excellent review papers are available (Carvalho et al., Ortiz et al., others); for example, "Glutathione in multiple sclerosis: more than just an antioxidant?" The overwhelming finding is that not only is oxidative stress elevated and glutathione levels reduced, but also, the measure of glutathione levels indicates the stage, severity and progression of the disease. Two papers by Choi et al (2017) clearly showed that glutathione levels were correlated with disability scales in MS, and they suggested that "GSH provides a distinct measure associated with the disease progression… possibly due to its dynamic alignment with pathogenic processes of MS related to oxidative stress."

Recent technological advances in radiology have allowed us to "look" into living human brains and witness them at work. An offshoot of MRI (Magnetic Resonance Imaging) is MRS (Magnetic Resonance Spectroscopy). MRS can be tuned in to glutathione content in the brain. This technology has confirmed that glutathione levels are indeed lower in MS patients.

Singh and his researchers at the University of South Carolina looked for the fundamental tissue abnormality in multiple sclerosis and found that myelin breakdown results mainly from strong inflammatory chemicals called cytokines that generate huge numbers of free radicals. Pre-treating neurological tissues with NAC (N-acetylcysteine) to raise glutathione levels protected these tissues from demyelination. Conversely, when GSH was chemically depleted, demyelination worsened.

What can be done to address this problem, particularly as it relates to glutathione and dietary intervention?

Polish researchers (Socha et al.) have published several studies looking at the dietary and lifestyle habits of MS patients. Some of their findings revealed that poor dietary habits "significantly" decrease selenium concentrations (see below). At the same time, glutathione levels fell while markers of oxidative stress rose. It was interesting to note that cigarette smoke was correlated with disease severity; cigarettes are an enormous source of free radicals.

Dietary sources of cysteine have shown some promise, but well-controlled studies are still lacking. A small European study examined the potential of a garlic extract (a glutathione precursor called "S-allyl cysteine") which showed promise in an experimental model. Others have looked at other glutathione precursors such as NAC, methionine and whey protein.

Selenium and multiple sclerosis

Some research suggests that low selenium levels are connected to the development of MS. Selenium is an essential part of the GSH peroxidase enzyme, and low selenium levels certainly decrease GSH effectiveness. Mai's team in Denmark supplied high-dose antioxidant supplements to MS patients, composed of 6 mg of selenium, 2 g of vitamin C and 480 mg of vitamin E. These patients showed few side effects, and glutathione peroxidase activity increased by a factor of five within five weeks.

Conclusion

MS is difficult to study because its spontaneous remissions and relapses make it very unpredictable. That means improvements in a patient's condition can't be reliably attributed to a particular treatment. In order to be statistically believable, trials would have to include hundreds of subjects.

However, certain findings have been demonstrated consistently in multiple sclerosis patients. The breakdown products of oxidative stress are present in large numbers, and the level of free radical formation corresponds directly to the severity of the MS attack. Glutathione activity is clearly impaired in this disease. This has been confirmed by cutting-edge brain-imaging procedures.

In MS, individual tissues suffer less free radical damage when antioxidants and glutathione therapy are used. Although this is not a cure, numerous authors have suggested that reduced oxidative damage would help MS patients, and advocate the helpful role of elevated GSH levels.

MULTIPLE SCLEROSIS

REFERENCES

Bačić Baronica K. et al. *Progression of multiple sclerosis is associated with gender differences in glutathione S-transferase P1 detoxification pathway.* Acta Neurobiol Exp (Wars) 74(3):257-65, 2014

Bystricka Z, Laubertova L, Durfinova M, Paduchova Z. *Methionine metabolism & multiple sclerosis.* Biomarkers 6:1-8, 2017

Calabrese V, Raffaele R, Cosentino E, Rizza V. *Changes in cerebrospinal fluid levels of malondialdehyde & GSH reductase activity in multiple sclerosis.* International Journal of Clinical Pharmacology Research 14(4):119-123, 1994

Carvalho AN, Lim JL, Nijland PG, Witte ME, Van Horssen J. *Glutathione in multiple sclerosis: more than just an antioxidant?* Mult Scler 20(11):1425-31, 2014

Choi IY, Lee SP, Denney DR, Lynch SG. *Lower levels of glutathione in the brains of secondary progressive multiple sclerosis patients measured by 1H magnetic resonance chemical shift imaging at 3 T.* Mult Scler 17(3):289-96, 2011

Choi IY et al. *In vivo evidence of oxidative stress in brains of patients with progressive multiple sclerosis.* Mult Scler 1:1352458517711568, 2017

Choi IY, Lee P, Hughes AJ, Denney DR, Lynch SG. *Longitudinal changes of cerebral glutathione (GSH) levels associated with the clinical course of disease progression in patients with secondary progressive multiple sclerosis.* Mult Scler 23(7):956-962, 2017

Clausen J, Jensen GE, Nielsen SA. *Selenium in chronic neurologic diseases. Multiple sclerosis & Batten's disease.* Biological Trace Element Research 15:179-203, 1988

Escribano BM. et al. *Dose-dependent S-allyl cysteine ameliorates MS disease-related pathology by reducing oxidative stress & biomerkers of dysbiosis in experimental autoimmune encephalomyelitis.* Eur J Pharmacol pii: S0014-2999(17)30607-6, 2017

Ferreira B, Mendes F, Osorio N, Caseiro A, Gabriel A, Valado A. *Glutathione in multiple sclerosis.* Br J Biomed Sci 70(2):75-9, 2013

Gironi M. et al. *Oxidative stress is differentially present in multiple sclerosis courses, early evident, & unrelated to treatment.* J Immunol Res 2014:961863, 2014

Guy J, Ellis EA, Hope GM, Rao NA. *Antioxidant enzymes reduce loss of blood-brain barrier integrity in experimental optic neuritis.* Archives of Ophthalmology 107(9): 1359-63 1989

Jenner P. *Oxidative damage in neurodegenerative disease.* Lancet 344:796-798, 1994

Jensen GE, Clausen J. *Glutathione peroxidase & reductase, glucose-6-phosphate dehydrogenase & catalase activities in multiple sclerosis.* J Neurol Sci. Jan;63(1):45-53 1984

Karg E, Klivenyi P, Nemeth I, et al. *Nonenzymatic antioxidants of blood in multiple sclerosis.* J. Neurol. 246:533-539, 1999

Knight JA. *Reactive oxygen species & the neurodegenerative disorders.* Annals of Clinical Laboratory Science 27(1):11-25, 1997

Korpela H, Kinnunen E, Juntunen J, Kumulainen J, Koskenvuo M. *Serum selenium concentration, GSH peroxidase activity & lipid peroxides in a co-twin control study on multiple sclerosis.* Journal of the Neurological Sciences 91(1-2):79-84, 1989

Langemann H, Kabiersch A,

Newcombe J. *Measurement of low-molecular-weight antioxidants, uric acid, tyrosine & tryptophan in plaques & white matter from patients with multiple sclerosis.* European Neurology 32(5):248-252, 1992

Le Vine SM. *The role of reactive oxygen species in the pathogenesis of multiple sclerosis.* Medical Hypothesis 39(3):271-274, 1992

Lieben CK, Blokland A, Deutz NE, Jansen W, Hang G, Hupperts RM. *Intake of tryptophan -enriched whey protein acutely enhances recall of positive loaded words in patients with multiple sclerosis.* Clin Nutr pii:S0261-5614(17)30005-5, 2017

Lutsky MA, Zemskov AM, Razinkin KA. *[Biochemical markers of oxidative stress in different forms & phases of multiple sclerosis].* Zh Nevrol Psikhiatr IM S S Korsakova 114(11):74-7, 2014

Mai J, Sorenson PS, Hansen JC. *High dose antioxidant supplementation to MS patients. Effects on GSH peroxidase, clinical safety & absorption of selenium.* Biological Trace Element Research 24(2):109-117, 1990

Mazzella GL, Sinforiani E, Savoldi F, Allegrini M, Lanzola E, Scelsi R. *Blood cells GSH peroxidase activity & selenium in multiple sclerosis.* European Neurology 22(6):442-446, 1983

Morales Pantoja IE. et al. *Nrf2-dysregulation correlates with reduced synthesis & low glutathione levels in experimental autoimmune encephalomyelitis.* J Neurochem 139(4):640-650, 2016

Ortiz GG. et al. *Oxidative stress is increased in serum from Mexican patients with relapsing-remitting multiple sclerosis.* Dis Markers 26(1):35-9, 2009

Polidoro G, Di Ilio C, Arduini A, La Rovere G, Federici G. *Superoxide dismutase, reduced GSH & TBA-reactive products in erythrocytes of patients with multiple sclerosis.* International Journal of Biochemistry 16(5):505-509, 1984

Rae CED, Williams SR. *Glutathione in the human brain: Review of its roles & measurement by magnetic resonance spectroscopy.* Anal Biochem 529:127-143, 2017

Ronquist G, Frithz G. *Adenylate kinase activity & GSH concentration of cerebrospinal fluid in different neurological disorders.* European Neurology 18(2):106-110, 1979

Schipper HM. et al. *Tolerability & Safety of Combined Glatiramer* Acetate & N-Acetylcysteine in Relapsing-Remitting Multiple Sclerosis. Clin Neuropharmacol 38(4):127-31, 2015

Shukla VK, Jensen GE, Clausen J. *Erythrocyte GSH peroxidase deficiency in multiple sclerosis.* Acta Neurology Scandinavia 56(6):542-550, 1977

Simonian NA, Coyle JT. *Oxidative stress in neurodegenerative diseases.* Annual Review of Pharmacology & Toxicology 36:83-106, 1996

Singh I, Pahan K, Khan M, Singh AK. *Cytokine-mediated induction of ceramide production is redox-sensitive. Implications to proinflammatory cytokine-mediated apoptosis in demyelinating diseases.* J. Biol. Chem. 273:20354-20362, 1998

Socha K. et al. *Dietary habits & selenium, glutathione peroxidase & total antioxidant status in the serum of patients with relapsing-remitting multiple sclerosis.* Nutr J 13:62, 2014

Szeinberg A, Golan R, Ben Ezzer J, Sarova-Pinhas I, Sadeh M, Braham J. *Decreased erythrocyte GSH peroxidase activity in multiple sclerosis.* Acta Neurology Scandinavia 60(5):265-271, 1979

Toshniwal PK, Zarling EJ. *Evidence for increased lipid peroxidation in multiple sclerosis. Neurochemistry Research 17(2):205-207, 1992*

Zivkovic M. et al. *The glutathione S-transferase T1 deletion is associated with susceptibility to multiple sclerosis.* J Neurol Sci 334(1-2):6-9, 2013.

31

Seizures

SEIZURES ARE A BROAD GROUP of neurological disorders, typified by muscle contractions, twitching and partial or complete loss of consciousness. Specific symptoms depend on the precise location in the brain of chaotic bursts of electrical activity. Seizures range from violent, uncontrollable contractions of the whole body to a subtle and momentary "loss of contact," that may seem like no more than daydreaming.

Seizures have been referred to as convulsions, fits and epilepsy, as well as by other names that do not accurately reflect the various disorders. Types of seizures include tonic-clonic (grand mal), absence (petit mal), complex-partial (psychomotor, temporal lobe), focal (Jacksonian), and status epilepticus[1] (intractable fits). Not all seizures are epileptic. The most common type of seizure in very young children is called a "febrile seizure," caused by the rapid onset of fever. Seizures may be caused by stroke, or result from injury, tumors, meningitis, hypoglycemia, alcohol withdrawal or other health complications.

The most common type of epilepsy is specific seizure with recurrent, unprovoked attacks. This affects close to three million Americans—about one in a hundred, half of them children or adolescents. Remarkably the worldwide figures are much higher, with estimates of almost 1 in 25 people being affected. Of these, one-half fortunately grows out of the disorder.

Treatment

Recurrent seizures usually require medication with such oral anticonvulsants as phenobarbital, valproic acid, phenytoin, rufinamide, carbamazepine and others. Patients may need to take these drugs indefinitely. Unfortunately, they are not a cure and can have many side-effects, some severe.

Nutritional supplements are used in both conventional and complementary medicine. B-vitamins, particularly B_6 (pyridoxine), are effective against certain seizures. Magnesium is also useful, especially in seizures related to high blood pressure. Selenium is used in epileptics, since deficiency of this mineral is thought to intensify the frequency and severity of seizures.

Free radical damage in seizures

Seizures are typified by tremendous bioelectrical activity in the affected area of the brain. This generates free radicals in large numbers. Convulsions that provoke loss of consciousness may be accompanied by breathing abnormalities and subsequent oxidative stress. When frequent and/or prolonged, oxidative stress damages brain cells. Many studies show that lipid peroxidation resulting from free radical formation can damage neurological cells. Moreover, the higher the level of oxidative stress in these tissues, the harder it is to treat. At a certain point, patients may react to the medication with further

---

[1] A continuous state of seizure.

epileptic activity. Canadian researchers at the University of Calgary have suggested that this continual free radical damage may result in certain types of brain tumor.

Glutathione levels in seizures

I wrote in earlier editions of this book, "Considerable research has demonstrated that GSH levels fall significantly in seizure conditions. What is less clear is whether this deficiency causes seizures, results from them, or both. Nevertheless, the total body glutathione levels of seizure patients are measurably lower than those of normal individuals, and this GSH deficiency is even more noticeable in the affected areas of the brain."

Since then, research has shed considerably more light on the actual roles of GSH in seizure. Studies describe a broad range of seizures sharing similar biochemical abnormalities. These generally include low antioxidant status, elevated free radical damage, high oxidative stress and—most salient to this discussion—low glutathione levels. Low levels of glutathione activity are present both in patients taking anti-epileptic medication and those not. Most patients on anti-seizure medication are unable to correct their antioxidant balance. This implies that the low glutathione is not necessarily a result of seizure but rather a cause or condition of it. (Menon 2014, Keskin 2016, others).

Further evidence that low glutathione levels are both a result and a cause of seizures can be found by focusing on the mitochondria—tiny structures within the neurons of each cell that produce the energy it needs. These phenomena are described in fascinating detail in Waldbaum 2010, Rowley 2013, Rowley 2015 (see references).

Swiss scientists led by Mueller studied three groups: patients with active epilepsy, those with controlled epilepsy and non-epileptics. They determined that low glutathione levels more often lead to seizures than result from them. Other research supports this theory by showing that seizures are more frequent or severe when glutathione levels are experimentally lowered. Whatever the specific mechanism, the overall picture shows that glutathione levels fall steadily as seizures progress.

Not only do seizures lower glutathione levels, the drugs used to treat them reduce glutathione levels even further. Japanese researchers Ono, Sakamoto and Sakura showed that both carbamazepine and phenytoin—popular anti-seizure medications—diminish glutathione and leave cells even more susceptible to oxidative damage. Turkish physiologists found the same of valproic acid, another anti-seizure drug. However, scientists at Harvard University studying childhood seizures found that glutathione levels improved after anticonvulsants were halted and patients were given selenium. Other scientists have made this link to selenium deficiency. Both Seven (2013) and Saad (2014) state that low selenium status is a causative factor in the development of seizures. As discussed in other places in this book, selenium's major action in our body is through its bonding with GSH to form active glutathione peroxidase, one of the most important enzymes in the regulation of oxidant/antioxidant balance.

Glutathione protects from seizures

Since glutathione directly affects the activity of brain cells, it is called a neuromodulator. Japanese scientists Abe, Nakanishi and Saito were able to protect animals from drug-induced seizures by injecting glutathione directly into the fluid of their brains and spinal cords. Canadians at Toronto Western Hospital showed that combined vitamin E and glutathione reduced the number of brain cells damaged after seizure activity. In Texas, Jenkinson, Jordan and Duncan were able to protect laboratory animals from

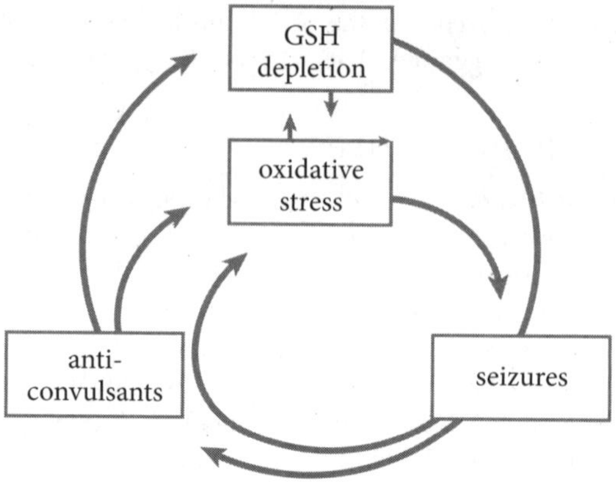

FIGURE 60: The vicious circles of seizure and glutathione loss

seizures and death by injecting them with glutathione, and Italians at the University of Milan successfully prevented seizures caused by isoniazid—a tuberculosis medication—by administering glutathione beforehand.

Several scientists have used N-acetylcysteine (NAC, see Chapter 4), a powerful glutathione precursor, to treat seizures. Swedish researchers led by Ben-Menachem applied it to patients suffering from progressive myoclonic epilepsy—a particularly hard-to-treat disease that gradually destroys the nervous system. Patients on a daily dose of 6 grams showed marked improvements, and an American team from Gainesville, Florida used NAC, vitamin E, vitamin B_2, zinc and selenium to treat this type of seizure, with similarly positive results.

Currently, studies are underway to address low GSH levels in seizures, using the glutathione precursor NAC as a complementary therapy alongside the standard pharmaceutical drugs. Pauletti and his team wrote in the journal "Brain" (2017) that "targeting oxidative stress…significantly improves long-term disease outcomes."

Conclusion

Free radical formation and oxidative stress can be seen as both a cause and a result of seizures, and conditions that diminish glutathione levels—including the use of anti-seizure drugs themselves—may further lower glutathione levels. Since glutathione is also an anticonvulsant, it is useful as a complementary therapy to both treat and prevent seizures, as well as to lessen the adverse effects of conventional drugs.

SEIZURES

REFERENCES

ABBOTT LC, NEJAD HH, BOTTJE WG, HASSAN AS. *Glutathione levels in specific brain regions of genetically epileptic (tg/tg) mice.* Brain Res Bull 1990 Oct;25(4):629-31

ABE K, NAKANISHI K, SAITO H. *The anticonvulsive effect of glutathione in mice.* Biol Pharm Bull 1999 Nov;22(11):1177-9

ABE K, NAKANISHI K, SAITO H. *The possible role of endogenous glutathione as an anticonvulsant in mice.* Brain Res 2000 Jan 31;854(1-2):235-8

BELLISSIMO MI, AMADO D, ABDALLA DS, FERREIRA EC, CAVALHEIRO EA, NAFFAH-MAZZACORATTI MG. *Superoxide dismutase, glutathione peroxidase activities & the hydroperoxide concentration are modified in the hippocampus of epileptic rats.* Epilepsy Res 2001 Aug;46(2):121-8

BEN-MENACHEM E, KYLLERMAN M, MARKLUND S. *Superoxide dismutase & glutathione peroxidase function in progressive myoclonus epilepsies.* Epilepsy Res 2000 Jun;40(1):33-9

Beutler E, Curnutte JT, Forman L. *Glutathione peroxidase deficiency & childhood seizures.* Lancet 1991 Sep 14;338(8768):700

Cárdenas-Rodriguez N, Coballase-Urrutia E, Pérez-Cruz C, et al. *Relevance of the glutathione system in temporal lobe epilepsy: evidence in human & experimental models.* Oxid Med Cell Longev 2014:759293, 2014

Cengiz M, Yuksel A, Seven M. *The effects of carbamazepine & valproic acid on the erythrocyte glutathione, glutathione peroxidase, superoxide dismutase & serum lipid peroxidation in epileptic children.* Pharmacol Res 2000 Apr;41(4):423-5

Cock HR, Tong X, Hargreaves IP, Heales SJ, Clark JB, Patsalos PN, Thom M, Groves M, Schapira AH, Shorvon SD, Walker MC. *Mitochondrial dysfunction associated with neuronal death following status epilepticus in rat.* Epilepsy Res 2002 Feb;48(3):157-68

Devi PU, Saraogi P, Manocha A, Vohora D. *Pharmacological & biochemical analysis of interactions between N-acetylcysteine & some antiepileptic drugs on experimental seizures in mice. CNS Neurosci Ther* 18(5):406-13, 2012

Dominiak A, Wikaniec A, Wroczyński P, Adamczyk A. *Selenium in the Therapy of Neurological Diseases. Where is it Going?* Curr Neuropharmacol 14(3):282-99, 2016

Erakovic V, Zupan G, Varljen J, Radosevic S, Simonic A.Electroconvulsive shock in rats: changes in superoxide dismutase & glutathione peroxidase activity. *Brain Res Mol Brain Res 2000 Mar 29;76(2):266-74*

Frantseva MV, Perez Velazquez JL, Tsoraklidis G, Mendonca AJ, Adamchik Y, Mills LR, Carlen PL, Burnham MW. *Oxidative stress is involved in seizure-induced neurodegeneration in the kindling model of epilepsy.* Neuroscience 2000;97(3):431-5

Frantseva MV, Velazquez JL, Hwang PA, Carlen PL. *Free radical production correlates with cell death in an in vitro model of epilepsy.* Eur J Neurosci 2000 Apr;12(4):1431-9

Gluck MR, Jayatilleke E, Shaw S, Rowan AJ, Haroutunian V. *CNS oxidative stress associated with the kainic acid rodent model of experimental epilepsy.* Epilepsy Res 2000 Mar;39(1):63-71

Günes S, Dirik E, et al. *Oxidant status in children after febrile seizures.* Pediatr Neurol 40(1):47-9, 2009

Hiramatsu M, Mori A. *Brain glutathione & seizures.* Folia Psychiatr Neurol Jpn 1980;34(3):363

Hiramatsu M, Mori A. *Reduced & oxidized glutathione in brain & convulsions.* Neurochem Res 1981 Mar;6(3):301-6

Hurd RW, Wilder BJ, Helveston WR, Uthman BM. *Treatment of four siblings with progressive myoclonus epilepsy of the Unverricht-Lundborg type with N-acetylcysteine.* Neurology 1996 Nov;47(5):1264-8

Jenkinson SG, Jordan JM, Duncan CA. *Effects of selenium deficiency on glutathione-induced protection from hyperbaric hyperoxia in rat.* Am J Physiol 1989 Dec;257(6 Pt 1):L393-8

Jiang D, Akopian G, Ho YS, Walsh JP, Andersen JK. *Chronic brain oxidation in a glutathione peroxidase knockout mouse model results in increased resistance to induced epileptic seizures.* Exp Neurol 2000 Aug;164(2):257-68

Kalapos MP. *Carbamazepine-provoked hepatotoxicity & possible aetiopathological role of glutathione in the events. Retrospective review of old data & call for new investigation.* Adverse Drug React Toxicol Rev 21(3):123-41, 2002

Keskin Guler S, Aytac B, Durak ZE et al. *Antioxidative-oxidative balance in epilepsy patients on antiepileptic therapy: a prospective case-control study.* Neurol Sci 37(5):763-7, 2016

Kürekçi AE, Alpay F, Tanindi S, et al. *Plasma trace element, plasma glutathione peroxidase, & superoxide dismutase levels in epileptic children receiving antiepileptic drug therapy.* Epilepsia 36(6):600-4, 1995

Kurekci AE, Alpay F, Tanindi S, Gokcay E, Ozcan O, Akin R, Isimer A, Sayal A. *Plasma trace element, plasma glutathione peroxidase, & superoxide dismutase levels in epileptic children receiving antiepileptic drug therapy.* Epilepsia 1995 Jun;36(6):600-4

Liang LP, Patel M. *Plasma cysteine/cystine redox couple disruption in animal models of temporal lobe epilepsy. Redox Biol* 9:45-49, 2016

Liu CS, Wu HM, Kao SH, Wei YH. *Serum trace elements, glutathione, copper/zinc superoxide dismutase, & lipid peroxidation in epileptic patients with phenytoin or carbamazepine monotherapy.* Clin Neuropharmacol 1998 Jan-Feb;21(1):62-4

Lores Arnaiz S, Travacio M, Llesuy S, Rodriguez de Lores Arnaiz G. *Regional vulnerability to oxidative stress in a model of experimental epilepsy.* Neurochem Res 1998 Dec;23(12):1477-83

Louw DF, Bose R, Sima AA, Sutherland GR. *Evidence for a high free radical state in low-grade astrocytomas.* Neurosurgery 1997 Nov;41(5):1146-50; discussion 1151

Menon B, Remalingam K, Kumar RV. *Low plasma antioxidant status in patients with epilepsy & the role of antiepileptic drugs on oxidative stress.* Ann Indian Acad Neurol 17(4):398-404, 2014

Mueller SG, Trabesinger AH, Boesiger P, Wieser HG. *Brain glutathione levels in patients with epilepsy measured by in vivo (1)H-MRS.* Neurology

2001 Oct 23;57(8):1422-7

OGITA K, KITAYAMA T, OKUDA H, YONEDA Y. *Effects of glutathione depletion by 2-cyclohexen-1-one on excitatory amino acids-induced enhancement of activator protein-1 DNA binding in murine hippocampus.* J Neurochem 2001 Mar;76(6):1905-15

ONO H, SAKAMOTO A, SAKURA N. *Plasma total glutathione concentrations in epileptic patients taking anticonvulsants.* Clin Chim Acta 2000 Aug;298(1-2):135-43

PAULETTI A, TERRONE G, ET AL. *Targeting oxidative stress improves disease outcomes in a rat model of acquired epilepsy.* Brain 140(7):1885-1899, 2017

PEACOCK MD, SCHENK DA, LAWRENCE RA, MORGAN JA, JENKINSON SG. *Elimination of glutathione-induced protection from hyperbaric hyperoxia by acivicin.* J Appl Physiol 1994 Mar;76(3):1279-84

PINELLI A, TRIVULZIO S, COLOMBO-ZEFINETTI G, TOFANETTI O. *Anti-convulsant effects by reduced glutathione & related aminoacids in rats treated with isoniazid.* Toxicology 1988 Jan;48(1):103-7

RAMAEKERS VT, CALOMME M, VANDEN BERGHE D, MAKROPOULOS W. *Selenium deficiency triggering intractable seizures.* Neuropediatrics 1994 Aug;25(4):217-23

RAVIKUMAR A, ARUN P, DEVI KV, AUGUSTINE J, KURUP PA. *Isoprenoid pathway & free radical generation & damage in neuropsychiatric disorders.* Indian J Exp Biol 2000 May;38(5):438-46

ROWLEY S, LIAN LP, FULTON R, SHIMIZU T, DAY B, PATEL M. *Mitochondrial respiration deficits driven by reactive oxygen species in experimental temporal lobe epilepsy.* Neurobiol Dis 75:151-8, 2015

ROWLEY S, PATEL M. *Mitochondrial involvement & oxidative stress in temporal lobe epilepsy.* Free Radic Biol Med 62:121-31, 2013

RUMIÀ J, ET AL. *Oxidative stress markers in the neocortex of drug-resistant epilepsy patients submitted to epilepsy surgery.* Epilepsy Res 107(1-2):75-81, 2013

SAAD K, HAMMAD E, HASSAN AF, BADRY R. *Trace element, oxidant, & antioxidant enzyme values in blood of children with refractory epilepsy.* Int J Neurosci 124(3):181-6, 2014

SANTAVUORI P, HEISKALA H, WESTERMARCK T, SAINIO K, MOREN R. *Experience over 17 years with antioxidant treatment in Spielmeyer-Sjogren disease.* Am J Med Genet Suppl 1988;5:265-74

SCHWEIZER U, BRAUER AU, ET AL. *Selenium & brain function: a poorly recognized liaison.* Brain Res Brain Res Rev 45(3):164-78, 2004

SEVEN M, BASARAN SY, CENGIZ M, UNAL S, YUKSEL A. *Deficiency of selenium & zinc as a causative factor for idiopathic.* Epilepsy Res 104(1-2):35-9, 2013

SINGH R, PATHAK DN. *Lipid peroxidation & glutathione peroxidase, glutathione reductase, superoxide dismutase, catalase, & glucose-6-phosphate dehydrogenase activities in FeCl3-induced epileptogenic foci in the rat brain.* Epilepsia 1990 Jan-Feb;31(1):15-26

SOLOWIEJ E, SOBANIEC W. *[The effect of antiepileptic drug therapy on antioxidant enzyme activity & serum lipid peroxidation in young patients with epilepsy].* Neurol Neurochir Pol 37(5):991-1003, 2003

SUDHA K, RAO AV, RAO A. *Oxidative stress & antioxidants in epilepsy.* Clin Chim Acta 2001 Jan;303(1-2):19-24

TUPEEV IR, KRYZHANOVSKII GN, NIKUSHKIN EV, BORDIUKOV MM, IUZEFOVA SM. *The antioxidant system in the dynamic combined treatment of epilepsy patients with traditional anticonvulsant preparations & an antioxidant – alpha-tocopherol.* Biull Eksp Biol Med 1993 Oct;116(10):362-4

VISHNOI S, RAISUDDIN S, PARVEZ S. *Glutamate Excitotoxicity & Oxidative Stress in Epilepsy: Modulatory Role of Melatonin.* J Environ Pathol Toxicol Oncol 35(4):365-374, 2016

WALDBAUM S, PATEL M. *Mitochondrial dysfunction & oxidative stress: a contributing link to acquired epilepsy?* J Bioenerg Biomembr 42(6):449-55, 2010

WEBER GF, MAERTENS P, MENG XZ, PIPPENGER CE. *Glutathione peroxidase deficiency & childhood seizures.* Lancet 1991 Jun 15;337(8755):1443-4

WEI YH, LU CY, WEI CY, MA YS, LEE HC. *Oxidative stress in human aging & mitochondrial disease-consequences of defective mitochondrial respiration & impaired antioxidant enzyme system.* Chin J Physiol 2001 Mar 31;44(1):1-11

YÜKSEL A, CENGIZ M, SEVEN M, ULUTIN T. *Changes in the antioxidant system in epileptic children receiving antiepileptic drugs: two-year prospective studies.* J Child Neurol 2001 Aug;16(8):603-6

YÜKSEL A, CENGIZ M, SEVEN M, ULUTIN T. *Erythrocyte glutathione, glutathione peroxidase, superoxide dismutase & serum lipid peroxidation in epileptic children with valproate & carbamazepine monotherapy.* J Basic Clin Physiol Pharmacol 2000;11(1):73-81

YÜKSEL A, CENGIZ M, SEVEN M, ULUTIN T. *Erythrocyte glutathione, glutathione peroxidase, superoxide dismutase & serum lipid peroxidation in epileptic children with valproate & carbamazepine monotherapy.* J Basic Clin Physiol Pharmacol 11(1):73-81, 2000

32

Traumatic brain injury

An injury to the head can be complicated and devastating. There are many types of injury, as well as different symptoms and outcomes. Following head trauma it's not uncommon to experience a ringing in the head, only to recover shortly afterwards. Others suffer immediate deficits that last a lifetime. What is being increasingly recognized is that some of these injuries do not fully reveal their damage for months, or even years.

Traumatic brain injury (TBI) is typically a sudden event. Unlike a broken leg, however, the damage may extend beyond the obvious head injury itself. Personality, mood, cognition, attention span and much more can be adversely and permanently impacted. In recent years we've become cognizant of subtle brain injuries that accumulate over time and may not show symptoms until later in life. The sports of boxing and football have unfortunately, but frequently, contributed to a condition once called "punch drunk," and now known as Chronic Traumatic Encephalopathy (CTE).

TBI follows a bump, jolt or strike to the head. When the force is great enough, the brain itself is injured. Millions of North Americans suffer from brain injuries every year, and about half of these injuries are severe enough to warrant a visit to the hospital. In all likelihood, many more go unreported than are documented in official figures.

The most commonly reported causes of TBIs are motor vehicle accidents, but these are not the only ones. Countless hospital admissions result from injuries in sports, the military and industry. Of great concern is concussion, which can go temporarily unnoticed. In recent years, the general public, and especially the sporting community, have become more vigilant about the onset of concussion. Parents are more likely to

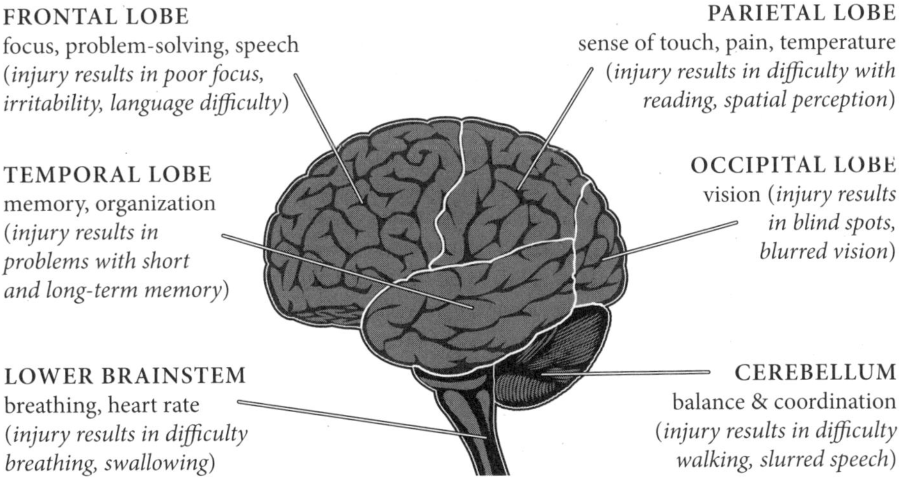

Figure 61: Consequences of Traumatic Brain Injury (TBI)

monitor their children after a blow to the head, and the days when a football player was given 'smelling salts' and sent back to the game after being knocked out are over.

An in-depth discussion of the various types of brain injuries is beyond the scope of this chapter. The topics of epidural hematomas, subdural hematomas, deceleration injuries, contrecoup injury, diffuse axonal injury and mechanisms all are important, but we will focus on their common after-effects, rather than each type of injury.

Oxidative stress and free radicals in brain injury

One organ that is particularly vulnerable to oxidative stress and free radical damage is the brain. It exhibits tremendous metabolic activity and receives 20% of the body's oxygen, despite representing only 2% of total body weight. Antioxidants in the brain are in great demand and run out easily, commonly leading to low antioxidant availability. Being mostly composed of lipids (fats), the brain is prone to the oxidation of these fats. This is 'lipid peroxidation.' When brain cells are injured, these fats or lipids are more exposed than ever to oxidation and free radical damage.

Oxidative stress and lipid peroxidation have been widely studied in experimental traumatic brain injury since the 1970s. Hall and associates, at various neurotrauma research centers with access to human subjects, have published extensively since the 1990s. They and others have shone great light upon the biochemical events following brain injury, among which the cascade of lipid peroxidation products has been established as a primary mechanism of ongoing injury.

Glutathione levels in brain injury

If glutathione is the 'master' antioxidant, it follows that it would be part of the body's response to the lipid peroxidation that follows brain injury. In fact, GSH levels not only fall after TBI, but also after other brain insults, including stroke, spinal cord injury and more. In experimental models, levels fall dramatically in the six to 24 hours following initial injury. In otherwise healthy individuals, the body makes great efforts to restore GSH.

Looking closer at the cascade of oxidative substances and the response of antioxidants, Ansari's group determined that depleted antioxidant systems following trauma could harm synapse function in the brain and nervous system, and that the opportunity for effective treatments following TBI is relatively short-lived. This implies that time-sensitive restoration of antioxidant function is critical.

This appears to be even more so the case in young children. It is known that under-four-year-olds suffer worse outcomes following traumatic brain injury. One determination is that their brains lack the ability to rapidly regenerate glutathione levels.

A study over twenty years old illuminates the importance of glutathione in protecting injured brain cells from secondary free-radical damage. In a laboratory, brain cells were grown in culture and subjected to mechanical trauma. Three groups of cell cultures were compared. In the first, GSH was depleted chemically; in the second, GSH levels were raised; in the last, GSH levels were untouched or 'normal.' The results were decisive: the less glutathione, the worse the injury; the more glutathione, the better the cells fared.

Studies looking at GSH levels in humans take this point further. A 2016 article in the publication World Neurosurgery suggested that the measurement of glutathione levels could be used to predict outcomes after head injury. A Chinese team gathered blood samples from 88 patients admitted within 24 hours of a TBI. Glutathione was measured first on admission, then after four days and finally at the end of one week. Patients' GSH levels were correlated with their levels of consciousness (on the Glasgow Coma Scale). The study concluded that higher glutathione levels were associated with better prognosis.

Head injuries in sports tend to be understated, but mild traumatic brain injuries (mTBI) that happen again and again lead to cumulative long-term consequences. The growing awareness of repetitive mTBI has raised awareness of another diagnosis—chronic traumatic encephalopathy (CTE). CTE causes nerve damage that can result in persistent cognitive, behavioral and psychiatric problems. Its exact prevalence is unknown, but is generally presumed to be higher than clinically reported, since many such injuries go undiagnosed. CTE is most commonly reported in American football and boxing, although CTE awareness is growing in other sports such as hockey, wrestling, soccer, rugby and baseball.

Two recent studies have looked at athletes in these sports with a new sort of brain scanner that can actually determine relative glutathione levels in the brain. Using magnetic resonance spectroscopy (MRS), evidence of glutathione depletion has been reported in mild head injuries that did not even lead to concussion.

Raising glutathione in brain injury

Efforts to raise glutathione levels after acute brain injury have shown promise, through human studies are lacking since researchers cannot inflict deliberate injury on a normal brain. However, controlled brain injury studies in rodents have been underway for at least twenty years. Xiong, Peterson and Lee demonstrated in 1999 that brain-injured rats given NAC (N-acetylcysteine) experienced better mitochondrial function—as long as the NAC was delivered within one hour of the trauma. One problem with NAC is its limited ability to efficiently cross the blood-brain-barrier (BBB). Researchers at the University of Kentucky slightly altered the NAC molecule to improve its access to neurons. Testing in rats showed clinical improvement in cognition, although once again the medication had to be given soon after injury to succeed. Other experimental drugs, such as gamma glutamyl cysteinyl ethyl ester (GCEE) also led to improvement in behavioral and histologic outcome in mice.

More recently, a novel approach has employed a specially-prepared whey protein isolate. Dan Linseman and his team at the University of Denver showed microscopic changes including improvement in brain glutathione and cognitive function after feeding mice a cysteine-rich glutathione precursor. This is one of very few studies demonstrating pre-treatment as an effective strategy. They concluded that this approach holds promise to prevent traumatic brain injury in some high-risk populations, such as athletes and military personnel.

Dozens of other studies on animals have been done using NAC. Results are mixed, but improvements following brain injury have been documented, ranging from biochemical improvement, to microscopic improvement, to improved clinical outcomes. Almost universally, these papers have called for further animal research and look forward to establishing human studies.

Remarkably, there have been placebo-controlled studies using antioxidants in both children and adult humans who have undergone brain trauma. One study was carried out by the United States military, which enrolled soldiers who had been exposed to a significant 'blast' injury (including explosions) and were admitted to a field hospital in Iraq. Participants were given either a placebo or the glutathione precursor NAC. After seven days, they were reevaluated for dizziness, hearing loss, headache, memory loss, sleep disturbance and cognitive function. The statistical analysis showed a clear benefit for those receiving the glutathione precursor. Surprisingly, even after 24 hours, the NAC group showed an 86% chance of symptom resolution as compared to the placebo group's likelihood of 42%—essentially doubling their chance of recovery.

Conclusions

TBI (traumatic brain injury), whether severe, mild or even unnoticed, has been repeatedly shown to increase oxidative stress and decrease glutathione levels. Levels of glutathione also have been correlated to the severity of clinical outcome. Finally, early studies show that increasing glutathione levels either prophylactically or as immediate treatment shows promise.

TRAUMATIC BRAIN INJURY

REFERENCES

AL NIMER F, STROM M, LINDBLOM R ET AL. *Naturally occurring variation in the Glutathione-S-Transferase 4 gene determines neurodegeneration after traumatic brain injury.* Antioxid Redox Signal 18(7):784-94, 2013

ANSARI MA, ROBERTS KN, SCHEFF SW. *Oxidative stress & modification of synaptic proteins in hippocampus after traumatic brain injury.* Free Radic Biol Med 45(4):443-52, 2008

ANTHONYMUTHU TS, KENNY EM, BAYIR H. *Therapies targeting lipid peroxidation in traumatic brain injury.* Brain Res 1640(Pt A):57-76, 2016

AZBILL RD, MU X, BRUCE-KELLER AJ ET AL. *Impaired mitochondrial function, oxidative stress & altered antioxidant enzyme activities following traumatic spinal cord injury.* Brain Res 765(2):283-90, 1997

BAYIR H ET AL. *Assessment of antioxidant reserves & oxidative stress in cerebrospinal fluid after severe traumatic brain injury in infants & children.* Pediatr Res 51(5):571-8, 2002

CALDERÓN-GUZMÁN D, OSNAYA-BRIZUELA N, GARCIA-ALVAREZ R ET AL. *Levels of glutathione & some biogenic amines in the human brain putamen after traumatic death.* Proc West Pharmacol Soc 51:27-9, 2008

CHEN G, SHI J, HU Z, HANG C. *Inhibitory effect on cerebral inflammatory response following traumatic brain injury in rats: a potential neuroprotective mechanism of N-acetylcysteine.* Mediators Inflamm 2008:716458, 2008

CLARK RSB ET AL. *Phase I randomized clinical trial of N-acetylcysteine in combination with an adjuvant probenecid for treatment of severe traumatic brain injury in children.* PLoS One 12(7):e0180280, 2017

DASH PK, HERGENROEDER GW, JETER CB ET AL. *Traumatic Brain Injury Alters Methionine Metabolism: Implications for Pathophysiology.* Front Syst Neurosci 10:36, 2016

DU L, EMPEY PE, JI J, CHAO H ET AL. *Probenecid & N-Acetylcysteine Prevent Loss of Intracellular Glutathione & Inhibit Neuronal Death after Mechanical Stretch Injury In Vitro.* J Neurotrauma 33(20):1913-1917, 2016

EAKIN K, BARATZ-GOLDSTEIN R, PICK CG ET AL. *Efficacy of N-acetyl cysteine in traumatic brain injury.* PLoS One 9(4):e90617, 2014

FAN P, YAMAUCHI T, NOBLE LJ, FERRIERO DM. *Age-dependent differences in glutathione peroxidase activity after traumatic brain injury.* J Neurotrauma 20(5):437-45, 2003

GARDNER AJ, IVERSON GL, WOJTOWICZ M, LEVI CR ET AL. *MR Spectroscopy Findings in Retired Professional Rugby League Players.* Int J Sports Med 38(3):241-252, 2017

GIDDAY JM, BEETSCH JW, PARK TS. *Endogenous glutathione protects cerebral endothelial cells from traumatic injury.* J Neurotrauma 16(1):27-36, 1999

GÜNTHER M, DAVIDSSON J, PLANTMAN S ET AL. *Neuroprotective effects of N-acetylcysteine amide on experimental focal penetrating brain injury in rats.* J Clin Neurosci 22(9):1477-83, 2015

HALL ED. *The role of oxygen radicals in traumatic injury: clinical implications.* J Emerg Med 11 Suppl 1:31-6, 1993

HALL ED. *Free radicals & CNS injury.* Crit Care Clin 5(4):793-805, 1989

HALL ED, ANDRUS PK, SMITH SL ET AL. *Neuroprotective efficacy of microvascularly-localized versus brain-penetrating antioxidants.* Acta Neurochir Suppl 66:107-13, 1996

HALL ED, VAISHNAV RA, MUSTAFA AG. *Antioxidant therapies for traumatic brain injury.* Neurotherapeutics 7(1):51-61, 2010

HICDONMEZ T, KANTER M, TIRYAKI M, PARSAK T, COBANOGLU S. *Neuroprotective effects of N-acetylcysteine on experimental closed head trauma in rats.* Neurochem Res 31(4):473-81, 2006

HOFFER ME, BALABAN C, SLADE MD, TSAO JW, HOFFER B. *Amelioration of acute sequelae of blast induced mild traumatic brain injury by N-acetyl cysteine:* a double-blind, placebo controlled study. PLoS One 8(1):e54163, 2013

IGNOWSKI E, WINTER AN, DUVAL N ET AL. *The cysteine-rich whey protein supplement, Immunocal preserves brain glutathione & improves cognitive, motor, & histopathological indices of traumatic brain injury in a mouse model of controlled cortical impact.* Free Radic Biol Med S0891-5849(18)31117-1, 2018

Jin W, Wang H, Yan W et al. *Role of Nrf2 in protection against traumatic brain injury in mice.* J Neurotrauma 26(1):131-9, 2009

Kasprzak HA, Wozniak A, Drewa G, Wozniak B. *Enhanced lipid peroxidation processes in patients after brain contusion.* J Neurotrauma 18(8):793-7, 2001

Khan M et al. *S-nitrosoglutathione reduces oxidative injury & promotes mechanisms of neurorepair following traumatic brain injury in rats.* J Neuroinflammation 8:78, 2011

Koerte IK et al. *Altered Neurochemistry in Former Professional Soccer Players without a History of Concussion.* J Neurotrauma 32(17):1287-93, 2015

Lai Y et al. *Autophagy is increased after traumatic brain injury in mice & is partially inhibited by the antioxidant gamma-glutamylcysteinyl ethyl ester.* J Cereb Blood Flow Metab 28(3):540-50, 2008

Lok J et al. *Y-glutamylcysteine ethyl ester protects cerebral endothelial cells during injury & decreases blood-brain barrier permeability after experimental brain trauma.* J Neurochem 118(2):248-55, 2011

McKee AC, Daneshvar DH, Alvarez VE, Stein TD. *The neuropathology of sport.* Acta Neuropathol 127(1):29-51, 2014

Ozbal S, Cankurt U, Tugyan K et al. *The effects of α-lipoic acid on immature rats with traumatic brain injury.* Biotech Histochem 90(3):206-15, 2015

Pandya JD, Readnower RD, Patel SP et al. *N-acetylcysteine amide confers neuroprotection, improves bioenergetics & behavioral outcome following TBI.* Exp Neurol 257:106-13, 2014

Patel SP, Sullivan PG, Pandya JD, Goldstein GA et al. *N-acetylcysteine amide preserves mitochondrial bioenergetics & improves functional recovery following spinal trauma.* Exp Neurol 257:95-105, 2014

Potts MB et al. *Traumatic injury to the immature brain: inflammation, oxidative injury, & iron-mediated damage as potential therapeutic targets.* NeuroRx 3(2):143-53, 2006

Reed TT, Owen J, Pierce WM et al. *Proteomic identification of nitrated brain proteins in traumatic brain-injured rats treated postinjury with gamma-glutamylcysteine ethyl ester:* insights into the role of elevation of glutathione as a potential therapeutic strategy for traumatic brain injury. J Neurosci Res 87(2):408-17,2009

Rodriguez-Rodriguez A, Egea-Guerrero JJ, Murillo Cabezas F, Carrillo-Vico A. *Oxidative stress in traumatic brain injury.* Curr Med Chem 21(10):1201-11, 2014

Senol N, Nazıroğlu M, Yürüker V. *N-acetylcysteine & selenium modulate oxidative stress, antioxidant vitamin & cytokine values in traumatic brain injury-induced rats.* Neurochem Res 39(4):685-92, 2014

Shen Q, Hiebert JB, Hartwell J, Thimmesch AR, Pierce JD. *Systematic Review of Traumatic Brain Injury & the Impact of Antioxidant Therapy on Clinical Outcomes.* Worldviews Evid Based Nurs 13(5):380-389, 2016

Slemmer JE, Shacka JJ, Sweeney MI, Weber JT. *Antioxidants & free radical scavengers for the treatment of stroke, traumatic brain injury & aging.* Curr Med Chem 15(4):404-14, 2008

Thomale UW, Griebenow M et al. *The antioxidant effect of N-acetylcysteine on experimental contusion in rats.* Acta Neurochir Suppl 95:429-31, 2005

Thomale UW, Griebenow M et al. *The effect of N-acetylcysteine on posttraumatic changes after controlled cortical impact in rats.* Intensive Care Med 32(1):149-55, 2006

Tsuru-Aoyagi K, Potts MB, Trivedi A et al. *Glutathione peroxidase activity modulates recovery in the injured immature brain.* Ann Neurol 65(5):540-9, 2009

Tyurin VA, Tyurina YY, Borisenko GG et al. *Oxidative stress following traumatic brain injury in rats: quantitation of biomarkers & detection of free radical intermediates.* J Neurochem 75(5):2178-89, 2000

Wang HC, Lin YJ, Shih FY et al. *The Role of Serial Oxidative Stress Levels in Acute Traumatic Brain Injury & as Predictors of Outcome.* World Neurosurg 87:463-70, 2016

Xiong Y, Peterson PL, Lee CP. *Effect of N-acetylcysteine on mitochondrial function following traumatic brain injury in rats.* J Neurotrauma 16(11):1067-82, 1999

Xiong Y, Shie FS, Zhang J, Lee CP, Ho YS. *The protective role of cellular glutathione peroxidase against trauma-induced mitochondrial dysfunction in the mouse brain.* J Stroke Cerebrovasc Dis 13(3):129-37, 2004

Yi JH, Hazell AS. *N-acetylcysteine attenuates early induction of heme oxygenase-1 following traumatic brain injury.* Brain Res 1033(1):13-9, 2005

Yi JH, Hoover R, McIntosh TK, Hazell AS. *Early, transient increase in complexin I & complexin II in the cerebral cortex following traumatic brain injury is attenuated by N-acetylcysteine.* J Neurotrauma 23(1):86-96, 2006

33
Sleep

Sleep is a fascinating brain state, essential in all mammals and many other life forms. In humans, it is characterized by lessened consciousness of the external environment and virtual paralysis of voluntary muscle movement. It recurs daily due to the "circadian rhythm"—a built-in process driven by daylight/nighttime cycles through regulatory hormones like melatonin. Sleep is a critical time for the body to restore biochemical and physical equilibrium, and to focus on muscle repair, detoxification and quenching free radicals.

Without getting into a detailed discussion of sleep patterns and physiology, it is enough to say that disruption of sleep results in a long list of potential physical and mental problems. Many sleep disorders have been described, including essential insomnia, sleep apnea, restless leg syndrome, narcolepsy and others. This chapter examines the role of glutathione.

Certain tissues are more sensitive to glutathione depletion than others. Measuring glutathione levels in specific areas of the brain of sleep-deprived animals, researchers find that the thalamus and hypothalamus are particularly susceptible. The vulnerability of these tissues may account for some of the functional effects of sleep deprivation.

Oxidized glutathione (GSSG) is an active component of the neurochemical SPS (sleep promoting substance). Researchers at Tokyo Medical University showed that high levels of oxidized glutathione promote sleep and affect other hypothalamic functions, such as temperature control. The same team also suggests that GSH detoxifies neuronal tissues more actively during certain periods of sleep. This may explain why people taking GSH precursors like CRWPI (cysteine-rich whey protein isolate) often report less need for sleep, yet feel more energetic.

Case study

Benjamin, a 44 year-old physician, always wanted a 36-hour day so he'd have time to see his patients, do his research, practice his music, stay in shape and spend more time with his wife and children. Like many other professionals, time and energy were at a premium. Aware of the effects of glutathione on the immune system, he took a course of vitamins, selenium and amino acids in the hope of more easily fighting off the viral illnesses to which he was exposed daily. He incorporated a bioactive whey protein isolate into his regimen, and was soon waking up from 30 to 60 minutes before his alarm went off, and feeling just as refreshed. Now he regularly works later into the evening.

Circadian rhythm

The hormone that has received the most attention in regards to sleep regulation has for many years been melatonin. Melatonin doesn't only keep us aligned with the day and night cycles of the circadian rhythm. It also acts as an antioxidant itself. Raising melatonin levels indirectly raises glutathione levels in the brain by relieving GSH of some of the work of soaking up free radicals. Not surprisingly, glutathione in turn affects melatonin function. It must be emphasized that GSH in the brain is not only its master antioxidant—it does more. Other functions include maintenance of neurotransmitters, membrane transport, detoxification, and modulation of signal transduction. Much attention has been paid to the interactions between the glutathione and melatonin systems.

As discussed elsewhere in this book, the ratio between "reduced" or "active" glutathione (GSH) and "oxidized" glutathione (GSSG) determines the level of oxidative stress. This GSH/GSSG ratio is referred to as the "redox state"—a reflection of free radical activity. Closer examination of the redox state reveals that it clearly follows a day/night (diurnal) pattern. Interestingly, this diurnal pattern is exaggerated as we get older, implying that the older brain may be more prone to oxidative damage.

Writing in the journal "Chronobiology International," which specializes in study of the circadian rhythm, German researchers suggested that elevated oxidative stress may indeed interfere with normal sleep patterns. Other research teams have proposed that following these redox states might provide a tool to measure the health of our internal circadian clocks.

An interesting study shows up in the "International Archives of Occupational and Environmental Health" journal, where nurses on night shift were measured for glutathione activity. They demonstrated significant differences in protection depending on the intensity of the night shifts.

Because of the profound effects of sleep on so many other biological systems—including obesity, diabetes, cardiovascular health, and metabolic syndrome—scientists have suggested that normalizing oxidative stress signals in sleep patterns may indirectly address some of these health issues.

Primary insomnia

Primary insomnia is poor sleep with no obvious medical, physical, or psychological cause. This is quite common, affecting about 10% of adults and a good quarter of the elderly. The cause remains elusive but the results are all too apparent—sleep deprivation leads to a cascade of other health issues. One reason that has come to the forefront is variation in oxidative stress, and specifically glutathione depletion. This appears to be a feature of sleep deprivation, whether short-term or chronic primary insomnia.

Sleep apnea

Imagine what would happen if you were to stop breathing dozens—even hundreds—of times each day. Whatever functions you were trying to carry out would be impaired, given the obvious fact that your body and brain require oxygen to continue functioning. Recast this scene to night time and you have sleep apnea—where individuals actually stop breathing ("apnea") multiple times during the night. This intermittent deprivation of oxygen has very serious long-term consequences, both medically and mentally.

Apnea can affect anyone at any age, but tends to be concentrated in two main groups. "Obstructive Sleep Apnea" is a partial blockage of the upper airway causing the soft tissues in the throat to collapse. This can be the result of large tonsils or of sinusitis, but in the majority of cases the cause is excess weight. In "central sleep apnea" the airway is not compromised. Rather, the brain's respiratory control center fails to send breathing signals. Obstructive sleep apnea is usually easier to treat. A weight loss of 5 to 15% of bodyweight often cures the problem.

By measuring the breakdown products resulting from free radical damage, researchers have established the connection between oxidative stress and sleep apnea. In the forefront is measurement of total glutathione alterations, including levels of glutathione peroxidase, GSH/GSSG ratios and other specific subgroups of GSH enzymes. All are reported to be greatly affected in obstructive sleep apnea. This has led several researchers to suggest that glutathione measurements be integrated into the diagnostic and prognostic parameters.

Several other findings have been made. Glutathione levels are more severely affected as the apnea worsens. Overweight people with apnea are particularly prone to free radical damage. Sleep apnea paired with low glutathione may predispose patients to dementia. Finally, levels of glutathione abnormalities seem to correlate to cognitive decline in apnea patients.

Glutathione augmentation in sleep disorders

A 2016 literature review published in the journal "Sleep and Breathing" examined studies of the potential treatment value of antioxidant therapy, concluding that it is warranted. Most treatment interventions were conducted with the glutathione precursor, NAC (N-acetylcysteine).

A closer look at some of these studies using NAC—particularly in sleep apnea—is encouraging. Not only were glutathione levels improved and oxidative stress reduced, in addition, sleep measurements like "Sleep Percent Time," "Slow Wave Sleep" and "Sleep Efficiency" all improved.

Conclusion

Sleep disorders are a major contributing factor to a long list of medical problems, including cardiac disease, neurodegenerative disease, obesity, diabetes, metabolic syndrome and more. Glutathione plays several roles. GSH and melatonin work together in both the circadian rhythm and antioxidant functions of the brain. Glutathione levels fall in most of the sleep disorders described here. This in turn tips the scales toward increased oxidative damage in the brain and subsequent functional and cognitive decline. It has been shown that reestablishing glutathione levels is beneficial.

SLEEP

REFERENCES

Alzoubi KH, Khabour OF, Salah HA, Abu Rashid BE. *The combined effect of sleep deprivation & Western diet on spatial learning & memory: role of BDNF & oxidative stress.* J Mol Neurosci 50(1):124-33, 2013

Arent CO et al. *The effects of n-acetylcysteine &/or deferoxamine on manic-like behavior & brain oxidative damage in mice submitted to the paradoxal sleep deprivation model of mania.* J Psychiatr Res. 65:71-9, 2015

Asker S, Asker M, Sarikaya E, Sunnetcioglu A, Aslan M, Demir H. *Oxidative stress parameters & their correlation with clinical, metabolic & polysomnographic parameters in severe obstructive sleep apnea syndrome.* Int J Clin Exp Med 8(7):11449-55, 2015

Blanco RA et al. *Diurnal variation in glutathione & cysteine redox states in human plasma.* Am J Clin Nutr 86(4):1016-23, 2007

Chen PC, Guo CH, Tseng CJ, Wang KC, Liu PJ. *Blood trace minerals concentrations & oxidative stress in patients with obstructive sleep apnea.* J Nutr Health Aging, 17(8):639-44, 2013

D'Almeida V, Lobo LL, Hippolide DC, et al. *Sleep deprivation induces brain region-specific decreases in glutathione levels.* Neuroreport 9: 2853-2856, 1998

Duffy SL et al. *Association of Anterior Cingulate Glutathione with Sleep Apnea in Older Adults At-Risk for Dementia.* Sleep 39(4):899-906, 2016

Gromadzinska J et al. *Relationship between intensity of night shift work & antioxidant status in blood of nurses.* Int Arch Occup Environ Health, 86(8):923-30, 2013

Gulec M, Ozkol H, Selvi Y, Tuluce Y, Aydin A, Besirogly L, Ozdemir PG. *Oxidative stress in patients with primary insomnia.* Prog Neuropsychopharmacol Biol Psychiatry 37(2):247-51, 2012

HARDELAND R, COTO-MONTES A, POEGGELER B. *Circadian rhythms, oxidative stress, & antioxidative defense mechanisms.* Chronobiol Int 20(6):921-62, 2003

HONDA K, KOMODA Y, INOUE S. *Oxidized glutathione regulates physiological sleep in unrestrained rats.* Brain Res. 636: 253-258, 1994

INOUE S, HONDA K, KOMODA Y. *Sleep as neuronal detoxification & restitution.* Behav. Brain Res. 69: 91-96, 1995

JOUETT NP ET AL. *N-Acetylcysteine reduces hyperacute intermittent hypoxia-induced sympathoexcitation in human subjects.* Exp Physiol 101(3):387-96, 2016

KIMURA M, KAPAS L, KRUEGER JM. *Oxidized glutathione promotes sleep in rabbits.* Brain Res. Bull. 45: 545-548, 1998

KONIG K, GALLIARDT H, MOORE M, TREFFON P, SEIDEL T, DIETZ KJ. *Assessing redox state & reactive oxygen species in circadian rhythmicity.* Methods Mol Biol 1158:239-71, 2014

LAMBERT AA, PARKER AM, MOON KK. *High-dose N-acetylcysteine in chronic obstructive pulmonary disease, prone positioning in acute respiratory distress syndrome, & continuous positive airway pressure & exhaled nitric oxide in obstructive sleep apnea.* Am J Respir Crit Care Med 189(2):223-4, 2014

LEE SD, JU G, CHOI JA, KIM JW, YOON IY. *The association of oxidative stress with central obesity in obstructive sleep apnea.* Sleep Breath 16(2):511-7, 2012

LIMÓN-PACHECO JH, GONSEBATT ME. *The glutathione system & its regulation by neurohormone melatonin in the central nervous system.* Cent Nerv Agents Med Chem 10(4):287-97, 2010

LIRA AB, DE SOUSA RODRIGUES CF. *Evaluation of oxidative stress markers in obstructive sleep apnea syndrome & additional antioxidant therapy: a review article.* Sleep Breath 20(4):1155-1160, 2016

MANCUSO M ET AL. *Oxidative stress biomarkers in patients with untreated obstructive sleep apnea syndrome.* Sleep Med 13(6):632-6, 2012

MÉNDEZ I, VÁSQUEZ-MARTÍNEZ O, HERNÁNDEZ-MUÑOZ R, VALENTE-GODÍNEZ H, DÍAZ MUÑOZ M. *Redox regulation & pro-oxidant reactions in the physiology of circadian systems.* Biochimie 124:178-186, 2016

NTALAPASCHA M ET AL. *Oxidative stress in patients with obstructive sleep apnea syndrome.* Sleep Breath 17(2):549-55, 2013

RADHA E, HILL TD, RAO GH, WHITE JG. *GSH levels in human platelets display a circadian rhythm in vitro.* Thromb Res 40(6):823-31, 1985

RADHA E, HALBERG F. *Rhythms of isolated platelet glutathione, aging, & the internal evolution of species.* Prog Clin Biol Res 227A:173-80, 1987

REY G, REDDY AB. *Interplay between cellular redox oscillations & circadian clocks.* Diabetes Obes Metab 17 Suppl 1:55-64, 2015

SADASIVAM K, PATIAL K, VIJAYAN VK, RAVI K. *Antioxidant treatment in obstructive sleep apnoea syndrome.* Indian J Chest Dis Allied Sci 53(3):153-62, 2011

SALES LV ET AL. *Cognition & biomarkers of oxidative stress in obstructive sleep apnea.* Clinics (Sao Paulo), 68(4):449-55, 2013

SERRA A ET AL. *Assessment of oxidative stress markers & hearing thresholds in patients with obstructive sleep apnea-hypopnoea treated with cysteine & superoxide dismutase therapy.* Acta Biomed 87(3):253-258, 2017

STANGHERLIN A, REDDY AB. *Regulation of circadian clocks by redox homeostasis.* J Biol Chem 288(37):26505-11, 2013

TRIVEDI MS, HOLGER D, BUI AT, CRADDOCK TJA, TARTAR JL. *Short-term sleep deprivation leads to decreased systemic redox metabolites & altered epigenetic status.* PLoS One 12(7):e0181978, 2017

VILLAFUERTE G, MIGUEL-PUGA A, RODRIGUEZ EM, MACHADO S, MANJARREZ E, ARIAS-CARRION O. *Sleep deprivation & oxidative stress in animal models: a systematic review.* Oxid Med Cell Longev 2015:234952, 2015

WANG P, LI J, CAO H, SHEN Y. *The effect of oxidative stress on obstructive sleep apnea-hypopnea syndrome combined with hypertension.* Lin Chung Er Bi Yan Hou Tou Jing Wai Ke Za Zhi 28(9):604-6, 2014

YILDIRIM T, ALP R. *The role of oxidative stress in the relation between fibromyalgia & obstructive sleep apnea.* Eur Rev Med Pharmacol Sci 21(1):20-20, 2017

34
Psychiatry

As our understanding of the brain has evolved, we have begun to appreciate the intricate interweave of psychiatry, neurology and biochemistry. These fields have overlapped and melded into psychoneurobiology, an integrated medical science that has already yielded important advances in the recognition and treatment of many brain disorders, including many well known psychiatric problems.

Psychoneurobiologists have recognized that free radicals and oxyradicals play an important role in the development and progression of many of these disorders. The brain is particularly susceptible to free radical attack because it generates more oxidative by-products per gram of tissue than any other organ. The brain's main antioxidant is GSH. Its importance cannot be overstated.

Canadian scientists Gawryluk, Young and their team obtained post-mortem brains from deceased psychiatric patients and found abnormally low glutathione levels in those affected by MDD (major depressive disorder), SCZ (schizophrenia), and BD (bipolar disorder).

Oxidative stress and glutathione are important factors in various other brain disorders such as brain injury, neurodegenerative disease, Huntington's disease, ALS (amyotrophic lateral sclerosis / Lou Gehrig's disease), Down syndrome and other pathologies dealt with here and in other chapters.

This chapter enters a realm usually addressed by psychiatry rather than neurology. A partial list of psychiatric pathologies linked to glutathione abnormalities is shown in Table 39.

Schizophrenia

The Greek meaning of schizophrenia—"split mind"—is misleading. The disorder should not be confused with split personality or multiple personality disorder. It is a different illness characterized by psychosis—a severe disturbance of normal thought, perception, speech and behavior. In mood disorders like anxiety and depression, the ability to discern the real from the imagined is relatively intact. A schizophrenic patient on the other hand often suffers from delusions, auditory or visual hallucinations and paranoid thoughts not based on reality.

Although there is no consensus as to the causes of schizophrenia, most specialists agree that its symptoms stem from a disturbance of normal brain chemistry. Schizophrenia seems to run in families, and yet no single schizophrenia gene has been identified. Psychotherapy alone is not enough.

ADD/ADHD	obsessive compulsive	autism
bipolar disorder	schizophrenia	panic disorder
depression	addiction	mental stress
impulse control	anxiety	mania

Table 40: Psychiatric Disorders of the brain linked to abnormal GSH function

Antipsychotic drugs have been able to reduce relapses by 50%, and to considerably shorten the periods of hospitalization. However, these drugs have significant side effects and long-term complications.

It has long been known that glutathione levels are lower in schizophrenic patients. Researchers have consistently demonstrated increased oxidative stress and decreased glutathione status in their brains. GSH levels fall as the disease grows more severe. The Russians NV and AV Govorin showed that during an acute phase of their disease, schizophrenics suffer higher levels of lipid peroxidation than when they're in remission. Research scientists such as Yao and Reddy of the Veteran's Administration Healthcare System, University of Pittsburgh suggest that oxidative stress plays an important pathophysiological role in schizophrenia.

A group of neurochemicals called catecholamines are normally produced by the body, but over-produced in schizophrenia as well as Parkinson's disease. The catecholamines break down into ortho-quinones—a group of powerful oxidants. Baez's team at the Department of Biochemical Toxicology in Stockholm University examined glutathione's ability to detoxify these metabolites. They concluded that GSH enzymes provided critical protection against the neurodegenerative diseases that are caused or conditioned by these dangerous oxyradicals.

Buckman and Kling at UCLA School of Medicine conducted a fascinating study in which CT-scans of schizophrenic patients revealed brain atrophy (shrinkage), suggesting damage to nerve tissue. They correlated the extent of atrophy to the degree of glutathione peroxidase deficiency. This suggests a unique function of GSH in preserving the brain from tissue damage in schizophrenics. These findings were corroborated at other centers, such as Hahnemann University in Philadelphia.

More recently, researchers have demonstrated that determining a patient's glutathione status could be helpful for diagnosing schizophrenia. Since it's already established that abnormally low GSH levels go along with schizophrenia, a multinational team (from Australia, Austria, Germany and Korea) measured glutathione levels to determine patients' long-term prognosis. After following their group of patients for seven years, they were able to successfully predict the development of their psychosis.

Taking advantage of recent developments in brain scanning, a Japanese team used Magnetic Resonance Spectroscopy (MRS)[1] to measure glutathione brain levels in living patients. As expected, lower GSH levels correlated with the severity of the schizophrenic symptoms.

Until about 2008 the question remained, "Will raising glutathione levels in humans improve the condition of schizophrenia?" The researcher at the cutting edge of this strategy was Australian doctor Michael Berk who initiated a series of studies using the glutathione precursor NAC (N-acetylcysteine). Initially, he combined this intervention with standard schizophrenic antipsychotic medications. His success was evident in the results, and subsequent studies have added to the validity of his approach. A good review of NAC and schizophrenia can be found in the Annals of Clinical Psychiatry (Chen et al 2016).

Antipsychotic drugs require long term use and cause a number of side-effects. Haldol, Thorazine and other neuroleptics cause a movement disorder called tardive dyskinesia.[2] This results in involuntary puckering of the lips and a writhing of the arms and legs that disfigures a large number of patients. It's possible that lipid peroxidation accounts for neuronal damage in this disorder. Scientists have put this theory to the test.

A Scottish team led by Brown and Reid measured oxidative breakdown products and antioxidant depletion in diskenetic patients.

[1] A version of Magnetic Resonance Imaging (MRI).

[2] Also known as uncontrolled movement disorder.

pessimism	anxiety	interpersonal friction
irritability	dysphoria (sadness)	inhibited communication
poor attitude	hopelessness	asthenia (low energy)
guilt	insomnia	hypersomnia
sexual disinterest	fatigue	anhedonia (inability to feel happy)
suicidal thoughts	loss of interest	lack of motivation

TABLE 41: Some Symptoms of Depression

They confirmed the relationship between lipid peroxidation and tardive diskinesia. Other researchers have shown that lipid peroxidation and GSH depletion are aggravated by antipsychotic drugs. Sagara at the Salk Institute in La Jolla, California said that treatments resulting in decreased intracellular GSH would aggravate haloperidol (a neuroleptic antipsychotic) toxicity, and may increase any tendency to tardive dyskinesia.

Researchers Cadet and Kahler from the National Institute of Health in Baltimore, as well as Mahadik and Scheffer from the Department of Health Behavior, Medical College of Georgia and others, have suggested that antioxidants should be used to prevent side effects in patients taking antipsychotics. The Georgia team also showed that oxidative injury increases and GSH-peroxidase levels fall even at the earliest stages of psychosis, and that antioxidants may prevent or slow deterioration.

It appears that sustained GSH levels may slow the progress of schizophrenia, improve symptomatology,[3] and decrease side effects of some of the drugs used against this disease.

Obsessive compulsive disorder

OCD (obsessive compulsive disorder) shares many features found in other psychiatric disorders, including the brain changes that occur in individuals exhibiting addictive behavior. Other studies report biochemical changes such as increased oxidative stress/free radical production, decreased glutathione and glutathione peroxidase, and overall impairment in oxidative status. Even more dramatically, these alterations have been correlated to the severity of obsessive-compulsive symptoms.

Currently, very few prospective studies have been carried out demonstrating the effects of raising glutathione in OCD, but they should be forthcoming.

Depression

MDD (major depressive disorder) is a serious debilitating illness that affects persons of every age, sex, cultural/racial background and economic status. Everyone can relate to "being depressed" but MDD is a severe condition with prolonged symptoms that interferes with life's daily functions. Symptoms of depression vary. A partial list appears in Table 40.

The NIMH (National Institute of Mental Health, USA) estimates that upward of 20 million adults have at least one bout of major depression per year. That's about 7% of the population experiencing depression in any one year. But when looking at how many adults will be affected by depression within their lifetime, the figure is a staggering 20%. Just as concerning is that one fifth of these may develop psychotic symptoms including hallucinations, delusions or paranoia. Moe

[3] The determination of characteristic symptoms.

recently recognized that 10 to 15% of women will develop postpartum depression. A shocking 15% of seriously depressed patients will die by suicide. This does not include those with suicidal thoughts and unsuccessful attempts, both of which are far more common.

The biological basis of depression is still being worked out. We can comfortably say that it includes neurotransmitter abnormalities, hormones, genetics and epigenetics, external stressors, environmental factors and neurodegenerative disorders. Also apparent in the past three decades is that oxidative stress, free radicals, antioxidants and GSH all play their parts in this disorder.

A handful of articles linked antioxidant dysfunction with depression in the 1980s, but only in the 1990s was this connection established. Initially it was shown that patients with MDD had higher levels of both lipid peroxidation and breakdown products of oxidative stress and free radical damage. This was followed by measurement of actual antioxidant function—which naturally includes an examination of glutathione status. It was no surprise to find that glutathione abnormalities were abundant.

Many more nuances of antioxidant dysfunction in depression were uncovered as other researchers elaborated on this foundational work. It seems that the more depressed the patient, the greater the free radical damage and the lesser the antioxidant protection. As expected, this held true for glutathione—the master antioxidant. Conversely, as patients' conditions improved, their oxidative stress markers improved too. By the turn of the millennium two groups—Bilici et al and Khanzode et al—showed that the use of SSRI[4] antidepressant drugs improved measurements of oxidation. Lukash et al were eventually able to correlate improvement in oxidative stress with positive response to SSRI antidepressants.

As mentioned earlier, post-mortem brain samples from psychiatric patients were found to be glutathione deficient. Today, scientists are able to measure glutathione levels in the brains of living patients with a specially-tuned "magnetic resonance spectroscopy" brain scanner. With it, a 2017 study by Freed et al examined glutathione levels in subjects aged 12 to 21 and suffering from major depression. This study validated older biopsy studies showing a significant decrease in GSH in the brain of depressed patients.

Clearly, low GSH levels are correlated with major depression. This begs the question: can raising glutathione levels improve symptoms of depression? Australian Michael Berk has been at the forefront of investigating the use of the glutathione precursor NAC (N-acetylcysteine) in psychiatric illness. A 2014 study of over 250 patients by his group showed improvement in many symptoms using this drug. Patients continued their usual medications but were also given either NAC or a placebo. According to multiple scales of depression, results showed an improvement in symptoms. This will certainly lead to more investigation of this approach as a complementary therapy for major depression.

Bipolar disorder

BPD (bipolar disorder), or BPAD (bipolar affective disorder), once called "manic-depressive illness" differs from pure depression in several ways. Patients suffer not only from depression, but also from periods of the contrary—a "manic" mood feeling "up", "wired", "elated" or "energized," usually beyond normally accepted behavior. Another, less severe form of bipolar disorder in which symptoms are not as extreme, is called "cyclothymic disorder" or "cyclothymia." Several forms of bipolar disorder range from people who swing between severe depression and severe mania to those whose symptoms are mostly depressive and only occasionally and mildly manic ("hypomania"). Mania or

[4] Selective serotonin reuptake inhibitors (SSRIs) used in the treatment of major depressive and anxiety disorders.

manic disorder is discussed in the next section. Bipolar disorder also tends to exhibit more of a genetic component than pure depression, and there is usually a strong family history. BPD figures vary somewhat, but statistics show that 1 to 3 percent of North Americans over 18 years of age are affected every year.

Not surprisingly, the findings of free radical damage, heightened oxidative stress, antioxidant abnormalities and decreased glutathione levels in BPD are also found in major depressive disorder. Additionally noted was a similar correlation between glutathione and the drugs used to treat the specific disorder. In Canada, Cuo, Shao, Young and Wang demonstrated that the pharmaceuticals Lithium and Valproate both increased glutathione activity in patients. A group at Johns Hopkins University in Baltimore correlated glutathione levels to the severity of symptoms in both bipolar disorder and schizophrenia. The correlation was strong enough for them to suggest that GSH levels could be a good indicator of patients' progress. Following the lines of thought resulting from the MDD research, there was hope that improved antioxidant defenses and raised glutathione might lead to more positive outcomes in bipolar patients.

Again Michael Berk and his team in Australia committed themselves to a randomized double-blind, placebo-controlled study using NAC (N-acetylcysteine) to treat BPD patients. They measured symptoms according to a number of different scales for bipolar disorder. His team, as well as several other research groups, continued this vein of research and showed improvements in severity of symptoms, daily functioning and quality of life, cognition, and increased time between attacks. More recently, Berk's team attempted to improve cognition in a group of severely bipolar patients with psychosis. A randomized placebo-controlled study on more than 50 patients led to significantly better performance in working memory tests after 6 months.

Mania (manic disorder)

Mania is usually part of the bipolar condition, but occasionally it occurs alone—outside the normal cycle of mania and depression. A manic phase is characterized by a heightened state of arousal, both physically and mentally. There is great instability of mood. The patient can experience anything from pure euphoria to utter rage. Patients may hold themselves in high esteem and become grandiose. They are compelled to talk a lot. Their thoughts race. They are strongly goal-orientated and may achieve great things. However, all this high-level activity, combined with minimal sleep, eventually leads to a "crash." Other negative outcomes include excessive risk-taking with sex, drugs, shopping, gambling and inappropriate gift giving. Violent behavior is not uncommon.

As with other psychiatric disorders described in this chapter, increased oxidative stress and decreased glutathione levels are well documented. Studies using glutathione or GSH precursors in pure mania are rare. Berk's group has done some small randomized studies in mania with promising results, but much more work is needed to establish this as a viable treatment option.

Attention deficit disorder

ADD (attention deficit disorder) can also manifest itself as ADHD (attention deficit hyper activity disorder) when symptoms of excessive physical activity are also present. This is considered a neurodevelopmental disorder, implying that it usually starts in childhood and may persist into adulthood. As the name implies, it is characterized by problems paying attention, avoiding distraction, focusing and controlling behavior. The frequency of ADD and ADHD are on the rise. Whether this is due to an increase in actual cases or just that we only now recognize them as disorders is an ongoing debate among mental health professionals and the public. Due to this uncertainty, reported rates of ADHD in America vary from 5% (American Psychiatric Association) to 11% (CDC—Centers for Disease Control and Prevention).

Curiously, the most successful drug treatments for ADD and ADHD have been stimulants. You might wonder why stimulating an already-hyperactive individual would be helpful. The paradox is resolved by the fact that the area of the brain which governs hyperactivity has been discovered to actually underperform in ADD/ADHD. Stimulation "wakes up" the brain area that normally restrains one's behavior.

The links to oxidative stress were discovered late in ADD/ADHD research. Only after 2005 was antioxidant therapy seriously considered. In 2006 and 2007, Eastern European researchers used pycnogenols (a family of antioxidants) to ease the burden on glutathione levels, but failed to improve symptoms. The correlation between glutathione deficiency and ADD/ADHD grew stronger as other researchers entered the arena. Several teams noticed that children with genetic errors in glutathione metabolism were more prone to the development of ADD/ADHD. In addition, these GSH errors made the patients more susceptible to environmental pollutants, which may have made their immune status even worse.

I'm aware of only one study to date that tried to directly raise glutathione levels in ADD/ADHD patients using NAC (N-acetylcysteine). Although the results were favorable, it was done in patients who also suffered from the autoimmune disease Lupus, making the finding much harder to understand. This certainly takes away from the relevance of this research. More work needs to be done.

Anxiety and panic disorder

Anyone with the normal range of human emotions understands the word "anxiety," but in medicine and psychiatry it's more difficult to define and categorize. Current diagnostic systems allow for "general anxiety disorder," "panic disorder," "phobias," and many other groupings. Clearly the symptom of anxiety occurs in many different psychological conditions, making it likely that many factors are at play. In at least some anxiety disorders, it appears that oxidative stress and glutathione deficiency are related.

Starting with animal studies, researchers have shown that genetic manipulation can down-regulate antioxidant genes and provoke anxiety in a group of rodents. Hassan et al focused on the human condition in a 2014 literature review of oxidative stress in anxiety disorders, saying that it may be a common feature of general anxiety disorder, phobias, obsessive-compulsive disorder, post-traumatic stress disorder, agoraphobia and panic disorder.

A group of Turkish researchers has focused particularly on the down-regulation of antioxidant genes in panic disorder for the past two decades. They are firm in their opinion that oxidative stress, glutathione metabolism and inflammatory processes all play a role in panic disorder.

Considering that psychosocial stress might be a form of anxiety, an interesting experiment studying lipid peroxidation was carried out in older people—some of whom practiced transcendental meditation. Results showed that meditators not only suffered less mental stress but also significantly lower oxidative stress.

Addiction

Addiction is now considered a brain "disease" in which distinct biochemical and physiological processes change brain structure and function. Addiction is characterized by chronic, repetitive, compulsive behavior, including drug abuse, gambling—even shopping and sex—all with potentially disastrous results. Patients are compelled to continue this behavior, even when they understand the negative consequences.

Many addictive conditions have demonstrated similar biochemical changes—including lowered glutathione metabolism and increased oxidative stress. Examples include compulsive gambling, as well as abuse of cannabis (marijuana), cocaine, amphetamine, and nicotine (tobacco).

Cannabis

Several studies have tried using NAC to reduce marijuana use in adolescents and young adults. With some success, subjects also reported improved management of compulsive behavior, emotionality and purposefulness. All responses were recorded on the Marijuana Craving Questionnaire.[5] Although results were mixed from study to study, this strategy has produced sufficient evidence to warrant further investigation.

Nicotine (tobacco)

Raising glutathione in smokers offers two important benefits. As well as addressing addictive behavior, glutathione also limits the damage done by cigarette-induced oxidative stress. Literally billions of free radicals are released with each puff of smoke, wreaking havoc in the lungs and airways, often leading to lung disease and cancer. In 2015 Prado et al. showed significant differences between NAC and a placebo group in both cigarette consumption and exhalation of carbon monoxide gas. Although only a few small studies looked specifically at smoking from the addictive perspective, early indications suggest that larger trials are warranted.

Cocaine

Although still in its earlier stages of investigation, the research on raising glutathione to ameliorate cocaine addition shows promise. Small studies have demonstrated reduction in self-reported craving, as well as less money spent and fewer days using the drug. Larger, well-designed controlled clinical studies will be needed to validate these findings.

Pathological Gambling

A handful of scientists have attempted to control pathological gambling habits using glutathione precursors. Grant and colleagues studied 29 confirmed gambling addicts, using NAC over 3 to 4 months and compared to a placebo group. At the end of the study 83% of the NAC group were considered to have responded well, while only 28% of the placebo group responded positively.

Conclusions

Many neurological and psychiatric disease processes are characterized by high levels of oxidative stress and free radical formation, as well as abnormalities in glutathione metabolism and antioxidant defenses. Even mental stress has been shown to destabilize oxidant/antioxidant balance in the brain.

Both schizophrenia and the drugs used to treat it lead to GSH abnormalities. Supporting and sustaining glutathione levels may prevent or slow the damage to brain cells typical of this disease. Tardive diskinesia, a long-term side-effect of antipsychotic drug usage, has also been linked to free radical production and depletion of glutathione defense mechanisms. Researchers have proposed that elevated GSH levels may slow progression of schizophrenia and ease the side effects of medications used to treat it.

A common denominator seems to run through a variety of psychological diagnoses. The combination of high oxidative stress, free radical formation, lowered antioxidant potential and lowered glutathione activity characterize a large number of common pathologies. The ones discussed in this

[5] A 45-item, multi-dimensional questionnaire that assesses marijuana craving.

chapter include MDD (major depressive disorder), BP (bipolar disorder), manic disorder, schizophrenia, panic disorder, anxiety, OCD (obsessive-compulsive disorder) and others.

Other applications of GSH in neurodegenerative disease are discussed elsewhere in this book. See the chapters on Alzheimer's disease (Chapter 26), Parkinson's disease (Chapter 25), multiple sclerosis (Chapter 30), Autism (Chapter 29), and other brain pathologies (Chapters 27 and 28).

PSYCHIATRY

REFERENCES

ABDALLA DS, MONTEIRO HP, OLIVEIRA JA, BECHARA EJ. *Activities of superoxide dismutase & glutathione peroxidase in schizophrenic & manic-depressive patients.* Clin Chem 32(5):805-7, 1986

ANDREAZZA AC ET AL. *Oxidative stress markers in bipolar disorder: a meta-analysis.* J Affect Disord 111(2-3):135-44, 2008

ANDREAZZA AC, KAPCZINSKI F ET AL. *Nitrotyrosine & glutathione antioxidant system in patients in the early & late stages of bipolar disorder.* J Psychiatry Neurosci 34(4):263-71, 2009

AFSHAR, H., ROOHAFZA, H., MOHAMMAD-BEIGI, H., HAGHIGHI, M., JAHANGARD, L., SHOKOUH, P., SADEGHI, M., HAFEZIAN, H. *N-acetylcysteine add-on treatment in refractory obsessive-compulsive disorder: a randomized, double-blind, placebo-controlled trial.* J. Clin. Psychopharmacol. 32 (6), 797–803. 2012

AMEN, SL., PIACENTINE, LB, AHMAD, ME, LI, SJ, MANTSCH, JR, RISINGER, RC, BAKER, DA. *Repeated N-acetyl cysteine reduces cocaine seeking in rodents & craving in cocaine-dependent humans.* Neuropsychopharmacology 36 (4), 871–878. 2011.

ATMACA M, KULOGLU M, TEZCAN E, USTUNDAG B. *Antioxidant enzyme & malondialdehyde levels in patients with social phobia.* Psychiatry Res 159(1-2), 2008

BERK M, DEAN O, COTTON SM, ET AL. *The efficacy of adjunctive N-acetylcysteine in major depressive disorders: a double-blind, randomized, placebo-contolled trial* J Clin Psychiatry, 75:628-636, 2014.

BERK M, MALHI GS, GRAY LJ, DEAN OM. *The promise of N-acetylcysteine in neuropsychiatry.* Trends Pharmacol Sci. 34(3):167-177, 2013.

BER M, COPOLOV D, DEAN O ET AL. *N-acetyl cysteine as a glutathione precursor for schizophrenia –a double-blind, randomized, placebo-controlled trial.* Biol Psychiatry 64(5):361-8, 2008

BERM, JEAVONS S, DEAN OM ET AL. *Nail-biting stuff? The effect of N-acetyl cysteine on nail-biting.* CNS Spectr 14(7):357-60, 2009

BERRY T. *A selenium transport protein model of a sub-type of schizophrenia.* Med. Hypothesis 43: 409-414, 1994

BILICI M, ET AL. *Antioxidative enzyme activities & lipid peroxidation in major depression: alterations by antidepressant treatments.* J Affect Disord 64:43-51, 2001.

BROWN K, REID A, WHITE T, ET AL. *Vitamin E, lipids, & lipid peroxidation products in tardive dyskinesia.* Biol. Psychiatry 43: 863-867, 1998

BRADSTREET JJ, SMITH S, BARAL M, ROSSIGNOL DA. *Biomarker-guided interventions of clinically relevant conditions associated with autism spectrum disorders & attention deficit hyperactivity disorder.* Altern Med Rev 15(1):15-32, 2010

BUCKMAN TD, KLING AS, EIDUSON S, ET AL. *Glutathione peroxidase & CT scan abnormalities in schizophrenia.* Biol. Psychiatry 22: 1349-1356, 1987

BUCKMAN TD, KLING AS, SUTPHIN MS, ET AL. *Platelet glutathione peroxidase & monoamine oxidase activity in schizophrenics with CT scan abnormalities: relation to psychosocial variables.* Psychiatry Res. 31: 1-14, 1990

CADET JL, KAHLER LA. *Free radical mechanisms in schizophrenia & tardive diskinesia.* Neurosci. Biobehav. Rev. 18: 457-467, 1994.

CARVALHO AF, ET AL. *N-acetylcysteine augmentation to tranylcypromine in treatment-resistant major depression.* J Clin Psychopharmacol. 33(5):719-720, 2013.

CEYLAN M, SENER S ET AL. *Oxidative imbalance in child & adolescent patients with attention-deficit/hyperactivity disorder.* Prog Neuropsychopharmacol Biol Psychiatry 34(8):1491 – 4, 2010

CEYLAN MF, SENER S, BAYRAKTAR AC, KAVUTCU M. *Changes in oxidative stress & cellular immunity serum markers in attention-deficit/hyperactivity disorder.* Psychiatry Clin Neurosci 66(3):220-6, 2012

CHAKRABORTY S, SINGH OP, DASGUPTA A, ET AL. *Correlation between lipid peroxidation-induced TBARS level & disease severity in obsessive-compulsive disorder.* Prog Neuropsychopharmacol Biol Psychiatry 33:363-6. 2009.

CHEN AT, CHIBNALL JT, NASRALLAH

HA. *Placebo-controlled augmentation trials of the antioxidant NAC in schizophrenia: A review.* Ann Clin Psychiatry 28(3):190-6, 2016

Cui J, Shao L, Young LT, Wang JF. *Role of glutathione in neuroprotective effects of mood stabilizing drugs lithium & valproate.* Neuroscience 144(4):1447-53, 2007

Dean O, Giorlando F, Berk M. *N-acetylcysteine in psychiatry: current therapeutic evidence & potential mechanisms of action.* J Psychiatry Neuroscience. 36(2):78-86, 2011.

Deepmala et al. *Clinical trials of N-acetyl-cysteine in psychiatry & neurology. A systematic review.* Neuroscience & Biobehavioral Reviews. 55(294-321, 2015.

Dvoráková M et al. *The effect of polyphenolic extract from pine bark, Pycnogenol on the level of glutathione in children suffering from attention deficit hyperactivity disorder (ADHD).* Redox Rep 11(4):163-72, 2006

Dvoráková M et al. *Urinary catecholamines in children with attention deficit hyperactivity disorder (ADHD): modulation by a polyphenolic extract from pine bark (pycnogenol).* Nutr Neurosci 10(3-4):151-7, 2007

Ersan S, Bakir S, Erdal Ersan E, et al. *Examination of free radical metabolism & antioxidant defence system elements in patients with obsessive-compulsive disorder.* Prog Neuropsychopharmacol Biol Psychiatry 30:1039-42. 2006

Farokhnia, M., et al. *N-acetylcysteine as an adjunct to risperidone for treatment of negative symptoms in patients with chronic schizophrenia: a randomized,double-blind, placebo-controlled study.* Clin.Neuropharmacol. 36 (6), 185–192. 2013.

Fekkes D, Bode WT, Zijlstra FJ, Pepplinkhuizen L. *Eicosanoid & amino acid metabolism in transient acute psychoses with psychedelic symptoms.* Prostaglandins Leukot. Essent. Fatty Acids 54: 261-264, 1996

Fendri C, Mechri A, Khiari G et al. *Oxidative stress involvement in schizophrenia pathophysiology: a review.* Encephale 32(2 Pt 1):244-52, 2006

Freed Rd, Hollenhorst C et al. *A pilot study of cortical glutathione in youth with depression.* Psychiatry Res 270:54-60, 2017

Gawryluk JW, Wang JF, Andreazza AC, Shao L, Young LT. *Decreased levels of glutathione, the major brain antioxidant, in post-mortem prefrontal cortex from patients with psychiatric disorders.* Int. J. Neuropsychopharmacol. 14 (1), 123–130. 2011.

Govorin NV, Govorin AV, Skazhutin SA. *Significance of disorders of the processes of lipid peroxidation in patients with persistent paranoid schizophrenia resistant to the treatment.* Zh. Nevropatol. Psikhiatr. Im. S. S. Korsakova 91: 121-124, 1991

Grant JE, Odlaug BL, Kim SW. *N-acetylcysteine, a glutamate modulator, in the treatment of trichotillomania: a double blind, placebo-controlled study.* Arch Gen Psychiatry 66(7):756-63, 2009

Grant JE, Kim SW, Odlaug BL. *N-acetyl cysteine, a glutamate- modulating agent, in the treatment of pathological gambling: a pilot study.* Biol Psychiatry; 62:652-7. 2007.

Grant JE, Odlaug BL, Chamberlain SR, Potenza MN, Schreiber LR, Donahue CB, Kim SW. *A randomized, placebo-controlled trial of N-acetylcysteine plus imaginal desensitization for nicotine-dependent pathological gamblers.* J. Clin. Psychiatry 75 (1), 39–45. 2014.

Gray KM et al. *A double-blind randomized controlled trial of N-acetylcysteine in cannabis-dependent adolescents.* Am. J. Psychiatry 169 (8), 805–812. 2012.

Gray KM, Watson NL, Carpenter MJ, Larowe SD. *NAC in young marijuana users: an open-label pilot study.* Am. J. Addict. 19 (2), 187–189. 2010.

Hassan W, Silva CE et al. *Association of oxidative stress to the genesis of anxiety:* implications for possible therapeutic interventions. Curr Neuropharmacol 12(2):120-39, 2014

Hovatta I, Tennant RS, Helton R et al. *Glyoxalase 1 & glutathione reductase 1 regulate anxiety in mice.* Nature 438 (7068):662-6, 2005

Huey ED, Zahn R, Krueger F, et al. *A psychological & neuroanatomical model of obsessive-compulsive disorder.* J Neuropsychiatry Clin Neurosci; 20:390-408. 2008

Khanzode SD, et al. *Oxidative damage & major depression: the potential antioxidant action of selective serotonin re-uptake inhibitors.* Redox Report, 8(6):365-370. 2003.

Knackstedt LA, LaRowe S, Mardikian P, et al. *The role of cystine- glutamate exchange in nicotine dependence in rats & humans.* Biol Psychiatry 65:841-5. 2009.

Koob GF, Volkow ND. *Neurocircuitry of addiction.* Neuropsycho- pharmacology 2010 35:217-38. 2010.

Kodydková J, Vávrová L, Zeman et al. *Antioxidative enzymes & increased oxidative stress in depressive women.* Clin Biochem 42)13-14:1368-74, 2009

Kuloglu M, Atmaca M, Tezcan E, et al. *Antioxidant enzyme activities & malondialdehyde levels in patients with obsessive-compulsive disorder.* Neuropsychobiology 46:27-32. 2002.

Kuloglu M, Atmaca M, Tezcan E, et al. *Antioxidant enzyme & malondialdehyde levels in patients with panic disorder.* Neuropsychobiology 46(4):186-9, 2002

LaRowe SD, Mardikian P, Malcolm R, Myrick H, Kalivas P, McFarland K, Saladin

M, McRae A, Brady, K. *Safety & tolerability of N-acetylcysteine in cocaine-dependent individuals.* Am. J. Addict. 15 (1), 105–110. 2006.

LaRowe SD, Myrick H, Hedden S, Mardikian P, Saladin M, McRae A, Brady K, Kalivas PW, Malcolm, R. *Is cocaine desire reduced by N-acetylcysteine? Am. J. Psychiatry 164 (7), 1115–1117, 2007.*

Lavoie S, Berger M et al. *Erythrocyte glutathione levels as long-term predictor of transition to psychosis.* Trans Psychiatry 7(3):e1064, 2017

Lee JY, Hwang IW et al. *Association of glutathione S-transferases M1, T1 & P1 gene polymorphisms with attention deficit & hyperactivity disorder in Korean children.* Gene 586(2):228-33, 2016

Leffa DT, Bellaver B, de Oliveira C et al. *Increased Oxidative Parameters & Decreased Cytokine Levels in an Animal Model of Attention-Deficit/Hyperactivity Disorder.* Neurochem Res 10.1007/s11064-017-2341-6, 2017

Lohr JB. *Oxygen radicals & neuropsychiatric illness. Speculations.* Arch. Gen. Psychiatry 48: 1097-1106, 1991

Lohr JB, Browning JA. *Free radical involvement in neuropsychiatric illnesses.* Psychpharmacol. Bull. 31: 159-165, 1995

Lukash AI, et al. *Free radical processes & antioxidant system in depression & treatment.* Zh Nevrol Psikhiatr Im S S Korsakova. 102(9):41-44. 2002.

Mahadik SP, Scheffer RE. *Oxidative injury & potential use of antioxidants in schizophrenia.* Prostaglandins Leukot. Essent. Fatty Acids 55:45-54, 1996

Mahadik SP, Mukherjee S, Scheffer RE, et al. *Elevated plasma lipid peroxidases at onset of non-affective psychosis.* Biol. Psychiatry 43: 674-679, 1998

Mardikian PN, LaRowe SD, Hedden S, Kalivas PW, Malcolm RJ. *An open label trial of N-acetylcysteine for the treatment of cocaine dependence: a pilot study. Prog. Neuropsychopharmacol.* Biol. Psychiatry 31 (2), 389–394. 2007.

Matsuzawa D, Hashimoto K. *Magnetic resonance spectroscopy study of the antioxidant defense system in schizophrenia.* Antioxid Redox Signal 15(7):2057-65, 2011

McClure EA, Baker NL, Gray KM. *Cigarette smoking during an N-acetylcysteine-assisted cannabis cessation trial in adolescents.* Am. J. Drug Alcohol Abuse 40 (4), 285–291. 2014.

Morales E, Julvez J, Torrent M et al. *Association of early-life exposure to household gas appliances & indoor nitrogen dioxide with cognition & attention.* Am J Epidemiol 169(11):1327-36, 2009

Mukherjee S, Mahadik SP, Scheffer RE, et al. *Impaired antioxidant defense at the onset of psychosis.* Schizophr. Res. 19: 19-26, 1996

Ozdemir E, Cetinkaya S, Ersan S, et al. *Serum selenium & plasma malondialdehyde levels & antioxidant enzyme activities in patients with obsessive-compulsive disorder.* Prog Neuropsychopharmacol Biol Psychiatry; 33:62-5. 2009.

Ozdemir O, Selvi Y et al. *Comparison of superoxide dismutase, glutathione peroxidase & adenosine deaminase activities between respiratory & nocturnal subtypes of patients with panic disorder.* Neuropsychobiology 66(4):244-51, 2012

Ozcan ME, Gulec M, Ozerol E, Polat R, Akyol O. *Antioxidant enzyme activities & oxidative stress in effective disorders.* Int Clin Psychopharmacol. Mar;19(2):89-95, 2004

Pai BN, Janakiramaiah N, Gangadhar BN, Ravindranath V. *Depletion of glutathione & enhanced lipid peroxidation in the CSF of acute psychotics following haloperidol administration.* Biol. Psychiatry 36: 489-491, 1994

Pal SN, Dandiya PC. *Glutathione as a cerebral substrate in depressive behavior.* Pharmacol. Biochem. Behav. 48: 845-851, 1994

Prado, E. et al. 2015. *N-acetylcysteine for therapy-resistant tobacco use disorder: a pilot study.* Redox Rep. (Epub ahead of print).

Rapado-Castro M, Dodd S et al. *Cognitive effects of adjunctive N-acetyl cysteine in psychosis.* Psychol Med 47(5):866-876, 2017

LG Nucifora, T Tanaka, LN Hayes, M Kim. *Reduction of plasma GSH in psychosis associated with schizophrenia & bipolar disorder in translational psychiatry.* Transl Psychiatry 7(8):e1215, 2017

Reddy R, Sahebarao MP, Mukherjee S, Murthy JN. *Enzymes of the antioxidant defense system in chronic schizophrenic patients.* Biol. Psychiatry 30: 409-412, 1991

Reddy RD, Yao JK. *Free radical pathology in schizophrenia: a review.* Prostaglandins Leukot. Essent. Fatty Acids 55: 33-43, 1996

Roten, AT, Baker, NL, Gray, KM. *Marijuana craving trajectories in an adolescent marijuana cessation pharmacotherapy trial.* Addict. Behav. 38 (3), 1788–1791. 2013.

Rotrosen J, Adler L, Edson R, Lavori P. *Antioxidant treatment of tardive dyskinesia.* Prostaglandins Leukot. Essent. Fatty Acids 55: 77-81, 1996

Sagara Y. *Induction of reactive O2 species in neurons by haloperidol.* J. Neurochem. 71: 1002-1012, 1998

Schneider RH, Nidich SI, Salerno JW, et al. *Lower lipid peroxidase levels in practitioners of the Transcendental Meditation program.* Psychosom. Med. 60: 38-41, 1998

Selek S, Herken H, Bulut M, et al. *Oxidative imbalance in obsessive compulsive disorder patients: a total evaluation of oxidant-antioxidant status.* Prog

Neuropsychopharmacol Biol Psychiatry 32:487-91. 2008.

Smythies JR. *Oxidative reactions & schizophrenia: a review.* Schizophrenic Res. 24: 357-364, 1997

Tsuboi H et al. *Depessive symptoms are independently correlated with lipid peroxidation in a female population: comparison with vitamins & caratinoids.* J Psychosom Res, 56(1):53-58. 2004.

Van Schooten FJ, Besaratinia A, De Flora S, et al. *Effects of oral ad- ministration of N-acetyl-L-cysteine: a multi-biomarker study in smokers.* Cancer Epidemiol Biomarkers Prev. 11:167-75. 2002.

Verlaet AA, Ceulemans B et al. *Effect of Pycnogenol on attention-deficit hyperactivity disorder (ADHD): study protocol for a randomised controlled trial.* Trials 18(1):145. Doi: 10.1186/s13063-017, 2017

Yao JK, Reddy R, McElhinny LG, Van Kammen DP. *Effects of haloperidol on antioxidant defense system enzymes in schizophrenia.* J. Psychiatr. Res. 32: 385-391, 1998

Yao JK, Reddy R, McElhinny LG, Van Kammen DP. *Reduced status of plasma total antioxidant capacity in schizophrenia.* Schizophrenic. Res. 32: 1-8, 1998

Yao JK, Reddy R, Van Kammen DP. *Human plasma glutathione peroxidase & symptom severity in schizophrenia.* Biol. Psychiatry 45: 1512-1515, 1999

Zafir A, Ara A, Banu N. *Invivo antioxidant status: a putative target of antidepressant action.* Prog Neuropsychpharmacol Biol Psychiatry 33 (2):220-8, 2009

Index

D

E

F

G

N

O

P

U

V

W

Z